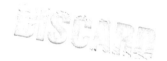

NO MORE
HOT FLASHES...
and even *more* good news

ALSO BY PENNY WISE BUDOFF, M.D.

No More Hot Flashes and Other Good News
No More Menstrual Cramps and Other Good News

NO MORE HOT FLASHES...

and even *more* good news

PENNY WISE BUDOFF, M.D.

WITH CONTRIBUTIONS FROM OTHER NOTED PHYSICIANS IN THE FIELD OF WOMEN'S HEALTH

WARNER BOOKS

A Time Warner Company

Warner Books, Inc., 1271 Avenue of the Americas, New York, NY 10020
Visit our Web site at http://warnerbooks.com

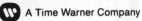 A Time Warner Company

Printed in the United States of America
First Printing: August 1998
10 9 8 7 6 5 4 3 2 1

Library of Congress Cataloging-in-Publication Data

Budoff, Penny Wise.
    No more hot flashes—and even more good news / Penny Wise Budoff.
        p.   cm.
    Includes index.
    ISBN 0-446-52236-8
    1. Menopause.   2. Menopause—Psychological aspects.   3. Middle
aged women—Diseases.   I. Title.
    RG186.B8   1998
    618. 1'75—dc21   97-51975
                                                            CIP

Book design and composition by L&G McRee

To the wonderful women who have been my patients. To their warmth and friendship, inquisitiveness, truthfulness, and to their tenacity and ability to learn medical facts. I have learned much from them and admire and respect their ability to make difficult choices and to face their problems with bravery and even a sense of humor.

A Note to My Readers

I hope that the information in this book will help you better understand your many medical and surgical choices. However, this book is not intended to be a substitute for individual medical diagnosis and advice from your doctor or health care professional. Always consult with your personal health care provider before implementing any program or therapy.

Contents

Acknowledgments

Without a doubt, my first acknowledgment goes to Sy, my wonderful and supportive husband. My handsome son and gorgeous daughter are grown and no longer live at home, so unlike with the first two books, I no longer felt guilty about taking time from them. My daughter, Cindy, has taken my small vitamin and skin care business, Bonne Forme ®, under her wing. She also helps me every time I have a computer question or problem. My son, Jeff, an orthopedic sports medicine and hand surgeon in West Palm Beach, Florida, wrote a chapter that I am positive will be one of your favorites.

This book has contributions from several special people, each with excellent credentials in her or his own right. While it is true that I started out to write this book on my own, it soon become clear to me that writing all of the chapters by myself would be much akin to trying to do women's health care as a solo practitioner. It can't be done. Medicine and surgery have just become too specialized and it is impossible for any one person to know all there is to know. Furthermore, new developments are taking place at such a rapid rate that even specialists have to really try hard just to keep up with their own specialties. Therefore, while I wrote portions of the book, portions of it were written with other physicians in different specialties.

Actually this book reconfirms the need for a group attempt to provide women's health care—that was the basis of the women's center I established in 1985. If primary care doctors practicing in a multispecialist group offer the best women's health care, this book offering advice on women's health is written on a similar basis. As with a women's center, there must be one physician in charge. The primary caregiver (or—in the case of this book—the author) must make sure that head to toe have been covered and nothing is left undone. In addition, she helps her patients understand their options and acts as an ombudsman making sure that information from these specialists is comprehensible and appropriate for the patients' individual physical and emotional needs.

There are many thank-yous to those whose work helped make this book special. The list is somewhat long; therefore, additional information on those who made major contributions to the writing appear where I think it will be most likely to be noted and read—at the beginnings of the various chapters. Also, you may consult "About the Contributors" at the end of the book. The participants are a scholarly group with long lists of degrees. However, don't let that scare you.

The following short thank-yous are in the order that chapters appear in the book:

James Simon, M.D., for his chapter on perimenopause. He is Clinical Professor of Obstetrics and Gynecology at George Washington University and a "Top Washington Physician" as well as one of the "Best Doctors in America." He is one of the foremost experts in the field of infertility and menopause.

Howard Fillit, M.D., for the chapter on estrogen and the brain. He is Clinical Professor of Geriatrics and Medicine at the Mount Sinai Medical Center in New York City. He was the first to report that estrogen replacement therapy improves cognition in women with Alzheimer's disease.

Jeffrey E. Budoff, M.D., "My son, the doctor!", for his chapter on the musculoskeletal system. He is a practicing orthopedic surgeon fellowship-trained in sports medicine and hand surgery. He specializes in surgery of the upper extremity (shoulder, elbow, wrist, and hand) and knees. His natural flair for writing plus a sense of humor makes this chapter fun to read. His mentor, Dr. Robert Nirschl, contributed to the manuscript and provided his own metaphors where emphasis was needed. Their fascinating chapter will effortlessly educate you about your muscles and joints.

Stuart Weinerman, M.D., for the chapter on osteoporosis. A practicing endocrinologist with expertise in osteoporosis, he heads the metabolic bone unit at North Shore University Hospital and practices at the North Shore University Hospital Women's Health Services in Bethpage, Long Island, New York.

Hemmi N. Bhagavan, Ph.D., F.A.C.N., for his help with the chapter on vitamins and calcium. He holds a master's degree in biochemistry and a Ph.D. in nutrition/biochemistry. He was elected Fellow of the American College of Nutrition many years ago. He worked as Senior Clinical Coordinator at Hoffman LaRoche in their vitamin division for many years. He is a wonderful source of solid information on vitamins and their therapeutic and preventive role.

John Miklos, M.D., and Lawrence Lind, M.D., are two urogynecologists who wrote the chapters on urinary tract infections and urinary incontinence. Their new specialty, urogynecology, will serve women better than ever before, offering both nonsurgical and minimally invasive surgical techniques. They will convince you that incontinence and bladder infections are not a normal part of aging!

Erna Busch, M.D., for the chapter on breast cancer. She has extensive fellowship training in cancer surgery and is a breast cancer surgeon at North Shore University Hospital in Manhasset, New York. Nearly at the end of her first pregnancy, she produced a wonderful chapter, and then a beautiful baby girl as well.

Burton Krumholz, M.D., for his help with the chapter on cervical cancer. Professor of Obstetrics and Gynecology at Long Island Jewish Hospital, he has been a friend for many years. He has devoted his entire career to the practice and teaching of colposcopy and gives courses all over the world. He is the past president of the American Society for Colposcopy and Cervical Pathology.

John Lovecchio, M.D., for his help with the chapters on ovarian cancer and hysterectomy. He heads the department of gynecological cancer surgery at North Shore University Hospital in Manhasset, New York, and is Professor of Clinical Obstetrics and Gynecology, New York University School of Medicine. He read my chapters on ovarian cancer and hysterectomy and delighted in making cryptic notes in the margin.

Seth Stern, M.D., added a page of notes on laparoscopic surgery, one of his favorite activities. Assistant Attending in the Department of Obstetrics and Gynecology, he is on full-time staff at North Shore University Hospital, and the only male gynecologist at the North Shore University Hospital Women's Health Services in Bethpage, Long Island, where I practice. He is considerate, patient, and an excellent gynecologic surgeon who is dedicated to his patients. He has a lovely wife and three children.

Joan Kasofsky, my bubbly red-headed friend, for her artistic help.

John Terzakis, M.D., of the Department of Pathology at Lenox Hill Hospital, who faxed me pathology information.

Jill Baron, M.D., a wonderful family doctor, who took excellent care of my patients while I was writing. And thanks to our head nurse, Marie Calandra, R.N., who is loved by patients and always remembers names and faces. More thanks to our wonderful staff who care and make patients feel comfortable.

My sister, Sheila, as well as Phyllis and all my dear friends for always being there.

Frances Jalet-Miller did all of the editing and queried any fuzzy passages.

And to Jane Freeman for her flying fingers over the keyboard that cleaned up the computer disks at the last moment.

And last but not least, to Maureen Egen, President of Warner Books, who believed in me and made this book possible.

PENNY WISE BUDOFF, M.D.
1998

Introduction

No More Hot Flashes and Other Good News was a *New York Times* best-seller in 1983. That was a special thrill for me, for it meant my theories about women and their health care were on target. Over the years, *No More Menstrual Cramps and Other Good News* (1980) and *No More Hot Flashes and Other Good News* (1983) have been considered classic books on women's health, helping to create the basis of the women's health movement. Indeed, a number of medical schools have assigned both books as required reading, and many universities today use the books in their Psychology of Women classes. Departments of radiation therapy and many physicians have also used the books for patient information.

It seems amazing that until 1996 *No More Hot Flashes and Other Good News* was selling steadily and remained very much up-to-date. Perhaps this was because it was ahead of its time. When the book was published, my views on hormone replacement therapy, lumpectomy and radiation therapy for breast cancer, and second opinions and medical alternatives to hysterectomies were considered radical by some. But lumpectomy and radiation therapy have become the procedure of choice for early breast cancer, many doctors now agree that some type of replacement therapy should be considered for the majority of postmenopausal women, and finally, there really were too many unnecessary hysterectomies.

Now we hear this information all the time, in magazines, on talk shows, television, and radio. However, I was publicizing women's health issues, and television and radio were airing my seminal research on menstrual pain,[1] all the way back in the seventies. In Seattle, I did the first television program ever on menstrual pain and had scores of women follow me back to my hotel room in hopes of getting more information. I did three separate solo hours on *Donahue*, was on *Oprah* three times, and did more television, radio, and print interviews than I care to remember.

I lectured throughout the United States and in London, Berlin, and Cape Town to physician audiences back when physician audiences were one hundred percent male and not very sympathetic to women's health issues. I have seen many changes in medical and surgical care over my thirty years in practice, and equally important, I have seen tremendous change in women as patients. Almost all of it is good. I cannot say that we do not have a way to go, to more equal research, to more equal care, but we are well on our way.

Those of us who are fifty or older share common experiences, for example, our mothers' secrecy about their age. Now women are more open about their age and often announce it while referring proudly to their well-toned bodies and muscular legs. Then there are the changing attitudes about marriage. When I was twenty-one, although I was a busy second-year medical student, I felt I was over the hill and overdue to get married. I married at twenty-two. Most of my patients today are well into their thirties and still single. And few of them feel guilty. In just three decades, mind-sets about an institution as basic as marriage have done a 180-degree turn.

I belong to a generation that has had to adjust to tremendous social change. Social values, morals, economic pressures, and feminist consciousness-raising have radically changed our everyday world. Our choice is either to accept change and forge ahead with our younger sisters or be left behind. New health issues have come to the forefront. AIDS has become a fact of life, not only for the younger single woman, but for the older woman who seeks a sexual relationship. I give virtually the same lecture on AIDS protection to the fifteen-year-olds and the sixty-year-olds in my practice. This information is equally relevant to both.

Heart disease in women is finally getting the attention it deserves as the number one killer of women. Give a lecture on menopause, and you will have a standing-room-only group of women and a few questioning men. The baby-boomer generation has had their first hot flashes and menopause has become an important issue to a new generation of women.

I was and still am dedicated to educating women about their health options and would like to share with you some of what I have learned in thirty-plus years of practice and twenty years of advocacy for better women's health.

Since my last book, my time has been filled with another all-consuming project. It was apparent to me by the late seventies, that women were at a double disadvantage: as the patient in the doctor/patient relationship, and the female in what was mostly a male/female role. Worse, their care was fragmented. The medical establishment had divided women's bodies into two parts, medical or reproductive. I was a family doctor and accustomed to thinking holistically: that women were total human beings, not thyroids, pelvises, or breasts. Not only were women not receiving comprehensive care, but also issues of special interest to women were neglected. In addition, it was important to have women participate in the treatment decisions that would affect their bodies and their lives. Women needed a place where their complaints would be taken seriously. In 1980, I began to plan a women's center where family doctors and specialists interested in women and women's health problems could pool their efforts to give women the best care available, a center where preventive medicine was key. There, women would have the results of their mammography, or sonography, within minutes.

It took five years to get a bank loan. Male bank presidents just couldn't understand how such a center could make any money when "we were eliminating half of the population right off the bat." But in 1985, the Penny Wise Budoff, M.D., Women's Health Center finally opened, because my husband finally found one bank president who believed in me and my idea.

Compliance is a major problem in the practice of medicine today. Having multiple services under one roof makes patient compliance more likely. It's hard to miss your mammography appointment when the doctor walks you down the hall to the X-ray technician. Perhaps equally important is the fact that each patient in the center has one chart, no matter how many physicians she may see over the years. One chart helps to ensure that there is no overprescription or medications that don't mix. A complete history of prior illnesses, therapies, and lab tests is on one chart so that duplication of lab tests or X rays is avoided. One chart helps to coordinate care between primary care doctors and subspecialists who may see the same patient.

In 1992, the center became part of North Shore University Hospital/New York University Medical Center. At about that same time, I had the privilege of speaking to more than five hundred CEOs and trustees of the major voluntary hospitals across the United States about the benefits of establishing multispecialty women's centers. In addition, since 1985 doctors and administrators from many states as well as Canada have toured the facility in order to learn how to set up their own centers. I have been happy to see this concept spread as I feel strongly that dedicated multispecialty centers offer the very best and most convenient care for women.

Meanwhile, I have gotten older. Haven't we all? Getting older is not easy. It's often been said that "the golden years are not for sissies." *No More Hot Flashes* is not a glossy, upbeat book about how fabulously happy postmenopausal women are, or how they have fantastic sex. This book is honest, written by a doctor who is also postmenopausal and who has cared for thousands of women and their physical and mental concerns for the past three decades.

I think that nearly all women who decide to take hormone replacement can have a positive experience. The problem is, few doctors have a major interest in menopause. They use one estrogen and one progesterone. When a patient complains of side effects, she is simply told to stick it out, or the dose of the same drug is increased or decreased. Well, that's not the way it should be. This is the art of medicine. By choosing the correct estrogen to begin with, and making modifications as needed, nearly every woman who chooses to take hormonal therapy should be satisfied.

You therefore need to know when you are in good hands, or equally as important, when you are not. How will you know? Basically, you have to work to become educated. You have to know what questions to ask to ascertain whether or not your care is up-to-date. This book was designed to help you do just that. Get educated about your body and learn what your choices are before you make decisions.

It used to be a lot easier. Doctors made all the decisions and patients complied. Part of the difficulty now is that women are asked to help make these decisions. How to become a partner in your care is the thrust of this book. It will take you from your physical examination to the intricacies of necessary lab tests. It also will arm you with in-depth knowledge about your health. If you have been diagnosed with one of the problems discussed in this book, you should read every detail in that chapter. Where chapters will give you more information than you need, use what you need today and save the rest for reference. I hope you'll never need it.

We have an enormous challenge ahead of us. We must give equal care to women . . . no longer is second-class research or second-class care acceptable. But the good news is, when we improve health care for women, we will improve health care for men as well. What is good for the goose is good for the gander. Coordinated care, easy access, instant results, preventive medicine plus time to talk are benefits that are not limited to women's health. We all know that.

I have always felt a keen responsibility for the precious seat I was granted in medical school. I have had tremendous energy, and for many years continued to see patients and do research during the day and write at night. I love what I do, and I love my patients and am thrilled that I had the chance to become a physician. And so I am excited to continue to type on my computer long into the nights until this book contains all that I think any mature woman needs to know about her body and how to take care of it.

For the first time, women have the clout that is needed to influence and shape their health care. This is the time to acknowledge that you really do have the ability to optimize your future. Read the book, take good care of yourself and enjoy.

Note

1. P. W. Budoff, "Dysmenorrhea, New Treatment," letter, *American Journal of Ob/Gyn,* September 15, 1977; idem, "Mefenamic Acid in the Treatment of Primary Dysmenorrhea," *Journal of the American Medical Association* 241, no. 25 (1979): 2713–16; idem, "Mefenamic Acid for Dysmenorrhea in Patients with Intrauterine Devices," *Journal of the American Medical Association* 2, no. 7 (1979); idem, "Zomepirac Sodium in the Treatment of Primary Dysmenorrhea Syndrome," *New England Journal of Medicine* 307 (1982): 714–19.

PART I

Health Issues for Every Woman

Chapter 1

FINALLY UNDERSTANDING PERIMENOPAUSE

James A. Simon, M.D., of Washington, D.C., has been a good friend. I know him from meetings of the North American Menopause Society, where his knowledge has always been much appreciated by the members of this fine organization. Jim can always be found in the middle of a large group of attentive female physicians. He is very gentle as he patiently explains his point of view on menopause or infertility. Even at home he is surrounded by women: his charming wife and three daughters.

Not only are his credits long and impressive, in addition, he has been kind, helpful, and willing to edit or give an opinion. I am most grateful for his graciousness and willingness to share his expertise. I hope you will appreciate our combined efforts to explain the perimenopause and why it presents women with so many unsettling ups and downs. After you have read the chapter, you will have better insight into what your body is experiencing and why.

What's all the fuss about? Why are forty-year-old women so interested in their hormones? What is so fascinating about the perimenopausal state? This is a chapter for women in their late thirties through mid-forties who have had even one hot flash. It is also for you who have had periods that are erratic from time to time, or all of the time. Not to fret. Welcome to your perimenopause!

Perhaps my awareness of this concentration on the loss of hormonal perfection began one day in my office when a forty-two-year-old patient complained to me that the night before, sex wasn't as good as usual. Was she becoming menopausal? she demanded. Upon further questioning, she denied hot flashes, night sweats, irregular periods, and vaginal dryness. Don't worry, I said, "all men have mediocre nights from time to time."

The majority of women sail through this phase of their lives with scarcely any notice. But some are aware of decreased libido that persists over time, some worry about increasing premenstrual mood swings, while others simply have new, confusing patterns of menstruation. If it helps, you have lots of company.

Furthermore, if you have hot flashes and your best friend doesn't, don't think, even for one minute, that she is in any way "better" than you. It's your body chemistry, not your mind. I am aware that some patients seem embarrassed by their symptoms and feel guilty about voicing complaints. It takes me back to the days when I did menstrual pain research. Women who had cramps seemed to be looked down upon by friends and sisters who had none. However, once the basis for cramps was known, emotional causes for their symptoms were discarded and there was acceptance of the physiologic differences between women. We have not quite arrived at this point in understanding perimenopausal symptomatology.

So the problem is that we all have a lot to learn. And until more research is done and there is better understanding of the entire process, you need to understand the basics and know that hot flashes will not go away with a paternalistic pat on the head.

LET'S BEGIN WITH A DEFINITION OF THE PERIMENOPAUSE AND MENOPAUSE

The perimenopause represents a time of hormonal transition, from "fertile cycles" with regular menstrual patterns and normal reproductive levels of hormones, to menopause and the absence of menstruation. It includes the time interval from the beginning of menopausal symptoms (also called climacteric symptoms) until one full year past the date of the last menstrual period when "menopause" has been reached.

Menopause is defined as a retrospective point in time and is not reached until an entire year has passed without a menstrual period. When a year has passed without a period, you can look back and say you are menopausal, or as some say, postmenopausal.

The climacteric refers to the years of *symptoms* that occur from the onset of ovarian decline to the time after menopause when symptoms stop.

Perimenopause: Its Essence Is Its Variability

Perimenopause seems to be a newly emphasized phenomenon, probably because of the sheer numbers of women in the baby-boomer generation who are entering this phase of their lives. An estimated twenty million women are in—or will enter—the menopausal transition in the next few years. With a population this large, there is inevitably an increased amount of new discussion and attention paid to issues specific to this group. Obviously, this will soon also include attention from both medical and consumer industries. Because of political pressures brought by these women, the perimenopause now has an identity. The U.S. government has launched several investigations into its biological basis and symptomatology in order to provide a scientific basis to our understanding. There are a myriad of problems, however, for as you will soon realize, the essence of the perimenopause is its variability, and that is what makes it so hard to study. Where do researchers begin when some women have symptoms at thirty-five, others at forty-nine, and others virtually never have symptoms at all?

To make matters worse, many physicians are ill prepared to assist their patients in this phase of their lives. In fact, our knowledge of the perimenopause is far weaker than that of the postmenopausal period. The void stems from the variability and lack of a clear-cut beginning and obvious end to the perimenopause. Individual differences confuse the matter further. For example, during her entire perimenopausal transition, a woman may have few symptoms although her estrogen levels may be normal, high, or in the low *normal range*. Other women have *intermittent* very low estrogen levels that are in the *postmenopausal range* with resulting severe hot flashes, sleep disturbances, and other symptoms of the "menopause" despite still having regular menstrual cycles. This becomes even more confusing when a perimenopausal woman, after three to four months of severe hot flashes and night sweats and even loss of menses, abruptly stops having symptoms and recovers with a normal estrogen level for no apparent reason.

Swings in hormone levels actually occur from day to day. Even normal twenty-year-olds have experienced that. In all age groups, estrogen levels are low in the beginning of the cycle after a period, and vaginal tissues are drier than they are later in the month. However, major hormonal fluctuations can be triggered by illness, stress, time zone travel (another form of stress), as well as by aging ovaries that are decreasing their estrogen production.

CULTURAL DIFFERENCES

To add to the confusion, cultural differences seem to affect the symptom experience of peri- and postmenopausal women. For example, while Canadian and American white women have a similar frequency of perimenopausal symptoms, Japanese women overall report a much lower frequency of symptoms. Differences in diet (see page 122), exercise, and even language may affect the reported incidence of these symptoms. For example, the Japanese word for "hot flash" is more like "blush" and therefore may have a slightly different connotation, leading to a difference in reporting their symptoms.

UNDERSTANDING THE BASICS: A REVIEW OF THE NORMAL MONTHLY CYCLE

We tend to think of our monthly cycles beginning the day we start to bleed. Actually, this is the end of the cycle. Bleeding marks the culmination of an approximately twenty-eight-day process, the sole purpose of which is to produce a fertilized egg and a uterine milieu in which it can grow. If fertilization does not occur, the endometrium sloughs off and appears externally as menstruation. As soon as menstruation ends, a new monthly cycle begins again.

Ovarian Cycle:

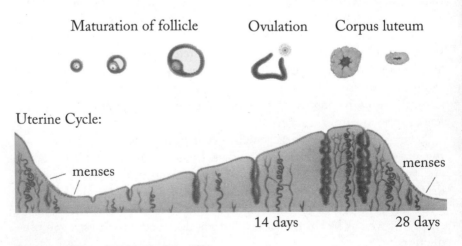

Maturation of follicle   Ovulation   Corpus luteum

Uterine Cycle:

menses   menses

14 days   28 days

Diagrams © Warner-Lambert Company 1981.

The Estrogen-Dominant, or First, Phase of the Cycle

The monthly cycle begins with a signal from the hypothalamus (the glandular control center in the brain) to the pituitary gland. The signal prods the pituitary to release FSH (follicle-stimulating hormone) into the bloodstream. When FSH reaches the ovaries, a follicle containing that month's dominant egg begins to develop. The cells that compose the follicle secrete estrogen (in a form called estradiol) and also protect the egg by bathing it in fluid and nourishing it. The follicle, growing from microscopic size to approximately two centimeters in diameter, pushes to the surface of the ovary with its precious contents, the egg. The surface of the ovary becomes thin and stretched over the follicle. After estrogen levels peak on about day 12, they drop slightly,* triggering the hypothalamus to signal the pituitary to start releasing LH (luteinizing hormone).

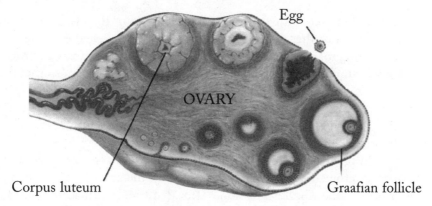

Diagram © Warner-Lambert Company 1981.

At the same time, estrogen circulating in the blood is preparing the uterus and fallopian tubes for the arrival of the egg and the act of fertilization (when sperm meets egg). The uterine lining, or endometrium, begins to thicken as estrogen causes the cells to multiply and increases the endometrial blood supply. The opening of the cervix dilates and the mucus it produces becomes copious and capable of supporting the transit of sperm. Estrogen enhances the capacity of the uterine musculature to contract rhythmically—another aid to the sperm—and it also increases the motility of the fallopian tubes, readying them to receive the egg.

*This small decline in estrogen can cause slight spotting or bleeding to occur at the time of ovulation.

Ovulation

LH stimulates ovulation and the subsequent secretion of both estrogen and progesterone in the second part of the cycle; LH causes the follicle to rupture through the cell layer at the surface of the ovary. Next the egg is propelled through the surface of the ovary with its accompanying follicular fluid.* Then, the egg can be "picked up" by the delicate open ends of the fallopian tubes, which will guide it on its way to the uterus. The ruptured follicle may now fill with blood. Under the continuing influence of LH, this blood rapidly dissipates, and the follicle cells are transformed and then mature into a bright yellow spot on the ovary known as the corpus luteum (yellow body). Although the corpus luteum still secretes estrogen, it now also secretes a second female hormone called progesterone, which is the predominant hormone in the second half of the cycle.

The Progesterone-Dominant, or Second, Phase of the Cycle

Progesterone governs the second, or luteal, phase of the cycle (see figure on page 15). It further develops and matures the thickened endometrium in preparation for pregnancy. It inhibits or reverses the effects of estrogen. It stops the multiplication of endometrial cells, matures them so that they are capable of nourishing the egg, reduces and thickens cervical mucus, and exerts a quieting effect on the uterine muscles. Progesterone also inhibits the hypothalamus from sending out instructions for more FSH, which would start a new cycle.

Should pregnancy occur, the corpus luteum will continue to produce the progesterone that is necessary to maintain the pregnancy for the first eight weeks following fertilization. After that time, the placenta normally takes over this function. If pregnancy does not occur, LH declines, the corpus luteum begins to degenerate, and progesterone production falls. As the levels of progesterone and estrogen rapidly fall, the matured endometrium, which no longer has their support, breaks cleanly away from the uterine wall and flows out as menstruation. The fall of progesterone also allows the pituitary gland to begin a new cycle.

And so you see that the hypothalamus, pituitary, and ovaries directly interrelate and depend upon each other. The relationship works through feedback. From one site, increasing or decreasing hormonal levels travel

---

*New cells, created to close the surface defect caused by ovulation, are thought to be the site where ovarian cancer originates. Therefore, for the 50 percent of ovarian cancer cases that are thought to be related to ovulation, the risk is believed to be higher in women who have had more cycles when ovulation has occurred, i.e., more ovulations.

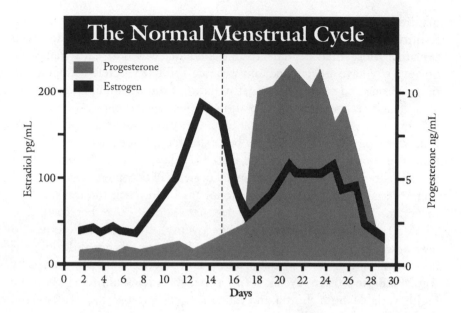

The Normal Menstrual Cycle

Adapted from C. B. Coulan, "Neuroendocrinology and Ovarian Function," in *Danforth's Obstetrics and Gynecology,* 6th ed., ed. J. R. Scott, P. J. DiSaia, C. B. Hammond, and W. N. Spellacy (Philadelphia, Pa.: J.B. Lippincott, 1990), 57–73. Reprinted courtesy of Pharmacia and Upjohn.

through the bloodstream and turn hormonal secretions on or off from the second site and vice versa.

The powerful influence of these hormones isn't confined to the reproductive organs. Because they are secreted directly into the bloodstream, they bathe all the cells and tissues throughout the body and brain. That means they influence many different aspects of our well-being.

UNDERSTANDING OUR CHANGING PHYSIOLOGY

Although some texts describe perimenopause physiology as a normal life process during a transition, other texts see perimenopause as a time of pathophysiology, a time of physiological change leading to disordered function or to disease. The truth probably lies somewhere in between.

The pathophysiology of the menopause becomes apparent long before the last menstrual period. There are several million eggs in the ovary during fetal life. This number has dwindled to only about one hundred thousand by the time of puberty, but by the late forties there are literally just hundreds. This decrease is associated with a fall in hormone levels and fertility. As the most hormone-sensitive and fertile eggs have already been ovulated, those that are left are like students who just can't make the grade. They have a decreased and variable ability to secrete estrogen and progesterone and require greater stimulation from the brain and pituitary gland (their teachers) to develop and complete ovulation.

This increase in variability results in alterations of the menstrual cycle from the typical 28 to 30 days to both shorter and longer cycles. (Count from the first day of flow to the next first day of flow.) Actually, most women anticipate that their menstrual cycles will become farther and farther apart and ultimately stop at menopause. However, the transition to menopause actually begins with cycles that are closer together. Instead of 28 to 30 days (median=28 days at age twenty), the median becomes 26 days at age forty, and then 24 to 25 days becomes the norm during this perimenopausal time. These shorter cycles sometimes are punctuated by regular 28- to 30-day cycles. With time, the cycles ultimately become highly variable, both shorter and much longer—even 45 days and longer. A change in menstrual cyclicity often occurs between the ages of forty-seven and forty-eight and lasts an average of 3.8 years until menopause.

So, if you are experiencing short cycles, long cycles, or increasing premenstrual syndrome, your doctor can usually reassure you that this is just one of life's transition times.

Commonly, women may begin to experience hot flashes and night sweats in their mid- to late forties that persist until a few years after menopause or until hormone replacement is begun. A hot flash is an abrupt episode of heat sensation marked by the anticipatory knowledge that something is about to happen—like the aura of a migraine headache. The heat sensation that occurs in the face and upper body is often accompanied by flushing, heart palpitations, and sweats. The core temperature of the body actually rises slightly before the aura of a hot flash. Then blood vessels dilate and blood flow and heart rate increase, flushing the skin of the upper body, with the result that heat is lost from the surface of the body and the body cools off. Many women note that they feel chilled as their body temperature drops after the flash. Hot flashes usually occur for two years after a natural menopause but may occur for ten or more years. Symptoms are usually worse at the beginning, then wane and occur less frequently and with less severity as time goes on. For perimenopausal women who have both ovaries removed surgically or for whom chemotherapy or radiation causes a more rapid loss of ovarian function, symptoms are more frequent, severe, and last longer (on average 8.5 years). Hot flashes are also more frequent and more severe in smokers.

Nuts and Bolts as to Why This Happens

The new variability in cycle length is largely due to changes in the first half of the menstrual cycle. Estradiol, the prime estrogen of the reproductive-age woman, and progesterone start to become more variable in their secretion.

As the ovarian follicles containing these last few hundred eggs become more resistant to stimulation (ovulation), the FSH levels begin to rise. The pituitary increases its hormonal output of FSH and LH to try to prod these aging eggs to develop. It is this subtle rise in FSH levels, despite regular menstrual cycles, that can give the first biological indication that the perimenopause and its reduced fertility are occurring.

Actually, perimenopausal cycles can be broadly grouped into three "patterns":

1. The first pattern consists of a normal-length cycle with normal hormone levels. This pattern is common at the beginning of the perimenopause and disappears the closer you get to menopause.

2. The second pattern resembles the first except that the cycles are slightly shorter, with higher FSH levels and *higher* estradiol levels early in the cycle. This tends to make ovulation occur 2 to 3 days earlier (i.e., on day 12 to 13). The second half of these cycles can be hormonally normal and of normal length. However, these cycles may be associated with increased premenstrual symptoms (bloating, breast tenderness, fluid retention, mood swings, etc.).

3. The third pattern is usually anovulatory. Here, the aging egg fails to respond to FSH. This cycle is associated with a high FSH level, lower or occasionally normal estradiol level, lack of ovulation with its absence of progesterone, and long cycle duration. These longer cycles can end in bleeding ranging from light spotting to hemorrhage. They seldom are associated with PMS-like symptoms.

How to Tell if You Are Perimenopausal, or How Old Are You Really?

Many women want objective evidence that *proves* what's causing these symptoms. One new approach comes from the early days of in vitro fertilization. Infertility doctors learned that certain infertile women, even though they were still having regular menstrual cycles, had a poor response to fertility drugs. This group of women failed to ovulate more than one egg when given fertility drugs, in contrast to other women of the same age. Infertility experts recognized that blood samples obtained from these infertile women early in the menstrual cycle (i.e., on day 3) had elevated FSH levels. This, they learned, signified a reduced number of follicles with eggs in the ovary. Not only were there fewer eggs, but also these eggs were less likely to respond to stimulation than those in younger women or even women of the same age with lower FSH levels! With time, measurement of FSH became standard for the assignment of an "ovarian follicular age" and took precedence over using chronological age ("How old are you?") in the assessment of a woman's probability of achieving a pregnancy with in vitro fertilization.

Prior to this "ovarian follicular age" discovery, doctors used the FSH assay (test) only to determine whether a woman was menopausal or not. If the FSH was greater than 40 mIU/ml (milli international units/milliliter), then the woman was told she was menopausal. The use of the menstrual cycle day 3 FSH test has enabled physicians and patients to better understand the gradation between normal reproductive age and menopause.

This, however, is still not an exact science. The day 3 FSH test tells a physician whether a woman is in the perimenopausal age range, but the value of the prediction is short lived. It works best for the menstrual cycle in which it is taken. Even the following menstrual cycle may have a different FSH level and a different assessment of both fertility and one's transition to menopause. Again, the issue is variability. However, if a series of FSH tests all performed on day 3 over a few months characteristically show levels above 20 mIU/ml, then a woman is on her way to menopause, even though she may still be having perfectly regular menstrual cycles. Her fertility is likely to be reduced (but not zero), and she may have some hot flashes.

Symptoms during the Perimenopause

Perimenopausal symptoms can be broadly grouped into four basic categories, originally described by Mastroianni and Paulson in 1986. These categories are:

1. *Menstrual irregularities and bleeding problems.* Bleeding problems can be variable. These include irregular cycles (both short and long), light periods, heavy periods, and occasional uterine hemorrhage.

2. *Hot flashes.* This category includes those pesky symptoms of hot flashes (really a sign of estrogen deficiency in the brain).

3. *Psychological and psychosocial disturbances.* Psychological symptoms include altered libido and sexual response, and commonly an increase in premenstrual symptoms. Psychosocial symptoms of stress and/or depression related to hormonal changes may be exacerbated or caused by changes in a woman's psychological and social environment.

4. *Estrogen deficiency symptoms.* These include atrophy of the vulva and vagina, diminished turgor and sagging of the breasts as they are replaced by fatty tissue, thinning of the skin with an increase in wrinkles, etc. There are a large variety of long-term medical consequences such as osteoporosis, heart disease, and Alzheimer's disease, which may have their roots in this period of time even if they are not present as diseases yet. Early accelerated bone loss and changes in the cardiovascular system also probably contribute to the increased risk of heart attack and stroke, which begins to increase during the perimenopause.

CATEGORY 1: MENSTRUAL IRREGULARITIES AND BLEEDING PROBLEMS

In the perimenopause, menstrual disturbances are very common and rival hot flashes in terms of their prevalence. The changes in menstrual pattern may be subtle in the beginning, but as time goes on, they become more profound and a woman may experience long cycles with delayed or absent ovulation. This may result in a thicker than normal uterine lining due to the prolonged estrogen stimulation, which causes heavy menstrual flow often accompanied by the passage of large clots. Occasionally no ovulation occurs and therefore no progesterone is produced—the so-called anovulatory cycle. As adequate progesterone seems critical for an abrupt end of menses, lack of progesterone may lead to heavy menstruation that fails to stop in the usual amount of time.

Absence of ovulation can also lead to other abnormal bleeding. When the endometrium (the lining of the uterus) is under only the influence of estrogen, the cells of the lining multiply and the lining becomes thicker and thicker with an increased propensity to spotting, staining, and bleeding. Occasionally, two or three menstrual cycles' worth of endometrium may accumulate followed by a hormonally normal cycle. Then, a large amount of bleeding from the shedding of this double- or triple-thick layer of endometrium may occur.

Occasionally, this delayed menstruation and buildup of endometrium can be profound. If no ovulation occurs over a long period of time (several months or years), the endometrium can become overgrown and disordered into a precancerous state. With time, this overgrowth can become more and more characteristic of endometrial cancer. (See chapter 13 for further information.) It is no wonder, then, that *most hysterectomies are done during this perimenopausal stage of life. It is estimated that as many as half of all hysterectomies performed during this interval of time could be avoided with appropriate hormonal management.*

In addition to hormonal problems, polyps,* fibroid tumors,† and adenomyosis‡ may also result in bleeding problems during this time. Whether they occur as a response to alterations in the hormonal environment or are "innocent bystanders" is not known. Fibroid tumors occur in as many as 40 percent of African American women and 20 percent of Caucasian women. They are the most common reason for hysterectomy. In addition to bleeding, they can cause pressure, pain, frequent urination, and other symptoms that are also described in chapter 13. Adenomyosis, a less common anatomic cause of bleeding, is present in 25 to 75 percent of all hysterectomy specimens. This disorder can now be diagnosed by MRI (magnetic resonance imaging). It has been found to be "familial." So if your mother or sister had a hysterectomy and her pathology report shows adenomyosis, it may be that your abnormal bleeding is aggravated by or complicated by this problem. (See page 379.)

CATEGORY 2: HOT FLASHES

Hot flashes occurring during the perimenopause are no different from those after menopause, except for the fact that they occur in a woman who is still menstruating. This response by the brain to low estrogen levels occurs in the perimenopausal woman when her estrogen concentration

---

*Polyps—grapelike projections of the uterine lining (caused by overgrowth).

†Fibroids—solid benign growths of tightly compacted muscle and fibrous tissue within the wall of the uterus.

‡Adenomyosis—an infiltration of the uterine wall by endometrial glands.

is at its lowest, or when the relative amount of estrogen compared with progesterone is at its lowest. Because of the variation in estrogen and progesterone through the normal menstrual cycle, it is no wonder that hot flashes in the perimenopausal woman occur most commonly at the very end of the cycle, i.e., just before or during menstruation. They also occasionally occur at midcycle when estrogen levels drop suddenly during ovulation.

While not proven yet, it is likely that midcycle flashes result from a more exaggerated fall in estrogen during ovulation. Women who have hot flashes during midcycle may not have flashes at any other time. The rapid fall in hormone levels at midcycle or before menstruation may create instability in the brain's thermostat and result in hot flashes. Hot flashes also differ among women and also vary in the same woman from cycle to cycle in intensity, frequency, and duration. Hot drinks, spicy foods, hot environments, alcohol, and stress may increase their occurrence and intensity. Thin women also tend to have more hot flashes than their more well-padded sisters.

It is always wise to remember that there are several medical conditions that also cause sweating and flushing. Hyperthyroidism, where there is an excess of thyroid hormone present, can cause excess sweating, sleepiness, fatigue, and flushing of the skin. These symptoms are secondary to a rapid heart rate and increased metabolic rate. Panic attacks may also be confusing because they typically produce sweating, flushing, and a rapid heart rate, which may make a woman think she is having hot flashes. Taking large doses of niacin can create flushes. Then there are two rarer problems known as carcinoid syndrome and pheochromocytoma that may produce symptoms similar enough to be confusing. In addition, several infectious diseases such as tuberculosis and Lyme disease may cause night sweats. If you seem to be having puzzling problems, always remember to seek good medical help.

CATEGORY 3: PSYCHOLOGICAL AND PSYCHOSOCIAL DISTURBANCES

Women in American society seem to have accumulated a variety of responsibilities which are unique compared to their male counterparts. The stress of a woman's combining full-time work, full-time housekeeping plus full-time motherhood is further complicated by the stresses of the menopausal transition. The hormonal shifts that occur at this time may be the straw that breaks the camel's back. Prior to menopause, women who may have had a tendency to be depressed may have been able to avoid obvious depression. But with fatigue from constant interruption of sleep due to night sweats, symptoms of depression may become apparent. Other psychosocial phenomena that often coincide with the perimenopause include the "empty nest syndrome," where a woman's sense of value may be diminished because she feels less needed to care for children now grown and gone and her household responsibilities are drastically reduced. Other women may sense their femininity waning as they are aging in a society that so highly values youth.

Finally, by the age of fifty, women are often saddled with the responsibility of caring for aging parents. As daughters, women seem to automatically be expected to care for aging parents while sons often are spared this burden. In addition, because husbands are often older than wives, many women find themselves caring for sick spouses.

On the other hand, many women in this age group have more power, money, experience, and drive than ever before in their lives. Menopause can be a time of new beginnings including reduced responsibilities for children, the wherewithal to cope with stresses, and an opportunity to explore new frontiers of personal growth. The mere fact that menopause can be a "beginning" is a revelation in itself. The end of menstruation can be liberating.

Mood Changes during the Perimenopause

In their investigation of mood changes during the perimenopause, doctors have been hampered by testing methods that were designed for diagnosing major clinical illness. The subtle changes prior to menopause may be impossible to quantify using these testing methods. That's why, all too often, information about psychological change in this period of time often lacks scientific documentation. The small degree of psychological change that occurs during perimenopause may be too tiny to pick up using our current standardized testing.

Many psychological symptoms occurring in this perimenopausal time are similar to premenstrual syndrome, or PMS, symptoms known to most menstruating women. They include but are not limited to fluid retention, bloating, breast tenderness, abdominal crampiness, heaviness in the legs, lack of energy, cravings for sweet or salty foods, and mood changes. Most mood changes consist of anxiety, irritability, or depression. However, these symptoms differ in intensity from cycle to cycle in the same woman, with few or very mild symptoms in some months to severe symptoms in other months.

However, each woman has her own constellation of symptoms that she experiences from month to month. Some women seem to have more physical symptoms, while others suffer from mental ones. Few, however, have symptoms that are severe enough to interfere with day-to-day activities. Not uncommonly, PMS tends to increase as a woman approaches menopause, especially during ovulatory menstrual cycles. The reasons for this are not clear. It may be related to waning hormonal secretion or to changes in hormonal balance.

We now know that progesterone is a potent "neurosteroid," a compound with profound impact on the cognitive and mood centers of the brain. *The rapid fall in progesterone at the end of the menstrual cycle may trigger events in the brain similar to "withdrawal" from narcotics or barbiturates.* Released from the quieting effect of progesterone, the brain may rebound with major mood changes. To date, the exact nature of progesterone's impact on the brain and PMS or depression in particular is not known. Clearly there is a complicated interaction between the changing hormonal environment and its biochemical and psychological effects.

Recently, the selective serotonin reuptake inhibitors (SSRIs) such as Prozac®, Paxil®, Zoloft®, Effexor®, and Luvox® have been shown to have a beneficial effect on PMS as well as depression. Some suggest that an increase in vitamin B_6 and exercise is helpful. In my own practice, I use a special diet plus vitamins and minerals that help give my patients relief. I have been especially interested in the eating habits of women with PMS. Although American women on the whole have inadequate diets, in my experience women with PMS have worse eating habits. They normally skip breakfast, eat a tiny or a fast-food lunch, and overeat at dinner. They also tend to have a poorly balanced diet. So in order to ensure a better diet, and to try to keep their blood sugar level, I devised the following diet and have used it with good success since 1980.

My PMS Diet

Each meal must contain a protein *and* a complex carbohydrate. Proteins are found in milk products such as yogurt, cottage cheese, pot cheese, and hard cheeses. If you have a local cheese shop, ask them for low-fat and/or low-salt cheeses. Lean meat, chicken, fish, tofu, and unsalted nuts in small quantities are other sources of protein. Complex carbohydrates are breads, crackers, pasta, pita bread, cereal, etc.

Breakfast: Most women never take time to eat breakfast. Cold cereal and low-fat milk with fruit is fast and satisfying. Or bread with vegetable pot cheese on top with a cup of coffee will do nicely. Or try a boiled egg and toast. Have you tried a low-calorie, no-cholesterol egg-white omelet? (Just be careful what you add to it.)

Mid-morning snack: Three hours later, a low-fat flavored yogurt and a small cracker; or a bland cheese and half-slice of bread; or turkey breast on a cracker; or a chicken leg and pita bread.

Lunch: Make sure it contains some protein and a complex carbohydrate. Salads should have some meat, chicken, rinsed tuna, or cheese in them. Remember, salad dressing is the fattening part. Try lemon squeezed over your salad, or plain balsamic vinegar. A turkey burger will do, using only half of the roll, and for a flavor boost, add a slice of raw onion.

Three-thirty snack: Tea plus lunch leftovers, or if you are at home, eat the first course of your dinner. Or try a piece of fruit and a small portion of a protein. This snack will get you over that tired feeling that comes in the middle of the afternoon and will prevent you from overeating at dinnertime.

Dinner: Eat what you normally would for dinner, but a little less than usual.

Bedtime snack: Drink a glass of skim milk and eat a rice cake or cracker. The tryptophan in the milk plus the carbohydrate will help you sleep. If you can't tolerate milk, then have water and a light snack along with your nighttime calcium supplement.

I am not suggesting that you eat a lot, rather that you eat small, balanced, frequent meals. This will decrease your food cravings for sweets and help you burn your food more efficiently. It will also help keep your blood sugar at a higher level throughout the day. Avoiding wide swings in blood sugar is important for maintaining your good mood.

Also, avoid alcohol (and save lots of calories too—why do women so often forget that alcoholic drinks have calories?). Finally, take a balanced, comprehensive vitamin and mineral supplement that contains vitamin B_1, B_2, B_6, vitamin E, magnesium, and calcium. Seventy percent of my patients have shown improvement using this diet and balanced A.M/P.M. vitamins—see page 392. Good luck!

Changes in Libido

The perimenopause may usher in a decrease in libido and sexual functioning. These changes are often thought to be psychological or psychosocial, but they have well-documented biological underpinnings. While it is difficult to document these changes with standardized testing methods, large studies from around the world have clearly demonstrated that women believe they will have a reduction in libido during the perimenopausal transition. Changes in PMS and bleeding patterns tend to increase concerns. In fact, a reduction in sexual contact and intercourse occurs commonly during this period of time, beginning as early as age forty. Studies have shown that even if a woman just believes that she is perimenopausal she is very likely to say that her sexual desire has decreased. While changes in libido have been classified as psychological or psychosocial in the past, these changes likely result from newly reduced levels of hormones circulating in the bloodstream.

The levels of the male hormone (testosterone) in the perimenopausal woman depend on both her ovaries and her adrenal glands. Toward menopause, testosterone production in the ovary falls as does estrogen production. After menopause, testosterone production falls precipitously, although it does continue to be produced for up to five years, in ever decreasing amounts. Interestingly, recent research by Swedish investigators has shown that androstenedione, a weak male-type hormone primarily made in the adrenal gland, is closely correlated to sexual desire, satisfaction, and arousal in perimenopausal women. Although this may seem odd, this same adrenal hormone has now also been implicated in the onset of sexual attraction and sexual fantasy which occurs in nine- and ten-year-olds.

Category 4: Estrogen Dependency

Most cells in the body are affected by estrogen in some way. Indeed, estrogen is a ubiquitous hormone in both men and women. When estrogen begins to wane, the organs most dramatically affected are those that depend highly and/or specifically on estrogen. These include the vagina, the bladder, the breast, the brain, and, to a lesser degree, other tissues such as skin, cartilage, muscle, and bone. Reproductive tissues, the vagina, uterus, bladder, urethra, and breast tissue are most commonly thought of as being estrogen dependent. They contain large numbers of submicroscopic elements known as estrogen receptors. The receptors provide a docking site for circulating estrogen molecules and bind them to the cell. The degree of effect is dependent on the estrogen itself, its concentration and potency, but most importantly, the amount of time it spends bound to the estrogen receptor.

The vulva and vagina are exquisitely sensitive to estrogen, which creates changes during the menstrual cycle in the quality and quantity of secretions. These facts are well known to most menstruating women. Needing a longer time to achieve sexual arousal and lubrication may occur during the perimenopause in some women as estrogen and testosterone levels fall. Some women may also experience some degree of vaginal dryness. Most women, however, have few sexual difficulties. If they do, an over-the-counter lubricant is normally very helpful. In my practice, I have found that vaginal dryness is a much more frequent complaint six to twenty-four months after the cessation of menses, or even later on in the postmenopausal phase. Some women may note an early subtle loss of pubic hair. The bladder and the urethra themselves are rich with estrogen receptors. A decrease in estrogen therefore may cause these tissues to lose their support and begin to sag. That is when lack of urinary control seems to manifest itself. (For an in-depth coverage of this topic please read chapter 9.)

The breast is obviously another estrogen-dependent organ. Falling estrogen levels cause some atrophy and loss of density as breast glandular tissue is replaced by fat. Women may experience a reduction in breast size and fullness. However, many of my patients find that their breasts seem fuller. These same women usually have also increased their weight.

Skin is also estrogen sensitive, although less directly than reproductive tissues. The French have known this for years, adding estrogen or estrogen-like compounds to cosmetics in an attempt to overcome the effects of reduced estrogen levels. In fact, estrogen, when applied directly to skin, increases the amount of elastic tissue, connective tissue, and water present in the skin. Together, these increases make the skin seem smoother and softer, and they also reduce wrinkles. When estrogen is taken orally or by patch, many of these same effects on the skin can be clearly demonstrated. One other effect is that estrogen tends to balance out increasing (relative to estrogen) levels of male hormones that occur after menopause. The predominance of male hormone after menopause is thought to result in increased facial hair, coarseness of the skin, and wrinkling (see page 93 for further comment).

Cardiovascular System

Estrogen has a profound impact on a woman's overall health by virtue of its many effects on the heart and blood vessels. While cardiovascular fitness was not as much of a concern to most women of previous generations, as women today become more invested in their own health, fitness has become paramount in terms of long life and good health. The effects of estrogen on the vascular system may not be obvious, but menstruating women rarely have heart attacks and strokes. In contrast, younger women who have had their ovaries removed and do not receive hormone replacement have the highest risk of cardiovascular disease.

Actually, if you are a type I (juvenile onset) diabetic, you may be at risk for premature menopause and therefore at increased risk of cardiovascular disease. A study by Janice Dorman, Ph.D., at the University of Pittsburgh of 122 type I diabetic women showed that they experienced menopause at age forty-two on average, an age much younger than their nondiabetic counterparts. She also found that they tended to be older at the time of their first period, and experienced longer menstrual cycles before age thirty. Dorman concluded that estrogen replacement therapy should be strongly considered in postmenopausal diabetics because their early loss of estrogen increases their already high risk of cardiovascular disease.

Bone

Although most women realize that estrogen deficiency *after* menopause leads to bone loss, it is not universally understood among women that this process begins *before* menopause, during the perimenopause. The first phase of bone loss occurs as a result of aging, and is present to similar degrees in both men and woman. This loss begins shortly after attaining skeletal maturity, between the ages of twenty-five to thirty. Believe it or not, it is downhill for your skeleton from this point on. The second phase of bone loss is due to falling estrogen in the perimenopausal years. This phase of loss begins at about age forty-five. It results in a reduced absorption of calcium from the diet, and increased loss of calcium from the urine, and a consequent "robbing" of calcium from your bones. This results in an intermediary level of bone loss that continues until after the last menstrual period—the menopause—when estrogen levels plummet and the rate of bone loss markedly accelerates.

Therapies for Perimenopausal Symptomatology

Bleeding pattern abnormalities are frequent during this time, but controlling them is not always simple. These problems result from the waning of normal ovarian function and the changes that this creates. One of the newer therapies offers low-dose 20 microgram estrogen oral contraceptives to women. I have mixed thoughts on the subject (see below), but for some women there may be more pros than cons. Again, individualization is key as well as careful watching.

PROS AND CONS OF ORAL CONTRACEPTIVES

Pros

1. Most women over age forty do not recognize their increased risk for unintended pregnancy. Actually, women in this period of life have a risk of unwanted pregnancy and abortion equal to that of adolescents! Natural family planning methods and timing of intercourse become more difficult because of erratic cycles. For this reason, oral contraceptives provide peace of mind during this time. They also decrease the incidence of ectopic pregnancy and functional ovarian cysts.

2. Most oral contraceptives provide good bleeding control with a reduction in the total amount of bleeding during menses and fewer days of spotting and staining. However, the first two to three months of their use may be marred by intermenstrual spotting and staining—most likely the result of irregular shedding of the lining of the uterus in response to the pill itself. However, decreased flow (and decreased menstrual pain and cramping) may also result in less iron-deficiency anemia.

3. Oral contraceptives have been found to be safe in women over the age of forty *unless* they are smokers. Smokers over age forty should not use oral contraceptives either for bleeding control or for contraception. It should be noted, however, that the data used in formulating this statement are not absolutely clear. Older studies using higher dose oral contraceptives have shown an unacceptably high risk of stroke and heart attack in women over the age of thirty-five who smoke. This is more likely due to the smoking than to the pills, but synergy between them does seem to exist. Data on the newer lower-dose pills and smokers over forty are less clear, but caution seems advisable. My advice is that if you want to use oral contraceptives and are a smoker who is over forty, stop smoking! I personally would not prescribe them to a smoker over the age of thirty-five.

4. Birth control pills provide other benefits, including a reduced risk of uterine (endometrial) and ovarian cancer. Taking them for just one year decreases the risk of ovarian cancer by 10 percent. Taking them for five years decreases the risk by 50 percent. They also decrease breast cysts and breast fibroadenomas, benefit bones, reduce PMS symptoms in some

women (although they increase it in others), and reduce the incidence of arthritic symptoms. These benefits have been associated with the use of birth control pills in younger women; however, it would seem that they may likely accrue to the perimenopausal woman, even though wide experience in this age group is not yet available.

Cons

Contraindications (i.e., conditions that make a specific treatment inadvisable) to birth control pills apply to perimenopausal women as well as all age groups. Women with a history of deep venous thrombosis or other blood clots may not be candidates for oral contraceptives. This fact is important, as many women who took part in the early oral contraceptive research trials some twenty to thirty years ago may have had blood clots as a complication of the high doses of estrogen used in these original birth control pills. These experiences, thirty years ago, *still* make these women "noncandidates" for birth control pills during their perimenopause.

Women with a history of active liver disease, cerebral vascular disease, cancer of the endometrium, jaundice with prior pill use, suspected pregnancy, and undiagnosed vaginal bleeding are not candidates for birth control pills. Women with a history of breast cancer, high blood pressure, high cholesterol, or with a history of heart attack or angina should not take birth control pills. (As you read about hormone replacement therapy later in the book, you will see that many of these major *contraindications* to birth control pills are major *indications* for encouraging hormone replacement; for example, history of heart attack, diabetes, and abnormal lipid levels.) Side effects in some women using oral contraceptives include bloating, fluid retention, depression or PMS-like symptoms, worsening of glucose control in diabetics or prediabetic states, gallbladder disease, possible adverse effects on lipid levels, worsening or beginning of hypertension, and benign liver tumors. In addition, some women have nausea, breast tenderness, and migraine headaches for several weeks until their body adjusts to the new hormonal milieu.

Although many physicians advocate birth control pills for nearly every perimenopausal woman, I do only when options such as those that follow have not worked. Again, there are exceptions and there are no hard and fast rules. There are patients who want the "pill" and need birth control. Everything must be individualized!

Progesterone-like Medications (PLM) for Cycle Control and Normalizing Bleeding Patterns

PLM use in the second portion of the menstrual cycle may prevent premenstrual spotting in women who have a deficiency of progesterone in the second half of the cycle and can also end prolonged or heavy menses (see page 369). Usually, ten days of PLM can be used prior to the onset of menses. The trick is to take the PLM in sync with your own cycle. Taking PLM is not like taking a birth control pill: PLM does not take over the cycle, it must mesh with an existing cycle. If given at the wrong time, it just makes things worse. On the other hand, if no regular cycle exists, PLM can help to create one. Therefore, a perimenopausal woman with erratic or prolonged cycles or very heavy bleeding may be able to achieve a monthly cycle with normal bleeding by using PLM in the following fashion.

First, I have my patient figure out when her period should be due. She then takes PLM for ten days, beginning the ten days so that the last, or tenth, pill is taken two days prior to the desired date of flow. (Bleeding normally occurs one to three days after discontinuing the PLM.)

After the first menses, regular monthly cycles can be created. This is how I instruct a patient who normally had a 28-day cycle: Counting from her last pill (not from when flow occurred), she takes no PLM for 18 days. Then she begins the pills and takes them for 10 days. She then continues—off for 18 days, on for 10—and in two to three months a regular cycle of 28 days is created. Other women who had shorter cycles (e.g., 26 days) may go off for 16 days and on for 10 days. Women are encouraged to stay on this regimen for three to four months, then stop to see if their periods resume a more regular cycle on their own. Sometimes they do. If irregular bleeding occurs, then it's back to cycling with PLM again, sometimes for years. Most women find that their cycles become regular, and that their bleeding, which in the past was heavy as well as unpredictable, becomes lighter on PLM.

This approach works because most perimenopausal women still have more than sufficient estrogen production. The real problem for most perimenopausal women with irregular bleeding is lack of ovulation or lack of sufficient progesterone production. Therefore, we are simply resupplying what these women lack, and are usually successful.

A number of perimenopausal women in my practice take cyclic monthly medroxyprogesterone acetate in 5 or 10 mg doses or norethindrone acetate in 2.5 or 5 mg doses until they become menopausal. When does the woman know she is menopausal? Simply when three sequential cycles of PLM do not result in bleeding. When there is no estrogen present, no lining grows. When there is no lining, obviously no flow is produced when PLM is stopped. At this point, blood FSH and estradiol levels should be checked to confirm that menopausal levels have been reached.

TYPES OF PROGESTERONE-LIKE MEDICATIONS AVAILABLE

Natural Progesterone

Not all progestational agents are equivalent. The parent compound—natural progesterone—contains twenty-one carbon atoms and is known as a C-21 carbon compound. Because of its structure, it is broken down rapidly by stomach acid, so that it is not usually suitable for oral use. More recently, natural progesterone has been milled into smaller particles (micronized), and this process has improved its absorption. In the U.S., until recently, women could only get micronized progesterone from "compounding druggists" who put the hormonal material along with fillers into capsules. Unfortunately, there was little or no uniform quality control across the U.S. of either the raw materials or the pharmacy practices. Therefore, most physicians were reluctant to prescribe micronized progesterone until it became available from a drug manufacturer with FDA approval. Patients and physicians alike must be careful when using these agents to make sure they are actually effective in preventing endometrial hyperplasia and balancing estrogen—especially the high estrogen levels that may occur in perimenopausal women.

One commercial preparation of oral micronized progesterone has been particularly well studied. In Europe it is called Utrogestan® and is made by Besins-Iscovesco (Paris, France); in Canada it is called Prometrium® and is made by Schering-Plough. By the time this book is published, Prometrium should be available in the U.S., marketed by Solvay. It was obtained and used in the PEPI (Postmenopausal Estrogen/Progestin Interventions) Trial in the United States recently and got high marks for lack of side effects and little to no adverse effects on blood lipids. It is most commonly used in 200 mg doses for twelve days each month. Aside from oral forms, natural progesterone is available in vaginal and rectal suppositories, and by injection.

Synthetic Progestational Agents

Synthetic agents tend to fall into two groups:

C-21 compounds. These are similar in structure to progesterone, derived from progesterone, and—like progesterone—contain twenty-one carbon atoms. Their structures, however, have been modified to improve oral absorption. The compound most frequently used in the U.S. is known as MPA, or medroxyprogesterone acetate (Provera®, Cycrin®, Amen®, etc.). It is most commonly used in 2.5, 5, or 10 mg doses. Another more potent compound in this same C-21 family is megestrol acetate, or Megace®. It is rarely used in hormone replacement but has an important role in the treatment of endometrial cancer.

C-19 compounds. These compounds are derived from testosterone (yes, testosterone). That a substance arising from a male hormone could have pregnancy progesterone-like hormonal activity seems incredible until you look at a diagram of the molecules (see page 42). At a glance, they seem to be very much alike. However, testosterone is a C-19 carbon compound. A slight change in the molecule produces compounds with progestational (pregnancy-like) activity. Known as 19-nortestosterone compounds, many of their names begin with the prefix "nor" (norethindrone, Aygestin® or norethindrone acetate, norgestrel, and others). Because it is more potent milligram for milligram than MPA, most physicians commonly equate the progestational effects of a 5 mg dose of norethindrone acetate (Aygestin®) to 10 mgs of MPA (Provera®). In my experience, when women cannot tolerate side effects of bloating and PMS-like symptoms from Provera®, I switch them to equivalent doses of Aygestin® (norethindrone acetate) or less often Micronor® (norethindrone) or Ovrette® (norgestrel), two progestin-only oral contraceptive pills, or Prometrium®. Often their symptoms are decreased. Aygestin® is also better in my experience for women with hard-to-control heavy bleeding problems. Although these "nor" compounds have a reputation for having adverse effects on blood lipids, I have generally not found this to be a problem. However, if I had a patient with a poor lipid profile, I would choose a C-21 compound, at least initially. And if a patient is on long-term 19-nor compounds, I watch her cholesterol, HDL, and LDL profile.

Fact: Only C-19 compounds are used in oral contraceptives to balance the potent synthetic estrogen called ethinyl estradiol, which is contained in most birth control pills in the United States.

Estrogen

For those women who have hot flashes as a result of waning estrogen levels yet are still in their forties, I usually advise them to stick it out for two to three months. Often their ovaries will "rev up" and go back to normal function with normal hormonal levels when their stress is reduced. That is why I'm not always in a rush to treat, even when estrogen levels are low and FSH is high. I have often seen low postmenopausal estrogen levels suddenly swing to high "thirty-year-old levels" without rhyme or reason. Remember: The essence of the perimenopause is its variability.

On the other hand, oral contraceptives will stop the flashes and control hormonal swings, or estrogen can be administered in either pill form or as a transdermal patch. A variety of types are available (see page 74). The application of these estrogen "supplements" can occur during the entire cycle, or simply during those phases when symptoms arise. For example, if a woman has hot flashes or premenstrual migraine just before her menstrual period and at no other time during her cycle, estrogen can be used just before menstruation in anticipation of symptoms. For women with premenstrual migraine headache I usually use a transdermal patch. Often a low dose of 0.375 or 0.05 mg for three to five days will suffice. This additional estrogen, at the time when estrogen and progesterone levels normally fall, will enable a patient's blood vessels to dilate, improve blood flow, and prevent the headache from occurring. On the other hand, I have also found that some women with premenstrual migraine respond beautifully to injectable *natural* progesterone, 100 mg in oil. The injection, which must be given in the buttock, is normally given seven to ten days before the onset of menses.

In those rare women with midcycle hot flashes, giving midcycle estrogen can result in abnormal bleeding because it may interfere with ovulation. Remember, no one ever died from hot flashes. If the above approaches don't seem right, you *can* always "tuff it out," at least for a while.

Several provisos must be included about the use of estrogen during perimenopause. First, careful studies of the perimenopause do not clearly demonstrate estrogen deficiency; in fact, some studies actually show increased estrogen levels (remember—variability). Second, as estrogen levels rise, the drive of the pituitary gland to stimulate and sustain the menstrual cycle is reduced. If supplementary estrogen is given in excess as a treatment for symptoms (such as hot flashes), it can lead to a cessation of the menstrual cycle. This is less likely when very low doses of estrogen are used as supplements. Should a woman's cycle cease with higher doses of estrogen supplementation and her symptoms persist, then either oral contraceptives or full hormonal therapy should be initiated (see chapter 2).

Nonhormonal Therapies for Vaginal Dryness

Vaginal dryness occurs one to two years postmenopause in most women. However, some perimenopausal women note some dryness. This can largely be reversed using a combination of lubricants and moisturizers that are available over the counter. It can also be reversed by using the Estring™ vaginal ring or by using small amounts of vaginal estrogen cream as described on page 88.

Nonhormonal Therapies, Designer Estrogens, and Alternative Therapy

See chapter 3 for information on phytoestrogens, vitamins, and other commonsense ideas for dealing with annoying symptoms.

Summary: Perimenopause and You

Few women in this perimenopausal stage of life need hormonal therapy. Most get through this transitional period just fine. Nonetheless, there are major changes coming in perimenopausal therapy for those women with irregular cycles and PMS-like symptoms. Much more medicalization soon will be offered by doctors and pharmaceutical companies in the form of low-dose, 20 microgram birth control pills or progesterone-type medication. For some women, this may be a good thing. The pills or progesterone-like substances will result in normal cycles, less monthly flow, and will probably help avoid some unnecessary surgery.

Unlike hormone replacement, where amounts of estrogen and progesterone-like substances given merely replace physiological hormone levels, birth control pills contain large amounts of hormones that override the woman's reproductive system. Although they contain four or more times the amount of estrogen used in replacement therapy, their secret is that the estrogen is constantly balanced by progesterone-like substances. Therefore they create their own steady, balanced hormonal milieu.

Every woman, by the time she reaches the perimenopausal years, brings her own personal baggage. Every woman enters this phase of life with her own genetic, medical, and social background. Some already have the onset of chronic illness, others jog four miles a day. Some women are dealing with tremendous financial and family stress, others may have supportive husbands and secure futures. Therefore, no two women can expect to have exactly the same perimenopausal experience. That is why each woman must have medical care tailored to her mental as well as social and physical needs.

Remember, most perimenopausal women require no therapy. Other women just need reassurance. Unfortunately, this chapter has had to dwell on therapy for the minority of women who actually require it. Although the emphasis seems to be on women who have problems, most women, once they are aware of the perimenopausal variations, accept the occasional blips without much concern. However, if you feel that you are experiencing problems, talk with your doctor. As you now should understand, it should be possible to get the individual therapy you deserve.

Hysterectomy and Replacement Therapy

Many women who have had a hysterectomy were started on hormone replacement in their thirties or forties. Many of my patients with this surgical history question the length of time they have taken estrogen. Often, they will say, "I've been on estrogen for ten years now. I'm worried about getting breast cancer." Many of these women are now only fifty-three or fifty-four. I remind them that, had they not had a hysterectomy and their ovaries removed, they would have had their own estrogen production until the average age of $51\frac{1}{2}$. So I tell them to count only from after the age of $51\frac{1}{2}$. Therefore, they should consider themselves to have been on estrogen for only two to three years. Few if any textbooks ever discuss this, but I think that it is a valid point. Furthermore, most of these women were placed on .625 mg or its equivalent of estrogen, which is less estrogen than their own ovaries would have produced during their perimenopausal years. If you are one of these women, I hope this makes you feel better.

References

Floter, A., et al. "Androgen Status and Sexual Life in Perimenopausal Women." *Menopause: The Journal of the North American Menopause Society* 4, no. 2 (1997): 95–100.

Treloan, Alan E., et al. "Variations of the Human Menstrual Cycle through Reproductive Life." *Interventional Journal of Fertility* 12, no. 2 (1967): 77–126.

WHO Scientific Group on Research on the Menopause in the 1990s. Geneva, Switzerland.

Chapter 2
MENOPAUSE

The postmenopausal time of life is a new phenomenon. Until recently, it only occurred for a tiny minority of women. The majority of women in 1900 died at about the time they would have become menopausal. The large number of women today who are entering menopause is startling. Doctors who went to medical school twenty to thirty years ago had little instruction in caring for the menopausal patient.

We all know generally what aging is about. Doctors as well as the general public, however, know very little about the specifics of aging and how various body systems fare with time and stress. There are actually few geriatricians in practice yet. Therefore, as we look at aging, for women in particular, there are many unanswered questions. We know basically that women live longer than men. We also know that women suffer more disability than men. This is not simply because they outlive them, but also because women have illnesses that are specific to women.

How can we be sure that women's health deteriorates just from the aging process itself, when it is a known fact that the sudden decrease in hormonal levels at menopause causes specific acceleration of some disease processes? It should also be apparent that problems usually do not happen overnight: For example, you do not have healthy bones one day then suddenly fracture your hip by stepping off a curb the next. Just because deteriorations are slow and silent does not mean that they are not occurring. It is only for the time being that they exist without causing symptoms.

And so the debate. Most of us want to believe that the majority of menopausal women in this country are healthy and function well. Indeed, we do more than our grandmothers ever did at the same age.

Leave us alone, some women say, menopause is a normal fact of life, and no one needs to do anything. But there may be a price for not doing anything.

Others feel that you must try to protect women through this period by giving them HRT (hormone replacement therapy) to ensure that they are protected. But there may be a price for taking hormones. Others want to take only herbs. But there may be a price here too for taking untested compounds, even those labeled "natural." Others will exercise and take lots of calcium. That too may have a price. What to do and how to do it best is what each one of us must decide for ourselves. Understanding the consequences is fundamental. I believe they exist for any decision you choose. Read on and make up your own mind. You really have to understand to be a partner in your health care. Make sure that your choices are made from an informed and knowledgeable point of view.

I believe in Margaret Mead's "postmenopausal zest." I only want it to last even longer and be 100 percent perfect.

This chapter will make you an expert on menopause. In my last book, in one especially technical passage, I exclaimed, "Can you believe—I'm trying to make you a doctor!" Well, when you have finished this chapter, you may be more savvy than some physicians. Sharing this information with other menopausal women is the best gift I can give and one of my greatest pleasures.

Putting Menopause into Perspective

When *No More Hot Flashes and Other Good News* was published in 1983, I thought that my book would be all the help that women would ever need to get through menopause. What I hadn't anticipated was that a whole new group of women, the baby boomers, would now have new questions to answer. In addition, women who are in their sixties and seventies now have questions about choices that never existed before. There is a lot more "good news" to share as we go into the next millennium.

Because of our sheer numbers (fifty million by the year 2000), postmenopausal women have become a very important segment of our society. Never have there been so many women entering the age of menopause. We are truly a twentieth-century phenomenon. In the 1400s women only lived to an average age of thirty-three. By 1900, women's life expectancy had increased to forty-eight years. Like other animals, women died when their ovaries stopped functioning and they could no longer reproduce.

However, a female infant born today can expect to live seventy-nine years or more and outlive her ovaries by one-third of her lifetime. Even more remarkable, you who are reading this chapter have an average life expectancy of nearly thirty-five years beyond your last menstrual period. That's because if you have already survived illness and childbirth and made it to the age of fifty, you should, on average, live to be eighty-five. The age at which menopause occurs has not significantly changed for centuries. However, the years you will live after menopause have suddenly increased. How we choose to live these additional years is what this chapter is about. Never have so many women entered menopause, been so well informed—and so confused!

One of the basic premises about menopause is that it is natural. All women go through it. Therefore, many women and some doctors feel it should not be altered in any way. However, evolution normally takes thousands of years. It cannot possibly adjust in such a short blink of time. So theoretical questions arise:

1. Is it natural to live so long? Because of better nutrition, sanitation, antibiotics, and attention to obstetrical and preventive health care, our life span has suddenly dramatically increased. Whether it is normal to live so long or not, we are there.

2. Should evolution have provided for a lifetime of hormonal output in women as it does in men? There are those who feel that menopause was originally evolutionarily necessary as it prevented childbearing by women who would be less able to care for offspring in the wild. Others believe it provided grandmothers to help care for youngsters in an extended family setting. Men, generally not involved with raising the young, retained their hormonal output and therefore their reproductive ability as well as their muscle mass for hunting and fighting ferocious animals and such.

3. Is it normal for women to live without some type of medical or hormonal support for thirty-five years after menopause? This will be answered as more and more observations are collected from various studies. I believe that the answer is probably no. Hormones, hormone-like medications, or specific plant foods, sometimes used in combination, will commonly be used to optimize this prolonged stage of life. Remember, there is no free lunch. There may be consequences to the decision not to take hormonal therapy just as there may be consequences to taking it or even to using alternatives.

The problems of individualizing therapy to those who will benefit most and omitting hormone-type therapy for those who will benefit least is what this chapter is about. Alternatives and other complementary therapies will be addressed in the next chapter. Whether you take hormones or not, I hope you will read it.

I know that my patients and I want similar things:

- To have our dreams fulfilled
- To have some leisure to enjoy
- To remain independent and in good health
- Not to depend upon others, including our children

How well you'll be able to fulfill your dreams will in large part depend on choices you make today. You have the power to affect the quality of your life. Menopause, a signpost along the road of life, suddenly has become a symbolic time for reevaluating and for entering a new era. As I have said before, it is not the "beginning of the end," but rather the "end of the beginning."

We must then understand all of our options, because in the final analysis, we are responsible for our own well-being. The decisions we make now may impact on our lives far into the future. On the other hand, I don't want to be too dramatic. Most of the decisions can wait a week, month, or several months to make. Furthermore, once again, all of the decisions you make today can be changed tomorrow, next month, or next year. Nothing is written in stone. I hope that as you learn more, the decisions will get easier and more perfect for you. That is not a collective you, I really mean *you*.

What Is Menopause?

The age at which menopause occurs is genetically predetermined. To the best of our knowledge, it does not seem to be influenced by age of menarche, number of pregnancies, number of live children delivered, use of birth control pills, height, weight, race, or economic status. It is well known, however, that smoking will hasten its arrival by two years or more, and juvenile diabetes even more so.

The word *menopause* is frequently used somewhat improperly to signify a range of time. It actually *refers to a single point in time,* namely the last menstrual period. The *climacteric refers to the symptoms* that occur during the years from the onset of premenopausal ovarian decline to the time after menopause, when its symptoms stop. The decline of ovarian function actually goes on for years, but the cessation of menses is an unmistakable biological marker for the loss of reproductive function. The average age at menopause in the United States is approximately 51.4 years.

Many factors contribute to how well we age, such as our genetic background. We all know women who are sixty and look forty, and we all know women who are fifty and look like sixty-five. It's not all genes, though, for the foods we eat, the exercise that we do or don't do, the alcohol and cigarettes we consume, the stress we undergo, the weight we gain, and the medications we take all impact on our lives. And then there are the psychological aspects of accepting aging and our general happiness.

MENOPAUSE, WHAT HAPPENS?

Even though menopause has occurred, estrogens are still present. Which ones and how much, however, depend on several factors. The human female has, besides estradiol, two other estrogen-type hormones—estrone and estriol. Estradiol is the most important and most powerful. It is the major female hormone of the premenopausal woman.

Estrone is less potent and is the principal estrogen of the postmenopausal woman. In the early postmenopausal time, estrone levels may be significant. Estrone is created in the postmenopausal woman from a weak, male-type hormone precursor known as androstenedione, which is secreted by the ovary (20 percent) and the adrenal gland (80 percent). Androstenedione is then converted in the body's fat cells to estrone. Estrone that results from this conversion may attain high levels, as it is outside the menstrual cycle control mechanisms that normally prevent excess buildup of estrogen in the younger woman. It is very important to also understand that because postmenopausal ovaries are no longer able to produce an egg, progesterone is not present to balance or oppose this estrogen.

The conversion rate of androstenedione in fat increases as we age and even more so with increasing obesity. Therefore, postmenopausal overweight women tend to have higher concentrations of estrone than their thinner sisters. This results in fewer menopausal symptoms. But because estrone is produced by these circuitous routes, and unopposed by progesterone, it may also place these women at higher risk for endometrial and breast cancer.

The third female hormone, estriol, is produced from estrone. It is not, therefore, directly secreted by the ovary. It is a weak hormone that has less effect than either estrone or estradiol. Although produced at high levels by the placenta during pregnancy, it is thought to be a breakdown product of the more potent or biologically active estrogens estradiol and estrone.

As time goes on in the postmenopausal period, the outer portion of the ovary no longer produces female hormone, yet its core retains its ability to produce androstenedione and a more powerful male hormone, testosterone. In the premenopausal woman, the ovaries' female hormones dominate. After menopause, the female hormonal output of the ovary plummets while male hormone production in the interior of the ovary drops by fifty percent, then declines over a few to many years depending on the individual. Because male hormone continues to be produced by the aging ovary as well as the adrenal glands, there is a change in the relative proportions of male to female hormones, which may upset their delicate balance. This can cause the growth of dark, coarse facial hairs on the chin as well as fuzzy facial hair that can sometimes be noticed on older women. Finally, however, all ovarian function is lost. This leaves the adrenal gland as well as our peripheral fat as the producers of estrone or its precursors.

It is fascinating to see from the diagrams of male and female hormones (see below) how slight is the distinction between male and female that we hold so sacred. Once you have seen these structures, it is easy to understand how readily they can be converted into one another. And they are constantly being interconverted. Progesterone is often the precursor for either male or female hormones; estradiol can be directly converted to estrone and vice versa; and testosterone can be converted into female hormone and vice versa. Male and female physiologies are not all that exclusive.

Estradiol Estrone Estriol

Testosterone Estradiol

MENOPAUSAL SYMPTOMS

As the menstrual cycle ceases and the hormones that have been saturating every cell of the body for more than forty years are withdrawn, a woman can experience conditions ranging from mild to nearly incapacitating. These are the most common and troubling symptoms of the climacteric, the bulleted items may be improved by the use of estrogen:

- Hot flashes that bring a sudden, unpredictable wave of heat and mild to drenching sweat over the upper body
- Night sweats, that is, hot flashes that occur in the night, disturbing sleep
- Vaginal dryness and atrophy/decreased sexual lubrication
- Vulvar atrophy/pubic hair loss
- Urinary incontinence
- Skin changes
- Psychological effects
- Cognitive changes (decreased concentration)
- Headache
- Decreased libido
- Sleep disturbances

In addition, women face other particularly serious conditions and chronic illness after menopause:

- Increased risk of heart attack
- Increased rate of bone loss
- Increased risk of arthritis/fibromyositis/chronic fatigue
- Increased risk of stroke
  Increased risk of breast cancer
- Increased risk of colon cancer
  Increased risk of endometrial cancer
- Increased risk of Alzheimer's disease
- Increased loss of muscle mass
- Increased risk of cataracts

Although the list is long, large numbers of older women do not remember menopause as a negative event.

In addition, there are positive events:

Loss of premenstrual syndrome symptoms
Freedom from worry over inadvertent pregnancy

Freedom from menses
Freedom from infant care, except for grandchildren
Time for yourself—to work or go back to school

Is It Aging or the Effect of Menopause, or Both?

Looking at the first two lists above, not one of the problems is one any of us would choose to have. Is this list the inevitable effect of aging, or is the event of menopause a separate and intensifying risk factor?

Consider this analogy. Many of us take antihypertensive medications although we have no obvious problems except for an elevated blood pressure reading. Yet these medications have to be taken daily and many have side effects that are troubling. We take them to prevent a future problem, even though we feel all right today. Antihypertensive drugs have helped to decrease the incidence of stroke, heart failure, and heart attack in the United States. They have literally saved and prolonged millions of lives by decreasing the rate of heart attack and stroke in this country.

Years ago we did not treat hypertension in older individuals. We thought that high blood pressure was a normal occurrence as we aged. We reasoned that higher blood pressure was necessary to push blood through older, stiffened arteries. What we did not realize was that silent progressive blood vessel damage was slowly occurring as a result of the high blood pressure. Increase in heart size, silent heart attacks, and increased deposition of LDL cholesterol into the arterial wall are complications of high blood pressure. We now know that with good blood pressure control, good diet, exercise, and sometimes cholesterol-lowering drugs we can reverse many of these silent vascular changes. We can actually make ourselves healthier and our blood vessels younger.

There are now new blood pressure guidelines instructing doctors to prescribe antihypertensive drugs to patients at even lower blood pressure levels. What was considered "normal" blood pressure years ago is now considered high. We now know that even mild blood pressure elevations take a progressive toll and damage our cardiovascular system.

"However," you may say, "hypertensive medications are given to patients with hypertension. Estrogen is being offered to healthy women to alleviate symptoms that they, their husbands, or friends basically think are really not all that important. Menopausal symptoms may make life miserable for a year or so, or four or five, but they are not life threatening."

It is easy to comprehend that hormone replacement will get rid of hot flashes and night sweats that are severe and interfere with life. It is less easy to conceptualize long-term hormonal replacement therapy (LTHRT) to help prevent future illnesses such as heart disease and osteoporosis. This is a new and difficult concept both for you and for your doctor.

And so it might be a good idea to look at the list of menopausal symptoms one more time. Are we using hormonal therapy to treat "healthy women"? As we begin to mull over this often raised objection, we need to ask, "Are we entering the postmenopausal age span already programmed for system failure?" Healthy today, but preprogrammed by our genetics and dietary and social flaws for deterioration? Are we less healthy than we think, slowly and imperceptibly getting older and less fit, brewing something akin to hypertension except that the final consequences are pathology such as heart attack, stroke, Alzheimer's, and fracture? Is it possible to circumvent or modify these problems? Is it possible to postpone these silent metabolic changes to a much later age so that we function, nearly at full capacity mentally and physically, until one night we die softly in our sleep? One day this will be possible. We stand only at the threshold.

Is it just the effect of aging that creates these problems, or does the actual event of menopause independently accelerate and adversely affect the problems? Just knowing who is at risk for which problems would be a great help. It is already possible to find out some of this information by careful determination of preexisting risk factors, present complaints, physical examination, and laboratory analysis.

Body Changes That Accompany Menopause and Aging

WEIGHT GAIN

Let us begin to look in detail at each item in our list. One of the biggest complaints I hear is weight gain at the time of menopause. I have the same complaint. Until several years ago I could still wear many of the clothes I wore in college. I have never been on a diet in my life. Never had to. I ate more than almost any man and never gained a pound. Everyone warned me that one day it would happen. It did. In the past few years, I have added ten pounds and I know exactly where they are. Is it because I take estrogen? I believe the answer is no. It's a fact of getting older and being post-menopausal and unless you try harder than most of us have been willing, you've joined us too. Losing those extra pounds is my next project after this book is completed!

We're not alone; men have the same problem. A 175-pound man at sixty-five does not have the same build that he had at thirty, even if his weight hasn't changed by one pound. Women are no different. Both men and women lose muscle as we age and most often replace muscle with fat. We lose some 30 to 40 percent of our muscle mass by the time we reach seventy. Just take an honest look in the mirror while in your bathing suit. Men have lost the muscle in their legs and thighs. "Little chicken legs" replace those muscular columns that carried them when they played football. Fat has accumulated in their bellies. Are these changes related to loss of testosterone? Trials of testosterone replacement in men have shown that this therapy can increase muscle mass and strength, bone density, give an added feeling of well-being, and increase libido. The effects of testosterone may depend upon the dosages used, but testosterone replacement has not had an adverse effect on the cardiovascular system, as we originally believed. In fact, some recent research suggests that testosterone replacement in men may benefit the heart and cardiovascular system. Men will have to be patient as studies are done. Their studies actually lag behind the research for women.

Women also have similar changes in body composition. As women age, the distribution of fat also tends to accumulate in a male-type central, or apple, pattern. This central abdominal fat distribution, which comes from large intra-abdominal fat stores, is associated with cardiovascular disease, stroke, diabetes, and hypertension. Actually, for women, increase in waistline measurement may be more important than weight gain itself. The female pattern, the pear shape, is thought to be safer and may be maintained by estrogen replacement if it is begun at an early enough date.

The loss of muscle means that we have to put out extra energy just to do what we used to. It also means that *muscle, which burns calories* efficiently, has been replaced by *fat, which stores calories* efficiently. Our metabolism changes. We eat the same amount, but we burn it less well. We are also, for some reason as we become postmenopausal, less active. And that is why, in 1997, the average dress size for women is now size 14!

Many women erroneously believe that estrogen makes you fat. I believe it doesn't. Many studies have shown that women who take hormones actually keep their weight under better control than those who do not take replacement therapy. It is possible, of course, that women who take hormonal therapy are more interested in health and eat better and exercise more. And in my own practice, when women stopped their hormones because of perceived weight gain, there was no weight difference afterward. And equal numbers of postmenopausal women, whether on or never on hormones, complain of weight gain. Some researchers feel that the metabolic rate, the rate at which we burn our food, is decreased by 4 to 5 percent after menopause. Compounding this, they feel that the lowering of estrogen may also be related to less energy expenditure.

Women who really are determined to keep the weight off must exercise. One possibility would be to walk at least thirty minutes four to five times a week. This is one of the important methods of controlling weight. I would also advise most women to lift light weights in order to maintain muscle, which will help burn calories. Unfortunately, many women have aches and pains in their joints and may not be able to walk and exercise due to physical discomfort. This is often one of the most difficult problems to deal with as this decrease in energy expenditure will make weight gain inevitable over time.

Women should also eat a low-fat, higher-fiber diet and always be sensible when it comes to food choices. Again, some of us are luckier than others. There are individual metabolic differences, and probably genetic programming to deal with. In fact, according to the ongoing Nurses' Health Study, overweight black and white women are more likely to have mothers who were overweight. Also, if you weighed more than ten pounds at birth you are more likely to be overweight. And if you are five feet one or shorter, in order to remain svelte, unless you do a lot of exercise, you probably will never be able to eat on average more than 1,200 to 1,400 calories per day without gaining weight. A rough guide to ideal weight is using a base of one hundred pounds for a five-foot woman; for every inch over five feet in height, add five pounds. Those of us who are taller can consume more calories, and also have the advantage of having more places to hide and distribute the weight.

One more note: while *one-third of white women are overweight, one half of black women have this problem.* That this higher rate of being overweight could be based in biology rather than on eating behavior was researched at the University of Pennsylvania by Dr. Foster. He studied sixteen overweight women while they were at rest and calculated the differences in calories utilized after allowing for body weight and muscle mass. He found that black women burned nearly one hundred fewer calories per day on average than white women. Unfortunately, in just thirty-five days, this one hundred calories adds up to an additional pound of unwanted fat. All this means is that women with low metabolic rates have to try harder to exercise and eat correctly. So be proud any month you don't gain weight!

CARDIOVASCULAR DISEASE

As women age their rate of coronary artery disease increases, making it the leading cause of death in women. One out of three women will die from heart disease, eight times more than die of breast cancer. In general, coronary disease begins later in women than in men. Age is the most important risk factor.

Several studies have led physicians to believe that estrogen has protective effects against aging of the arteries in general, and against atherosclerosis (deposition of fatty substances in the vessel wall causing narrowing), the major cause of heart attack, in particular. Rosenberg showed that young women who undergo surgical removal of both ovaries increased their risk of heart attack 7.2 times (720 percent) if the woman was younger than thirty-five years of age versus women who had no surgery or only their uterus removed. Between 1965 and 1973, the rate of hysterectomy almost doubled for women twenty-five to thirty-four years of age. We may only now be seeing for the first time the consequences of this surgery. On the other hand, replacing estrogen can cancel this risk.

More than thirty major studies have documented that there is a decrease in cardiovascular risk from taking postmenopausal estrogen. They generally show that if a postmenopausal woman used estrogen in the past, her risk of heart disease is reduced by 35 percent. For a woman currently using estrogen, there is a 50 percent decrease in cardiovascular disease. Other, more basic studies on animals confirm the human data. Adding progesterone-like medication, according to most experts, only minimally alters the benefit of estrogen. To sum up, these studies conclude that *estrogen reduces the risk of heart disease in women.* Furthermore, coronary arteriography studies have shown that *estrogen can prevent and reverse progression of blood vessel atherosclerosis.* Vitamin E, low-dose baby aspirin, exercise, a low-fat diet, maintaining normal weight, and low stress also help to lower this risk. Coronary artery disease is multifactorial; therefore, there are many ways to help prevent it. Do as much of it as your doctor recommends, and as much as you feel comfortable doing.

What about the woman who already has coronary artery disease (CAD)? Can estrogen make it better and prevent progression? Estrogen has a very important role in women who have already developed CAD. Risk reduction is even greater in these women, compared with women without CAD. This phenomenon has been seen time and time again. Reduction in the risk of *second* heart attack and angina, and increased survival rates have been well documented in women with CAD who are currently taking estrogen. Even after coronary artery bypass, or balloon angioplasty, estrogen improves survival. Smokers, of course, should stop smoking. But smokers who take estrogen are afforded cardiovascular protection equal to their nonsmoking friends. In addition, reduction in risk occurs equally in exercisers and nonexercisers, in women who follow good diets and those who don't, and that is good news too. Moreover, this is seen in all types of estrogens used here in the United States and around the world.

How Does Estrogen Decrease the Risk of Heart Attack and Stroke?

1. It improves lipids by raising HDL and lowering total cholesterol and LDL. It is often said that if a woman's HDL is more than 50, there is normally no increase in cardiac risk for several years in the future. HDL is very important in women. LDL, even when greater than 160, does not seem to adversely affect a woman's risk if her HDL is over 50. Estrogen also affects LPa, a lesser-known blood lipid that is correlated with coronary artery disease but is not measured routinely. Women, of course, can lower their blood lipids with lipid-lowering medications. In addition, aspirin decreases the risk of coronary artery disease because of its antiplatelet activity. Beta-blockers and ACE inhibitors also improve survival after MI (myocardial infarction, or heart attack). All of these medications have their own side effects. This would also seem to be the appropriate place to assure women who have a uterus and thus take estrogen and some form of progesterone-like medication that studies have shown that the combination still offers good cardiovascular protection. In the PEPI Trial, significant increases in HDL and decreases in LDL were seen in all groups that were treated with estrogen compared with those treated with a placebo.

2. Estrogen is a powerful antioxidant. Estrogen keeps LDL from becoming oxidized. It is thought that if LDL is not oxidized, its ability to enter and damage the blood vessel wall is decreased. Several studies have now shown that when women take estrogen, progression of blood vessel damage is either stopped or slowed.

3. Estrogen has been shown in multiple studies to dilate blood vessels by causing them to relax, thereby improving blood flow to the brain and heart. According to Philip Sarrel, M.D., of Yale University Medical School, vasodilation accounts for 60 to 70 percent of the protective effect of postmenopausal estrogens. For example, in a young woman with normal estrogen levels a stressful situation tends not to alter the blood flow to her heart. The same amount of stress in an older woman not on hor-

mone replacement may cause coronary artery spasm. This causes a narrowing of the blood vessels which decreases or may actually stop blood flow. Estrogen in the form of replacement therapy helps her blood vessels relax and protects her coronary arteries and brain during stress. Menopause without HRT puts women into a high-risk category for CAD.

Women with angina are at high risk for heart attack. Those who have already had a heart attack (myocardial infarct) are at high risk for a second heart attack. Angina may occur as pain, pressure, tightness or squeezing in the middle of the chest, or as back or neck pain. It may be associated with stress or exercise. It usually is gone in five minutes, and rest helps it go away. If it persists for hours or days, this is usually not pain from angina. If you can reproduce the pain by pressing over your chest wall or ribs near the center of your chest where they attach to your sternum, it's likely not heart pain.

Women in their fifties are generally at relatively low risk for heart attack. In women over sixty, the rate of asymptomatic and symptomatic coronary disease increases. When these women experience typical symptoms of angina they are 60 percent more likely to have coronary artery disease than women in their fifties who have pains in their chest. These women's workups may include an exercise treadmill test or the more accurate thallium stress test. Here a radioactive compound is injected into the bloodstream. It is taken up by healthy heart muscle but is absent from areas where muscle is damaged. A woman who tests positive has an 80 percent chance of having CAD. A negative stress test rules out major CAD at the time the test is performed. Exercise echocardiogram may be one of the best new tests for women. A negative exercise echocardiogram test nearly guarantees that the tested woman will not need surgical intervention or have a heart attack within the next year.

Is There Bias in Treating Women with Heart Disease Symptoms?

Why do women often not get good care when they show symptoms of heart disease? Is there bias against sending women for further testing once angina has been established? Or do women get the right amount of attention whereas men get too much testing? Older women are less likely than men to be discharged from the hospital with a prescription to take aspirin long term or to take beta-blockers, both of which are important means of secondary prevention. As for bypass surgery, women who undergo it are older, are referred later, have been sicker longer, and more often need emergency surgery than men who undergo bypasses. They are also more likely to have diabetes, hypertension, and/or congestive heart failure, and black women seem to have the worst statistics of all. Bypass surgery is often more difficult to perform on women just because generally they have tinier vessels than men do. Age, hypertension, prior surgery, and need for emergency surgery are all prime predictors of problems, as is small body size.

STROKE

Stroke is the third leading cause of death in the United States, and the leading cause of disability. Half of all stroke victims are women, meaning one out of five or six of us will have some form of cerebral vascular accident in our lifetime. Although women tend to have their strokes later than men, i.e., when they are in their seventies and eighties, the rate of stroke in women does increase after menopause. More than $30 billion is spent each year on this illness and on rehabilitation costs. Men and women often can no longer work after having a stroke, or need to be institutionalized.

Stroke has many causes when compared to heart attack, including weak blood vessels that rupture and clots that come from the heart or other parts of the body. Therefore, the role of estrogen is more difficult to ascertain. Two studies have found that women who have used estrogen have a decreased risk of stroke and death from stroke. Estrogen may be one preventive factor that can help.

Just as women may be insufficiently studied for heart disease, women are also less likely to be investigated for carotid artery disease. Your doctor should listen carefully with a stethoscope over the sides of your neck for carotid bruits at each annual physical. These bruits are whooshing sounds made by blood flow that becomes turbulent as it passes through narrowed arteries. This narrowing can be documented on ultrasound. If it is severe, you could be at high risk for stroke, and precautions and/or surgery can then be considered in order to avoid a stroke.

ALZHEIMER'S DISEASE

Alzheimer's disease is the main cause of dementia, and dementia is perhaps the most feared aspect of growing older. For a complete discussion of hormone replacement therapy in relation to dementia, please see chapter 4.

ARTHRITIS

Rheumatoid Arthritis

Women have more active immune systems than men. That is why autoimmune diseases such as rheumatoid arthritis, autoimmune thyroiditis, and systemic lupus erythematosus (SLE) predominate in women. Estrogen may influence these diseases. The risk of developing rheumatoid arthritis increases as we age. It is a serious disease that affects three times as many women as men. Studies have not definitely proven that estrogen improves this disease or that menopause worsens it. However, the Nurses' Health Study found that current use of estrogen was protective. A study from England found that even though estrogen had no obvious effect that could be observed by physicians, women's complaints of pain and joint swelling improved by 25 percent after being placed on HRT. Androgens may also be helpful. Studies show that male hormone may also help to suppress the overactive immune response in women.

One-third to more than half of women will suffer the onset of stiff and aching or swollen joints from osteoarthritis or rheumatoid arthritis during the climacteric between ages forty-five to fifty-five. In my own practice, I often find that starting patients on hormones greatly alleviates their discomfort. Women who for whatever reason go off hormones often note the recurrence of pain. When they begin hormone replacement again, their pain is gone or lessened. Arthritis pain is no small matter. It adversely influences all of your everyday activities. Actually, it has been known for years that women who take birth control pills are less likely to get arthritis.

Osteoarthritis, rheumatoid arthritis, as well as carpal tunnel syndrome, fibromyalgia, and Sjögren's syndrome, which is often associated with dryness of the eyes, mouth, and vagina, often begin with the onset of menopause. After menopause, women also have more rapid progression of osteoarthritic knee and hip problems. Rapidly progressing osteoarthritis, causing major deformity of fingers, can sometimes be mistaken for rheumatoid arthritis (unless X rays are taken and blood tests done) and occurs after menopause also.

Unfortunately, postmenopausal women who have rheumatoid arthritis are at increased risk for osteoporosis. This may be due in part to their use of steroid medication to control symptoms and pain, to their lack of mobility, or to the inflammatory effects of the disease that adversely affect bone metabolism, combined with estrogen deficiency. Studies have shown that women with rheumatoid arthritis increase their bone mass when treated with hormone replacement, compared with women who are not given replacement therapy. Women who have been on cortisone-type medication and have bone loss seem to benefit most from HRT. There is also new research that has found that bisphosphonates* also help to protect bone in patients on steroids.

Osteoarthritis

Osteoarthritis is the most common form of arthritis. Joints swell where the thin rim of cartilage at the end of the long bones has been damaged from either sports injury, repetitive use, or obesity, which constantly stresses the joint by making it bear more weight than was intended. All of these conditions result in damage to cartilage which may be exacerbated by the loss of estrogen. Cartilage is a lot like bone. Both tissues balance breakdown and repair in order to remain strong and healthy. Estrogen keeps this positive balance. There are estrogen receptors in cartilage, just as there are in bone. And estrogen appears to protect cartilage in the same way that it protects bone.

Several studies done in a retrospective manner have found that women on estrogen therapy have lower than expected risk of knee and hip arthritis. This association was even stronger in women with severe or bilateral disease. The Framingham study showed that women on long-term hormone replacement had lower rates of osteoarthritis.

While it seems that estrogen does protect against osteoarthritis, these are all epidemiological studies, rather than studies where one group of women is treated and another group of similar women is given a placebo. The results could be somewhat skewed because women who elect to take estrogen are often thinner, healthier, and more active. These are characteristics that may make these women less susceptible to osteoarthritis in the first place. Nevertheless, it seems that increasing numbers of studies show that women on hormone replacement have a lower than expected risk of osteoarthritis of the knee and hip.[1]

LOSS OF LIBIDO

Problems and worries about sexual functioning can manifest at this time. Although a woman may be concerned about a decrease in her sexual desire, her partner is probably becoming equally concerned about his capacity to perform sexually. After menopause, more women than is gen-

---

*New medications to treat bone loss (see chapter on osteoporosis).

erally known have an asexual marriage, often due to medical factors affecting the male partner's sexual abilities. Such matters should come to open discussion with both partners' doctors. There is help for nearly every male who suffers from impotence today.

It is important to emphasize that an enormous variety of prescription medications often decrease sex drive in both men and women. Over 1.5 billion prescriptions are written annually in the U.S. alone; it is an amazing list of many unsuspected prescribed, over-the-counter, and illicit drugs that can affect our sex drives. It would seem that medications would be the first culprits to rule out when first noticing loss of libido. Some are obvious in association, others would hardly ever be suspected. It is usually easy to change a medication or change a dose. The number of drugs that are associated with decrease in sex drive and erectile disorders took almost five pages in an article in the *Journal of Family Practice* (44, no. 1 [January 1997]). You could look up the reference, but in a nutshell, most antihypertensive medications, some more than others, interfere with male erection and may decrease desire in both sexes. Antidepressants are the next most likely culprits—again, some have this effect more than others. Antianxiety medications, a variety of medications in all categories, plus illicit drugs such as cocaine, marijuana, as well as tobacco and alcohol all take their toll.

Some women are relieved to no longer have sex. There are a myriad of reasons these women stop having sex that range from feeling that sex ends with menopause, or that it is primarily for conception purposes, to a fear of getting a sexually transmitted disease. On the other hand, many women enjoy a second honeymoon with the kids finally out of the house and peace and quiet. With no more fears of pregnancy, often there is new sexual freedom and pleasure.

To take a different tack, Gloria Steinem described how she felt once the preoccupation with sex was no longer a primary drive, proclaiming in her book *Moving Beyond Words* in the chapter "Doing Sixty": "Now I think: 'Why not take advantage of the hormonal changes age provides to clear our minds, sharpen our senses, and free whole areas of our brains?'"

SLEEP PROBLEMS

At the 1997 North American Menopause Society meeting, Drs. Woodward and Freedman reported on interruption of sleep in menopausal women. They studied women, monitoring their sleep and hot flashes. They found that on average, sleep was disturbed every eight minutes for fifteen seconds or so in symptomatic women and every eighteen minutes in asymptomatic women. They concluded that fragmentation of sleep is greater in women with hot flashes and that this may contribute to impairment of daytime functioning, daytime fatigue, and possibly mood change. I stated it this way in *No More Hot Flashes and Other Good News:* "Sleep deprivation can have a devastating effect on anyone. It can affect your personality—even your sexuality. It may be one of the prime factors in the emotional changes in menopausal women. It certainly can leave you chronically fatigued, tired, and unable to function, as well as depressed. Sleep deprivation is often used as a method of torture. If it disorients and breaks down the defenses of prisoners of war, women who are kept awake night after night by their sweats will also finally succumb."

SKIN CHANGES

Our skin often shows our age, although some women genetically seem to have better skin than others. Skin changes often seem to begin in the perimenopausal period. Estrogen and androgen both have a direct effect on skin through their receptors. Estrogen has been shown to increase the thickness of our skin and the formation of collagen, the portion of our skin that holds water and prevents dryness and wrinkles. It helps to preserve the elastic fibers that support skin tone and help it spring back into shape after being pinched. A study in the *Archives of Dermatology* (133 [1997]: 339–342) investigated 3,875 postmenopausal women and concluded after adjusting for weight, smoking, and sun exposure that those who were on estrogen had healthier skin. They found that the odds of having dry and wrinkled skin were reduced by 25 and 30 percent respectively in women who took estrogen as opposed to those who did not.

The collagen content of skin falls by 2.1 percent during each postmenopausal year, with the most rapid decline occurring in the years immediately after the menopause. (This occurs regardless of the age of menopause.) The total thickness of skin decreases by 1.2 percent per year in the first ten to fifteen postmenopausal years. These effects can be largely counteracted by taking hormone replacement with or without male hormone added.

As skin becomes thinner, more transparent, more friable, and looser in older women, there is a tendency to bruise and hemorrhage which leaves red discolorations over the arms and legs. In other women, the relatively high proportion of male hormone to remaining female hormone increases scalp hair loss while stimulating hair growth in unwanted locations, such as on the chin. As androgen receptors decrease in the skin with age there is a loss of pubic and armpit hair. Recently, researchers are assessing whether there is a correlation between thickness of the skin and bone density. This is because bone loss may be a part of general connective tissue disorder, as collagen composes 90 to 96 percent of the protein matrix of our bones.

I would like to add that smoking causes wrinkling of the skin. This is well known to many women who smoke. They hate their yellowish skin and the wrinkles around their mouth that age them and make it difficult for them to put lipstick on straight. Sun damage that results from sunbathing when we were young often haunts us now by causing brown spots, wrinkles, skin cancers, and little spider veins that show up where blood vessel damage occurred from ultraviolet rays. Use of sunblocks by adults and children over the age of six months can help. Staying out of the midday sun and wearing hats also helps. However, some sun is necessary for the skin to manufacture vitamin D.

COLON CANCER

To date, there are three studies that relate taking estrogen to a decrease in the risk of getting colon cancer. One large study reported in the April 1995 *Journal of the National Cancer Institute* found that the death rate from colon cancer was reduced in women who had taken estrogen for even as little as one year. Risk of dying decreased the longer they took estrogen. Women on estrogen for one year had a 19 percent decrease. Women on estrogen for eleven years who had stopped their estrogen had a 46 percent decrease, while current users had a 55 percent decrease if they had been on estrogen eleven years or longer! These results are most impressive. Two other studies showed similar results with a 50 percent decrease in colon cancer risk.

DIABETES

In a twelve-year follow-up of the Nurses' Health Study, nurses who were currently on estrogen—as compared with those who never used estrogen—were found to have a 20 percent decrease in the incidence of adult-onset diabetes after adjusting for weight and age. Women who have diabetes mellitus have a markedly increased risk of coronary artery disease. This risk is so dramatically increased that it obliterates the usual advantage of being female. Normally, the onset of menopause with its loss of estrogen support results in changes in insulin and glucose metabolism. After menopause, insulin levels tend to rise as "insulin resistance" develops as the tissues are less able to utilize insulin. This plus the deleterious changes in cholesterol, LDL, and HDL that normally occur with menopause put diabetic women at even higher risk for coronary artery disease once they are menopausal. Hormone replacement reduces this risk by 40 percent, and should be encouraged for all diabetic women to help overcome their additional cardiac risk factors. (See page 27 in the perimenopause chapter for information about diabetes causing premature menopause.)

CATARACTS

Women over 50 have a higher incidence of cataracts than men. This increases at menopause. Researchers in England feel that women who take estrogen may decrease their risk of developing cataracts.

The Estrogen Debate—Keeping an Open Mind

HOW TO LOOK AT RISK/BENEFIT

For many, thinking ahead ten to twenty years is difficult. When we first start to contemplate menopause, the very first question that is on every woman's mind is whether or not to take estrogen. Some women's groups feel that this is all about making some drug companies rich. They claim that corporations are medicalizing menopause for financial gain. Others are satisfied that with all this fuss, drug companies and the government are finally paying attention to women. Although there is no simple answer, there may come a simple prescription. Public policy may boil down to the bottom line, which is always money. Will hormonal therapy cut health costs for this ever growing segment of our population? If so, it will be encouraged. If not, it will not. Studies such as the Women's Health Initiative will try to determine benefits and risks. However, the study will not be finished until the year 2005, and the data will probably not be ready until 2007. Meanwhile, we are left in a dilemma.

Neither patients nor doctors have been well trained in preventive medicine. Doctors have been trained in crisis care—for example, to treat a broken hip. They're a lot better at fracture care than at preventing the fracture. Physicians are caught in the same dilemma as their female patients. Some feel that estrogen is the preventive medicine that will decrease the morbidity and mortality of the growing number of older women in this country. They are certain that hormone replacement therapy has the potential to improve the quality of life and to prolong life, and that estrogen replacement's potential impact is equal to or better than efforts to lower cholesterol and control hypertension. However, efforts to counsel patients about using estrogen continue to be widely divergent. Some of that depends upon the doctor, much depends on their specialty. Ob/gyns prescribe the most estrogen, internists and family doctors the least. Or it could depend on geography. California women are prescribed three times more estrogen than their counterparts on the East Coast, though I doubt they have three times more flashes. Female doctors also prescribe more estrogen than male doctors, and female doctors take more estrogen than the general population.

Therapy: What Do Women Really Want?

Not only do doctors behave differently depending on who and where they are, but also women have different agendas. Actually, only 25 percent of the four thousand women who become menopausal every day in the United States and Canada use HRT. Most women want to take hormones to get rid of bothersome symptoms such as hot flashes, sexual dysfunction, and emotional problems, whereas most doctors are more concerned about osteoporosis and heart disease. It seems that women from different countries actually take hormone replacement for different reasons. Dr. Lila Nachtigall reported that "French and South American women more often begin [hormone replacement] therapy to delay the effects of aging on physical appearance and also to improve the quality of their sex life. It was also found that HRT users were more likely to have had hysterectomies and were better educated and less obese than nonusers."

The most common reasons for discontinuing HRT are side effects (menstruation), fear of developing cancer, and fear of gaining weight. Some women believe erroneously that problems like osteoporosis spontaneously resolve after short-term therapy. This is a wrong assumption. Even women at high risk for osteoporosis, who already have had wrist or other fractures, often stop HRT, when they actually require long-term therapy. Much of the problem is that women do not have good information about HRT, a problem that rests squarely on the shoulders of their physicians.

Physicians must understand that counseling and education are needed before prescribing HRT. The "It's good for all women and therefore it's good for you" approach simply doesn't work. In today's health care environment time is difficult to find, however, investing time up front is essential. It is unrealistic to expect a woman to comply with hormone therapy if she doesn't comprehend the importance and the benefits of doing so. This is especially true when the long-term benefits seem abstract. For this reason, the benefits of HRT need to be related specifically to the woman's own health profile. Not taking enough time to inform a woman about the pros and cons of therapy on an individual basis, and not counseling about the occurrence of withdrawal bleeding, or the possibility of breast tenderness, often lead to early discontinuation of hormonal therapy or to her not even filling her original prescription.

The subject of withdrawal bleeding causes even more reluctance among women who as they grow older are less and less willing to start regimens that cause monthly bleeding. Bleeding, however, does not usually mean that anything is wrong. It is, in most cases, created by the therapy. Most women do not want to bleed, many simply stating that they have "done their time." By giving lower doses to start, or prescribing estrogen and progesterone together on a daily basis, this barrier to success can usually be overcome. Of course there are some women who do want to have their monthly flow return. In my long experience, these are usually women who are newly married to younger men! But a number of my patients simply don't seem to mind or state that they feel renewed when cycles restart.

"NATURAL" OVER-THE-COUNTER THERAPIES: BUYER BEWARE

I was recently sent an audiotape in which a woman was speaking about a natural cream containing progesterone which supposedly had the ability to improve your skin, sex life, and bones. She gave an example of how her elderly friend was discovered to have bone loss on an X ray, then used the cream. Three months later, her X ray was taken again and her bones were strong! First of all, it is not possible to tell anything about bone loss on a plain X ray until approximately one-third of the bone has been lost. Therefore, it is unlikely that anyone would use a plain X ray for accurate bone density measurement. By varying the amount of radiation used to take the X ray, bones can appear to be darker or whiter (denser). An enormous amount of inaccurate and misleading information is too often passed off as fact over our radio waves and in books and magazines.

I would like to say right here and up front that I am uncomfortable with my patients' using over-the-counter compounds that have never been tested in any substantive manner. It is important to know that a compound is safe and effective. Otherwise, we jeopardize our present and future health, and may also waste time and money with ineffective therapy. Worse, the substances may be harmful. Hearsay and anecdotal information should not replace scientific facts.

Recent studies have shown that the majority of women use herbal compounds and other alternative therapies. They willingly take an herbal product without ever having more than the salesperson's word that it works. Most important, there are almost no large well-controlled studies to back up these claims. In addition, more than half of these women do not inform their physicians of their alternative medications.

What does natural really mean? All of the menopausal estrogens used commercially by the large pharmaceutical manufacturers today are derived from plant or animal sources, or exactly mimic the 17 beta-estradiol molecule made by our ovaries. This sounds natural to me.

If you choose to use over-the-counter creams that contain estrogen, in general you should be aware that there is little or no testing done for content (amount of estrogen) or bioavailability (how readily the body can use it). However, there is a prescription estrogen gel (Estrogel®) that is standardized so that when a specific amount is rubbed into the skin, we have a pretty good idea of its effect and of the blood levels of estrogen that will be attained.

Some of my patients have taken capsules containing mixtures of "natural estrogens" obtained from compounding pharmacies. Several realized that these "natural" mixtures of estrone, estradiol, and estriol were more potent than their previously prescribed therapy, simply because they began to have side effects and bleed when they had never bled before on their usual hormone replacement. Interestingly, at a meeting I attended in September 1997, one of the companies that sells estriol capsules had information at its booth. Glancing down, I noted that the data the company was handing out were based on a *Journal of the American Medical Association (JAMA)* article from January 2, *1978!*

A full discussion of alternative therapies and new non-estrogen choices will be presented in the next chapter.

RISKS FROM HORMONE REPLACEMENT

The Endometrium: No Increased Risk if Hormone Replacement Is Done Correctly

Back in the 1970s, women on estrogen were found to be at higher risk for uterine cancer. This was confirmed in many studies. The problem was that much of the medical community did not realize the significance of progesterone, the second female hormone. To me, progesterone was basic. Mother Nature had found it necessary to balance estrogen with progesterone. I took my lead from her. From the mid-sixties, I always used both hormones for women with an intact uterus. My colleagues, most of whom were men in those years, often gave me a hard time. They couldn't understand why any doctor would cause patients to bleed again. I had private and public verbal disputes with other learned colleagues over the years, but these disputes are too old to go into now. Patience and common sense won out, however, and in 1983, the American College of Obstetrics and Gynecology issued a bulletin that stated that the "addition of progestin* for ten to thirteen days each cycle has been shown to reduce the risk of endometrial hyperplasia to near zero, and this should be accompanied by a significant reduction in the risk of developing endometrial cancer."

Because it is possible to offset the risk of endometrial cancer by the simple addition of a progesterone-like medication, the subject of endometrial cancer should virtually no longer cause concern when you are contemplating hormone replacement. (You should note the terms. Estrogen replacement signifies the use of estrogen alone, while hormone replacement means that both estrogen and a progesterone-like medication are used.)

There are a number of interesting studies on hormones and the endometrium. Collins from McMaster University in Canada reviewed survival data from women on unopposed estrogen who developed uterine cancer and those on hormone replacement who did not develop cancer. He found that both groups on hormones lived longer than matched

---

*A progesterone-type medication.

women who had never been given replacement! Their increase in life span was probably due to the cardiovascular and skeletal benefits of their therapy.

It is widely believed that endometrial cancer occurs after prolonged periods of unopposed estrogen (without progesterone), in the same way that it occurs in women who have a long history of anovulation, irregular menses, or late menopause. That is why birth control pills that give a monthly sufficient dose of progesterone-like medication are known to decrease the incidence of uterine cancer, even though they contain approximately three to eight times the amount of estrogen we use in hormone replacement.

Studies confirm that the progesterone component in hormone replacement therapy may reduce the risk of uterine cancer that can occur spontaneously in early menopause, because it counteracts *unopposed* estrogen that is sometimes secreted in low levels over prolonged periods of time, or in sudden large amounts by the early postmenopausal ovary.

The Breast Cancer Question: Are the Risks Higher on HRT?

The fear that HRT might increase the risk of breast cancer has caused many physicians to hesitate when advising their patients about menopausal therapy. It is the single most important reason why women either never start HRT or discontinue therapy. Breast cancer causes 17 percent of all cancer deaths in women, and will cause 31 percent of all new cancer cases in the United States this year.[2] Or to put it another way, a white woman between the ages of fifty and ninety-four has been estimated to have a 31 percent chance of dying from coronary artery disease, a 2.8 percent chance of dying from breast cancer, and a 2.8 percent chance of dying from hip fracture, according to S. R. Cummings.

Because breast cancer is such a prevalent disease, even a slight increase in its incidence could mean a large increase in the number of cancer cases in this country. Therefore, any increase in incidence that might be caused by administration of estrogen or of estrogen and progesterone must be considered in great detail.

All women are at significant risk for breast cancer, just because they are women. And the older we get, the greater our risk is. (See the SEER data from 1987–88. SEER stands for Surveillance, Epidemiology and End Results and is a program of the National Cancer Institute and the American Cancer Society.)

WOMEN'S RISK OF DEVELOPING BREAST CANCER
ACCORDING TO AGE

Age	Risk
25	1 in 19,608
30	1 in 2,525
35	1 in 622
40	1 in 217
45	1 in 93
50	1 in 50
55	1 in 33
60	1 in 24
65	1 in 17
70	1 in 14
75	1 in 11
80	1 in 10
85	1 in 9

How to interpret relative risk: To put our concern about hormone replacement's possible role in increasing the risk of breast cancer into perspective, I feel it is necessary to understand the relative risks of many other contributing factors to breast cancer. Some of these are under our control, some, like age, are not. Actually, *by the time we reach menopause, our breasts have already been subjected to half a century of hormonal, repro-ductive, and environmental influences. Each of these factors, separately or together, contributes to our susceptibility to breast cancer.*

HRT's influence, if any, on the risk of breast cancer varies in different studies. In general, studies show no increase in risk or that there is approximately a 1.3 to 1.4 times increase in risk, seen in women treated for more than five to ten years on hormones. Often doses were higher than those used today.

You should become acquainted with the term "relative risk." Basically, a relative risk of 1 refers to the "normal risk" of getting breast cancer for a woman with no known risk factors. Increased risk will raise this risk factor above 1, while things that decrease our risks will lower it to numbers below 1 (e.g., 0.6). In this way we can use numbers to weigh the influence of medications or lifestyle. For example:

1. Women who survive breast cancer are five times more likely to have another tumor, or putting it another way, their relative risk (RR) is 5, or they are 500 percent more likely to develop a second breast cancer.

2. A woman who started menstruating between ages eleven and fourteen is 1.3 times more likely to develop breast cancer than a woman whose menses started later. She has a 30 percent increased risk.

3. If you have your first child after age thirty, your risk is 1.9 times greater than a woman who had her first delivery before she was twenty. You would have a 90 percent increased risk. (Women who have never had children have a slightly lower risk, i.e., the same as women who first deliver between the ages of twenty-five and twenty-nine.)

4. If you have a late menopause, i.e., after fifty-five years of age, your risk is increased to 1.5, or a 50 percent increased risk compared with the woman who began menopause at $51\frac{1}{2}$ years.

5. A breast biopsy for benign breast disease also carries an increased relative risk of 1.5, or a 50 percent increase.

6. Having atypical cells on a previous breast biopsy increases this rate further, to 2.0 to 4.0 times relative risk, a 200 to 400 percent increase over women with no previous biopsy.

7. Consumption of alcohol at the rate of two to five drinks per day increases the relative risk of developing invasive breast cancer by 4 times, or 40 percent. Beer, wine, and liquor all pose the same risk.

8. Smoking for more than thirty years increases your relative risk to 1.6, or a 60 percent increase over nonsmokers. Smoking for more than twenty years increases risk by 1.3, or 30 percent.[3]

9. A high-fat diet may increase your risk, but this is not proven and continues to cause controversy.

10. Postmenopausal women who are overweight are at increased risk. Being overweight does not seem to affect risk for premenopausal women for some unknown reason.

11. Women who are sedentary—"couch potatoes"—seem to be at higher risk though the percent is not available.

12. Women who are taller than average are also are at increased risk for breast cancer.

13. Early removal of both ovaries with no replacement therapy is associated with a relative risk less than 1; the exact percent depends on the age you were when your ovaries were removed.

Obviously some risk factors are unchangeable, e.g., your age, time of first menstruation, height, family history. But you may be able to control other factors such as diet, exercise, smoking, and drinking. I hope this helps you put into perspective the risk that HRT may pose. Compared with two drinks of alcohol per day, it is much less. And unlike other factors, HRT provides benefits that may actually be more important statistically to you than any perceived risk of breast cancer, i.e., the protection of your heart, brain (from stroke and Alzheimer's), colon, and bones, which leads to a longer, more active life.

Nevertheless, it is crucial to understand that statistics are only statistics, and they never apply to you as an individual. It's somewhat like betting on a horse. You can read the horse's statistics on the racing sheet, and it may help you bet. But whether you place a bet that wins or loses depends on many factors, such as the track, the jockey, other horses, weather conditions, and a hunch.

Most women have a combination of interacting factors that modify her individual statistics. It may be possible for a woman to shave down some of her risks for breast cancer just by changing habits such as exercise, alcohol consumption, and smoking. On the other hand, a woman in a higher-risk category bears closer watching beginning at an early age. Any woman in a high-risk group would have to very carefully weigh the benefits she might get from hormone replacement against her already high risk of breast cancer.

So what do the experts say? I listened to Trudy Bush, Ph.D., lecture at the North American Menopause Society meeting in September 1995. She is perhaps one of the best-known epidemiologists on breast cancer and HRT. At the conclusion of her forty-five-minute lecture, which reviewed all the then recent studies, she paused for a moment then said, "Does HRT contribute to any increase in breast cancer? I don't know." Since then, I tell my patients, "If Trudy Bush doesn't know that answer, neither do I." In March of 1997, Roger Lobo, Chairman of the Department of Obstetrics and Gynecology at Columbia-Presbyterian Hospital, said that "if there was any increased risk, [his] gut feeling was that it would be no more than 20 percent, or a relative risk of 1.2 percent." Why we don't have a definite answer is simply that there are no good prospective studies completed to date. More important, however, the existing studies do *not* show consistent data that HRT increases breast cancer risk. If data were strong, then most studies would agree.

In contrast, there are a wide variety of studies that support the premise that HRT decreases heart disease. Basic science research, studies on animals, human data, as well as retrospective studies of large numbers of women all show a similar clear beneficial effect. Consistent data simply do not exist for breast cancer. That is good news, for it means quite simply that the risk, if any, is small.

When the major studies on hormone replacement and breast cancer are analyzed, results tend to center around the relative risk of 1 (which you now know means no increased risk). Some studies show more risk, others show a decreased risk. Most conclusions tend to be conservative, with risk factors near a 1.3 relative risk (or 30 percent increased risk). If this risk is real, because of the cardiac and bone benefits most doctors and statisticians still feel that the benefits outweigh the risk. Nonetheless, knowledge that there may be increased risk after five years (some studies say ten to fifteen years) on HRT makes many women uneasy. Women today are therefore put in a position where they must join the decision-making process and weigh their personal benefits and risks. In addition, everyone has different emotions about how much each risk factor means to her.

Assessing risk factors versus life expectancy: Let us try to understand the breast cancer/HRT question with yet another scenario. A research study by a group from Tufts University School of Medicine published in *JAMA* on April 9, 1997, addressed how hormone replacement might benefit life expectancy of an individual woman who has different risk factors for breast cancer, endometrial cancer, heart disease, and hip fracture. By taking the worst and most conservative estimates—the highest for breast cancer risk and the lowest for heart disease benefit—they created a personal decision pathway that any woman can use to help her decide whether or not to use hormone replacement.

Basically, their results showed that a fifty-year-old woman who has increased cholesterol, smokes, and has high blood pressure, even if she is at moderate breast cancer risk, will add two and a half years to her life if she decides to take estrogen. By measuring life expectancy as a way of looking at this problem they concluded that "hormone replacement therapy should increase life expectancy for nearly all postmenopausal women, with some gains exceeding three years, depending mainly on an individual's risk factors for coronary artery disease and breast cancer. For women with at least one risk factor for coronary artery disease, hormone therapy should extend life expectancy even for women having first-degree relatives (a mother, sister, or daughter) with breast cancer. Women without any risk factors for heart disease or hip fracture, but who have two first-degree relatives with breast cancer, however, should not receive hormone therapy." (Loss of life from stroke and colon cancer were not considered in this study.) In addition, the study concluded, "The benefit of hormone replacement in reducing the likelihood of developing coronary artery disease appears to outweigh the risk of breast cancer for nearly all women in whom this treatment might be considered. Our analysis supports the broader use of hormone replacement therapy." To state it one more time, they felt that *the only women who would not increase their longevity from hormone replacement were those who had the greatest risk for breast cancer and the least risk for coronary artery disease.*

To quote their article further: "Although patients confronting this decision often fear breast cancer more than heart disease, more American women die each year from heart disease than from any other cause, including breast cancer. While the 1-in-8 lifetime probability of developing breast cancer has been well publicized, 1 in 2 postmenopausal women will develop heart disease. Although breast cancer claims 43,000 lives per year in the United States, heart disease kills approximately 233,000 women annually, and nearly 65,000 women die each year from hip fracture." Erroneously, it is often said that young women die of breast disease, old women of heart disease. This statement, as a generality, is false. In every age category, more women die of heart attacks than of breast cancer. To quote an article by Malcolm Gladwell in the June 9, 1997, issue of *The New Yorker,* "For women between the ages of 45 and 54, death rates for heart disease are 1.4 times those of breast cancer. For women between 55 and 64, it's nearly 3 times the problem; for women between the ages of 65 and 74, it's $5\frac{1}{2}$ times the problem and for women 75 and older, it's almost 20 times the problem." Somehow women don't seem to realize that pain and suffering from cardiac disease can be fully as incapacitating and terrible as terminal breast cancer.

Because the risk of death is probably 26 percent lower in women on hormone replacement who develop breast cancer in contrast to women who develop breast cancer who are *not* taking hormone replacement, the Tufts researchers hypothesized that all women would likely live longer by taking hormone replacement.

Their research also found that gains in life expectancy were 10 to 25 percent less for black women on HRT. They also referred to the impact of other strategies; for example, a thirty-five-year-old woman who stopped smoking would increase life expectancy by 2.8 years, and if she lowered her cholesterol she would increase her life expectancy by 0.4 to 6.3 years. The article ended with the lament that although it is possible to wait for more data, randomized trials will not be concluded for "more than a decade while millions of women face this decision now."

Another study, the Nurses' Health Study, published in the *New England Journal of Medicine* in June 1997, came to similar conclusions. They found also that *there was an increased life expectancy in those nurses who took estrogen or estrogen and progestin therapy.* The 37 percent decrease in mortality, as compared with those nurses who never used hormones, was *not* due to differences in diet, alcohol intake, or vitamins, aspirin, or exercise between the two groups. Rather it was attributed to a *53 percent decrease in mortality due to heart disease, a 32 percent decrease in stroke, and a 29 percent decrease in mortality from cancer (a 64 percent decrease in death from colon cancer, a 24 percent decrease in death from breast cancer, and while fifty-eight nurses died of endometrial cancer, only five were on hormone therapy)*. Some of the decrease in breast cancer mortality is probably due to the fact that these women were diagnosed earlier than nonusers. However, the authors postulated, withdrawal of hormones after diagnosis of breast cancer might have a beneficial effect, making such *cancers less likely to be fatal than those breast cancers that arise in women not on hormones*. To quote the authors, *"Women taking hormones appear to be at a greater risk for the development of breast cancer than for death from the disease."* Again, the greatest reduction in mortality was found in women at highest risk for heart disease. Women at the lowest risk of coronary disease (who neither smoked nor had high blood pressure, high cholesterol levels, or diabetes; those who had no parental history of heart attack; and those who were near normal weight) had less benefit. They also noted that the protective benefits associated with hormones disappeared after not taking hormones for five years. *This study also demonstrated that women with a family history of breast cancer were not at any greater risk of death from breast cancer than women on hormone replacement without this history*. In summary, the benefits were found to outweigh risks, but the authors cautioned that the "risks and benefits vary depending on existing risk factors and the duration of hormone use and must be carefully considered for each woman." Although the authors found that there was an increased risk of breast cancer in women on hormones for ten years or more, *it is important to realize that if hormones protect women with the result that they live longer, they will be more prone to get breast cancer possibly only for the reason that they are older.* (See SEER data, page 63.)

Meta-analysis: Another way to look at risk: Many studies have looked at the subject of breast cancer and HRT. Except for two, all are retrospective studies, which means researchers gathered data from a woman's memory (rather than taking two similar groups of women, treating one with the hormones and treating the other with placebo, then evaluating both groups some set number of years later). Until new studies that are under way are completed (notably the CASH study and the WHI study), hard data are difficult to find. Nonetheless, researchers impatient for answers have devised a method known as meta-analysis. Using this method, the results of many different hormone replacement studies are pooled, or combined, in order to increase the numbers and hopefully get stronger data. Although such analyses of the data probably are helpful, they wind up pooling results of different studies that involved different estrogens and progesterone-like medications, different dosages, and possibly different methods of diagnosis and comparison. One of these meta-analyses, done by the Australians (involving twenty-three studies), found no increased risk of breast cancer in women who took HRT. Another by the Centers for Disease Control found no increased risk when women used estrogen for five years or less. After fifteen years, the risk increased by 30 percent (a 1.3 relative risk), a percent that many statisticians agree is not statistically significant. This study included subjects at increased risk: women who had family histories of breast cancer and personal histories of benign breast disease. Because of their inclusion, the results may be artificially higher. The third meta-analysis was done in Nashville, Tennessee. This study found no increased risk when .625 mg/day of conjugated estrogens (Premarin®) was used for several years, but a higher dose of 1.25 mg/day was associated with an increased risk.

Between the years 1973 and 1991, there was a 24 percent increase in invasive cancer rates in the United States. Actually, most doctors believe that the rates have been increasing since the 1940s. They feel that the increased cancer may be due to the fact that although estrogen and progesterone-type medication do not create cancer, they increase the rate of cell multiplication. This may increase the risk of a genetic error occurring that might not be noted and repaired by busy genetic mechanisms. The decreasing age at which menarche (the onset of menstruation) occurs, the later age of childbirth, and increasing postmenopausal obesity all increase the length of time a woman is exposed to estrogen or unopposed estrogen. This could theoretically increase the risk of breast cancer. In addition, in spite of the increased use of hormone replacement therapy, there has been a drop in breast cancer mortality by 1.6 percent for white women during the years 1989 to 1992, according to the *American Journal of Public Health* (87 [1997]: 775–781). However, this decline was not shared by black women, who showed a tiny increase in mortality. Almost all other cancers show a decline in mortality. For a bit of good news, look at the figure on page 70.

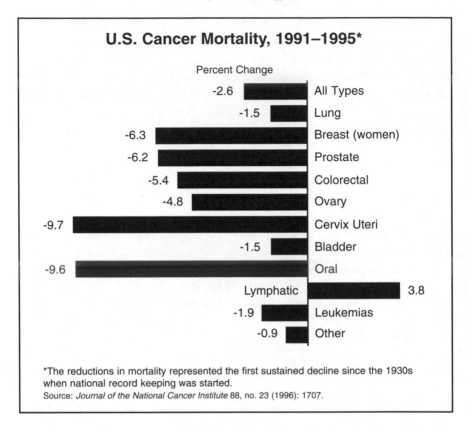

U.S. Cancer Mortality, 1991–1995*

Percent Change

	Percent Change
All Types	-2.6
Lung	-1.5
Breast (women)	-6.3
Prostate	-6.2
Colorectal	-5.4
Ovary	-4.8
Cervix Uteri	-9.7
Bladder	-1.5
Oral	-9.6
Lymphatic	3.8
Leukemias	-1.9
Other	-0.9

*The reductions in mortality represented the first sustained decline since the 1930s when national record keeping was started.
Source: *Journal of the National Cancer Institute* 88, no. 23 (1996): 1707.

Women with a personal history of breast cancer: Can they try hormonal therapy? Women with a personal history of breast cancer often suffer terribly from menopausal symptoms. In the past, we nearly always refused hormonal therapy for these women, but there are *no* clinical studies to support this point of view. Scientific thinking was based on old therapy where removing the woman's ovaries caused a remission in some cancer patients. It was also based on the fact that often breast cancers have receptors for estrogen and progesterone.

However, other facts seem to lead us to believe that hormone therapy in breast cancer patients may not be contraindicated. For example, during pregnancy, which is a time of very high estrogen and even higher progesterone levels, the prognosis for breast cancer diagnosed at that time is not worse, and termination of pregnancy is no longer routinely recommended. In addition, prospective studies have shown that removal of the ovaries has *no* effect on the outcome of breast cancer. Furthermore, women who develop breast cancer while on oral contraceptives have no worse prognosis.

The problem is that there are increasing numbers of young women who are diagnosed with breast cancer. Often, their cancers have been found early and it would seem that many of these women may be cured. After chemotherapy, 86 percent of breast cancer patients who are under the age of forty experience loss of ovarian hormone output and early menopause. Therefore, they suffer with hot flashes, and are at high risk for heart disease and osteoporosis. Tamoxifen, used as adjuvant (supplementary) therapy, may provide some protection against heart disease and osteoporosis, but it may not be as effective as estrogen and often triggers hot flashes. Similarly, raloxifene may also increase hot flashes. However, it offers cardiac and bone protection. Studies in cancer patients are not completed (see page 112).

The question for women with a history of breast cancer is: Do the benefits of estrogen outweigh the risks of taking it? Unfortunately there is, to date, no clear answer. However, a study that appeared in the summer 1995 issue of *Menopause, the Journal of the North American Menopause Society* sheds some light on the subject with a study from Australia. There were 901 women who had had surgically confirmed breast cancer; 90 were given estrogen for relief of menopausal symptoms beginning five years after their diagnosis and treatment for breast cancer. For seventy-two of the women, their cancer was only in their breast; the remaining had had cancer that had spread to their axilla (armpit). Most were placed on continuous combined therapy, i.e., estrogen with progesterone-like medication on a daily basis. Controls selected were women who were matched for age at diagnosis, axillary spread, tumor size, and disease-free interval. Therefore, women who had been disease free five years prior to starting HRT were matched to women who were also five years disease free but took no therapy. The results showed that *among the 90 HRT users, there were no deaths. Only 7 percent of the hormone users developed a recurrence of their cancer compared with 17 percent of the nonusers.* The authors concluded that "short-term use of combined continuous therapy by women with a personal history of breast cancer may be safe, and might even reduce the risk of recurrence."

There are also other studies from the U.S. and Europe that demonstrate improved survival in women with a history of breast cancer who went on HRT. Although this is interesting and probably good news, we still are unsure of the effects of estrogen on women who have had breast cancer. You and your physician may decide that the benefits of estrogen may outweigh the risks, or may make your life that much better, or you may feel more secure avoiding unknown risks. Either way, this is not an easy decision. To date, *most physicians feel that a personal history of breast cancer is a contraindication to hormone replacement.* However, physicians are beginning to realize that opinion is shifting, and *the woman who survives breast cancer has to consider not only her breast cancer, but the overall quality of her life as well as her risk of mortality.* It is possible that estrogen receptor–negative cancers (cancers that do not respond to estrogen) may have less risk than estrogen receptor–positive tumors. The bottom line remains; we really don't have the answers. However, women who have had breast cancer need and deserve counseling to make them aware that HRT is no longer a black-and-white issue. One last thought: Breast cancer or any other cancer can recur whether a woman takes hormone therapy, tamoxifen, raloxifene or not.

Before we leave this subject, it should be obvious that women with a history of breast cancer—depending on their risks for osteoporosis and cardiovascular disease—have choices other than estrogen. Potent medications that lower cholesterol more dramatically than estrogen does are available, although they do not relax arteries as does estrogen. Excellent therapy with Fosamax® is available for bone loss. Vaginal creams, lubricants, or the Estring™ ring works well for vaginal dryness. However, there are only moderately effective therapies for hot flashes, although a recent tiny study of ten women already on tamoxifen suggested that SSRI antidepressive medications such as Prozac®, Zoloft®, or Paxil® might help. And it goes without saying that exercise, a good diet, not smoking, vitamins, calcium, and good common sense should always be basic to your health. (Other suggestions for treating menopause without estrogen are offered in chapter 3, on alternative therapies.)

FIBROCYSTIC BREASTS

I do not think that fibrocystic breasts are a contraindication to taking HRT. In fact, I have had many patients who have long suffered with breast tenderness. Surprisingly, many felt relief when they began HRT. I think this was because these women finally had a normal balance of hormones. In my opinion, fibrocystic breast problems stem from disordered hormones, not necessarily too much estrogen, but rather too little progesterone. Again, it is important to evaluate and adjust doses or change the actual estrogen or progesterone-like medication in order to keep women comfortable.

HRT AFTER GYNECOLOGICAL CANCERS

It is important to know that it is usually all right to take HRT if you have a personal history of cervical cancer. Cervical cancer is not hormone dependent, and therefore there should be no increased risk. The few studies that exist on epithelial (the usual) ovarian cancer seem to show a better prognosis when patients take hormones. However, more studies are needed to prove or disprove this. In general, only women in early stages of endometrial cancer tend to be offered HRT. But three retrospective studies show that treated women may have better survival rates than women not offered HRT. However, these have been the only studies published to date. A new study has started that will enroll 2,200 women with endometrial cancer to see if estrogen affects prognosis of women with endometrial cancer. This important debate will finally be settled in several years. Women with a history of endometrial cancer who choose treatment, although they are posthysterectomy, usually take both estrogen and progesterone together daily. (See chapter 13 on hysterectomy for more information.)

HRT AFTER OTHER CANCERS

There is debate about taking estrogen after having a malignant melanoma. Some doctors feel it is okay, others feel that it may increase risk of recurrence. Colon cancer does not seem to be a contraindication to replacement therapy.

BIRTH CONTROL PILLS

It has been shown in the past that birth control pills do slightly increase the incidence of breast cancer that occurs before the age of forty-five. (Some felt that this was due to the fact that women on birth control pills were more likely to be examined more frequently and therefore more tumors were found.) New research has shown that the use of oral contraceptives may increase the risk of breast cancer for those women who have BRCA1* or BRCA2* mutations (see page 287). However, might there be some interaction for those women who took birth control pills and then take HRT? To date, no study has ever proved such an interaction, but someone should initiate a study to research this premise.

---

*Genetic mutations that increase the incidence of breast cancer.

Estrogen Choices: So Many to Choose From

Table 2.1 gives the trade names of the various hormonal compounds used in the treatment of menopause. It will make it easier for you to know which compounds you might be using, or other choices you may want to try.

TABLE 2.1

ingredients	trade name	manufacturer
Estrogens, oral		
conjugated estrogen	Premarin®	Wyeth-Ayerst Labs
conjugated estrogen/MPA	Prempro™	Wyeth-Ayerst Labs
esterified estrogens	Estratab®	Solvay
esterified estrogens	Menest™	SmithKline Beecham MPA
estropipate	Ogen®	Pharmacia & Upjohn
estropipate	Ortho-EST®	Ortho-McNeil Pharmaceuticals
micronized 17 beta-estradiol	Estrace®	Bristol-Myers Squibb
Estrogen patches		
17 beta-estradiol	Estraderm®	Novartis Pharmaceuticals
17 beta-estradiol	Climara®	Berlex
17 beta-estradiol	Vivelle™	Novartis Pharmaceuticals
17 beta-estradiol	Alora™	Procter & Gamble
17 beta-estradiol	FemPatch®	Warner-Lambert
Combination estrogen/ PLM patch		
17 beta-estradiol/ norethindrone acetate	CombiPatch®	Rhône-Poulenc Rorer
Estrogen, percutaneous		
estradiol gel*	Estrogel	Solvay
Estrogen, vaginal creams		
conjugated estrogens	Premarin® cream	Wyeth-Ayerst
17 beta-estradiol	Estrace® cream	Bristol-Myers Squibb
estropipate	Ogen® cream	Pharmacia & Upjohn
Dienestrol (synthetic)	Ortho® Dienstrol cream	Ortho-McNeil Pharmaceuticals

Estrogen-containing vaginal devices		
vaginal ring	Estring®	Pharmacia & Upjohn

Estrogens with testosterone		
esterified estrogens and methyltestosterone	Estratest H.S.®	Solvay
esterified estrogens and methyltestosterone	Estratest®	Solvay
esterified estrogens and methyltestosterone	Menest™	SmithKline Beecham

Progesterone, oral, vaginal, rectal		
micronized progesterone	generic	n/a
micronized progesterone	Prometrium®†	Solvay (U.S.)/Schering-Plough (Can.)
micronized progesterone, vaginal	Crinone‡	Wyeth-Ayerest Labs

Progesterone-like medications
C21 compounds (progesterone derived)

medroxyprogesterone acetate	Provera®	Pharmacia & Upjohn
medroxyprogesterone acetate	Amen®	Carnrick
medroxyprogesterone acetate	Cycrin®	Esi Pharma

C-19 compounds (nortestosterone derivatives)

norethindrone	Micronor®	Ortho-McNeil Pharmaceuticals
norethindrone	Nor QD®	Syntex
norethindrone acetate	Aygestin®	Esi Lederle
norgestrel	Ovrette®	Wyeth-Ayerst Labs

In addition to the intake methods listed, estrogen, testosterone, and progesterone-like medications are available by injection or implantable pellets.

*Pending FDA approval. Available in Canada and Europe.

†FDA approved for therapy of secondary amenorrhea (lack of menstrual flow caused by medical problems). FDA approval for HRT is pending.

‡Pending FDA approval for menopause therapy.

PERCEPTIONS ABOUT THE VARIOUS ESTROGENS

Natural forms of estrogen are most commonly used in hormone replacement therapy. However, there is little direct comparison of the various estrogens currently available. I presented the following material in table 2.2 at a meeting some years ago. It was based on my opinions, but agreed with by most experts at the meeting.

TABLE 2.2. PERCEPTIONS ABOUT ESTROGEN FROM THE PATIENT AND PHYSICIAN VIEWPOINTS

The following table assumes equivalent doses: Premarin® 0.625 mg, Estratab® 0.625 mg; Ogen®/Ortho-EST® 0.625 mg, Estrace® 1 mg, Estratest® H.S. 0.625 mg with 1.25 mg methyltestosterone, and .05 mg of Alora™, Climara®, Estraderm®, or Vivelle™.

	Doctors' perceptions	*Patients' perceptions*
Orals		
Premarin®	Proven since 1940s	Household word
	Millions of doses used	Often only estrogen recognized
	Prescribed first	Natural—from horses' urine
	Good control of symptoms	Breast tenderness
	Therapy for osteoporosis	Moderate bleeding (with intact
	Prevents hip fracture	uterus)
	Possibly best for lipids	
Estratab®	"Generic Premarin"	Unsure, not what friends take
	Good symptom control	Not from horses
	Fewer side effects	Less bloating than Premarin®
	Less bleeding than Premarin®	Less breast tenderness
	For osteoporosis therapy	Plant source
	Plant source	
	Less well documented antioxidant	
Estrace®	17 beta-estradiol	Identical to human estrogen
	Rapidly absorbed	Hot flashes may happen before
	*Breakthrough symptoms	next dose
	Therapy for osteoporosis	Compact dispenser available
	Slightly less potent than Premarin®	Plant source

*Breakthrough symptoms—when symptoms such as hot flashes recur while a woman is on medication.

	Doctors' perceptions	*Patients' perceptions*

Orals

| Ogen®/
Ortho-EST® | Weaker estrogen, less
  bioavailable
Least side effects
Least bleeding
Therapy for osteoporosis
Possible use of less progestin | Inadequate relief if flashes
  are severe
Little breast tenderness, bloating
Often no menses
Good for older women
Good for women who don't
  want flow
Plant source |

Transdermals—skin patches, all contain 17 beta-estradiol

| Estraderm®
(first patch
sold in U.S.) | 17 beta-estradiol
Constant estrogen dose
Bypasses liver
Less lipid benefit than orals
Safer for headache
Safer for varicosities
Safer for clotting problems
20 percent experience skin
  problems
Falls off/washes off
Indicated for osteoporosis
Must change patch twice a
  week
0.05, 0.1 dose | Identical to human estrogen
Don't have to take by mouth
Easier on liver
Safer with varicose veins,
  headache
It shows, he knows
It often doesn't stick
It itches sometimes
Rash
Bleeding likely, similar to
  Premarin® |

| Climara® | Pure
Bypasses liver
Tiny, flat, rarely loosens
  or comes off
Must change patch once
  weekly
Safer for varicosities
Safer for headache
Safer for clotting problems
Less benefit for blood lipids
0.05, 0.1 dose |
Easier on liver
Rare rash, rare itching
Change once a week
It shows, he knows
Breast tenderness
Bleeding likely |

| Vivelle™ | Like Climara® but changed
  twice a week
New, replacing Estraderm®
Less breast tenderness than
  with Climara®
0.0375, 0.05, 0.075, 0.1 dose | Rare skin problems
Minimal breast tenderness
Light to moderate bleed in some
  women |

| Alora™ | Like Vivelle™, in .05, .075,
  and .1 mg doses | |

| | *Doctors' perceptions* | *Patients' perceptions* |

Transdermals—skin patches

FemPatch®	Changed once weekly	Few side effects
	For older women	
	For women unable to tolerate full dose	
	Uses 0.025-mg dose (low dose)	
	For bone maintenance	

Orals, combination of estrogen with androgen

Estratest® H.S.	Alternative for patients:	For women with no uterus or ovaries
	When symptoms are not controlled	Helps hot flashes not controlled previously
	Who have had hysterectomy and oophorectomy	Helps sex drive
	Who are depressed	Improves mood
	Who have breast tenderness	May cause more assertive behavior
	Who have poor libido	
	Concerns:	May cause weight gain
	Less good for lipids	May cause hair loss (reversible)
	Weight gain	May cause acne
	Hair loss	
	Increased facial hair/acne	

Combination of estrogen and progestin

Prempro™: Contains both Premarin® and medroxyprogesterone acetate in combined continuous dose

	One daily pill	Easy to take
	No separate progestin	No forgetting progestin
	Decreases bleeding for some	No bleeding for some
	Erratic bleeding at first in younger patients	bleeding/spotting for others
	Possible less vascular benefit	

Premphase®: contains both Premarin® and medroxyprogesterone acetate in cyclic doses

| | Use for younger women | More bleeding for some |

Local therapies

Estring™ vaginal ring	Silicone ring with estrogen	For vaginal dryness
	Constant estrogen release	Possibly more convenient than creams
	Nonsignificant absorption	

	Doctors' perceptions	*Patients' perceptions*

Local therapies

Vaginal creams	†Local therapy in low dose	Used once weekly or as directed
	†Systemic therapy if higher dose	More like patch; may need added progesterone
	Estrace® vaginal cream, natural 17 beta-estradiol	
	Premarin® vaginal cream, natural estrogens	
	Dienestrol® cream, synthetic estrogen cream	

†When vaginal walls are atrophic, there is increased absorption of vaginal estrogen creams into the bloodstream. As vaginal tissues improve, less absorption occurs. Therefore, the amount of estrogen absorbed depends upon the dose and the condition of the vaginal tissues.

UNDERSTANDING THE DIFFERENT ESTROGEN PREPARATIONS

Pharmacokinetics

All non-oral methods for taking estrogen (patch, pellet, injection, or vaginal route) bypass the stomach, intestines, and the liver and allow estrogen to be absorbed directly into the bloodstream. This mimics the ovarian secretion of estrogen directly into the blood. The liver does not have to metabolize the oral hormones so that they can be absorbed. Non-oral methods are said to avoid the first pass through the liver. This benefits some patients, e.g., those with migraine, varicose veins, or hypertension. But for most women, a major benefit of the first pass is that orals more effectively lower serum cholesterol and raise HDL cholesterol.

Remember, *you should always take estrogen tablets after food or with a meal!* This will improve your body's ability to absorb it properly and will actually increase your total absorption. *You should never apply your transdermal patch within three hours of a bath or shower.* Moist skin, either because of water residue or moisturizing creams, is the most common reason for patches failing to adhere, skin reactions to the patch, and even poor absorption of the estrogen.

Generally, most estrogens are basically interchangeable, providing relief of symptoms and preventing osteoporosis in the average postmenopausal woman. Occasionally, a woman requires a specific estrogen preparation for her own particular symptomatology. Which estrogen may be best for her depends upon its pharmacokinetics, i.e., how it is absorbed into the bloodstream, its timing, and its rate of absorption as well as its total absorption. These basic factors often play a role in whether or not a woman will have side effects. They may also influence what her benefits will be from any given estrogen preparation.

Premarin®, for example, has led the estrogen market for fifty years. It is a formulation that is a modified-release preparation. This means that after a single dose, the active ingredients—mostly equilin (an equine estrogen) and estrone (the most common estrogen of the menopausal woman)—are released and absorbed more slowly into the bloodstream than most other oral products. This may be beneficial, as the more gradual rises and falls of estrogen may be better tolerated by some women.

On the other hand, Estrace®, a micronized estrogen, has rapid absorption and is quickly cleared from the body. Although most patients do well on this preparation, some find that the more rapid rise and rapid fall lead to a recurrence of menopausal symptoms or headaches before the next dose. Breaking the tablet in half and taking it twice a day usually overcomes this problem. Some patients with a history of migraine headache or menstrual headache, which seem to result from rapid withdrawal of estrogen, may do better on a patch that provides a more controlled release.

Potency

The active ingredient in Ogen® or Ortho-EST® is estrone, a weaker estrogen than the multiple estrogens that make up Premarin®. Because of this, most women have little to no bleeding and bloating-type side effects while on this preparation. Ogen® or Ortho-EST® therefore are especially liked by women who are older or simply cannot put up with side effects such as these. In addition, they are effective in preventing osteoporosis. No product-to-product comparisons (such as Ogen® or Ortho-EST® versus Premarin®) are published as of this date.

Differences in Patches

There are a wide variety of estradiol patches on the market for postmenopausal hormone replacement. They include Alora™, Climara®, Estraderm®, Vivelle™, and FemPatch®, and there are likely to be others in the near future. Although each of these provides safe and effective levels of estradiol for the treatment of menopausal symptoms, some but not all have gained FDA approval for the prevention of bone loss and osteoporosis. While all of these patches are similar, they may not all deliver exactly the same amount of estradiol. Climara®, for example, is used for an entire week at a time. While convenient, this patch does lose some of its potency by the end of the week. Similarly, Estraderm®, which contains its estradiol in a liquid layer of alcohol, may lose some of its potency by the fourth day of use, especially in hot dry weather. Dosing every third day, followed by every fourth day, may create minor symptoms during the fourth day when estradiol levels fall below the threshold for menopausal relief. Therefore, although these patches may appear to be interchangeable, some patients do better on one patch as opposed to the other. Sometimes too a patient may become sensitive to the particular adhesive of one patch, but not to the other, or may prefer a particular packaging or pricing.

Which Estrogen for Which Woman?

Now that there are so many different estrogens and progesterone-like compounds to choose from, how do you select the most appropriate one for you? Although most of the estrogens in the tables above have similar properties, there are nuances. Therefore, if you are not completely comfortable on your hormone replacement, your therapy can always be altered. I try to encourage patients, if possible, to wait four weeks for minor side effects to go away before changing their therapy, for it often takes that long for the estrogen's "steady state" blood levels to be reached. Your degree of comfort both mentally and physically will lead to your continuing hormonal therapy.

SPECIFIC SUGGESTIONS FOR SPECIFIC WOMEN

The following women could be you. Read through the list and see what my suggestions might be. I hope that you will find this helpful. Physicians have. It may be necessary for you to combine these theoretical women to adapt to your personal needs. Remember, however, that your own physician knows you best and should guide your final choices.

HRT FOR WOMEN WHO HAVE A UTERUS

A thirty-nine-year-old woman with premature ovarian failure
   The younger you are when you lose ovarian function due to surgery or

premature ovarian failure, the more critical hormone replacement becomes for cardiovascular and bone protection. This woman should be started on a higher dose of estrogen than the usual 0.625 mg, because if her ovaries were still functioning, she would have produced more estrogen than an average fifty-year-old. So an initial dose of Premarin® 0.9 or its equivalent might be tried first. She would also be given MPA (medroxyprogesterone acetate) for cycling probably in a 5 mg dose for twelve to fourteen days each month. If after four to six weeks she was still having symptoms, the dose of estrogen could be increased to 1.25 mg. It is likely that either dose will do nicely. Blood levels for estrogen could be checked to ensure that the amount of estrogen was adequate to protect her younger body. This amount of estrogen will likely bring back monthly menstrual cycling, which most younger women prefer. With time, as she ages, the estrogen dose should be lowered. If Premarin® is not well tolerated, almost any other oral could be substituted in equivalent doses. A transdermal would be fine too. Too little data is available on raloxifene in this age group.

Ten different fifty-year-old women who are approximately six months "postmenopausal"

The first woman has severe symptoms: She will do well on daily Premarin® 0.625 cycled with MPA 5 mg for ten to twelve days each month. This will probably result in a return of monthly bleeding for several months or years. Some of this just depends on her history. Women who have had heavy flow in the past are more likely to continue to have a monthly flow. With enough time, however, most women stop having periods. On the other hand, after an initial six to twelve months on cyclic therapy, this woman could be switched to Prempro™ 0.625/2.5 or any continuous combined estrogen/progesterone-type regimen and this might encourage her periods to stop.

If she felt too bloated on Premarin®, then Estratab®, Ogen® or Ortho-EST® 0.625, or Estrace® 1 mg could be tried and probably would have fewer side effects. A transdermal in .05 mg dose should also be fine.

If symptoms persist, she could try Estratest® H.S. (the H.S. stands for half strength) or increase the dose of estrogen for a few months. If premenstrual symptoms related to MPA are too severe, she might switch to Aygestin® 5 mg, in half-tablet dose (2.5 mg) for ten days each month to cycle, or to micronized progesterone 200 mg at bedtime for twelve days, or to a progesterone-containing IUD.

The second woman has few symptoms: This woman has more choices as to her estrogen. She could select Estratab®, Estrace®, Ogen® or Ortho-EST®, a lower-dose transdermal, or Premarin®, etc. Because we do not have to relieve severe symptoms, less potent preparations or lower doses could be considered. However, this choice and dose will be tempered by other factors such as presence of bone loss, smoking, hypertension, migraine, family history of Alzheimer's and colon cancer, etc. (See chapter on osteoporosis, p. 198.) However, if she has a good lipid profile and good bone density, perhaps this woman should choose not to take hormone therapy, at least not yet. We can then recheck this decision in twelve months. Remember, a decision to take estrogen or not to take estrogen need only last from visit to visit. Also, alternatives to estrogen, such as raloxifene, could be used (see chapter 3).

The third woman wants HRT but "refuses" to have menses again: It is hoped that this woman has none-too-severe symptoms and has had light menses in the past. Both of these factors will help. One choice would be to start on a weaker estrogen such as Ogen® or Ortho-EST® in 0.625 dose either cycled with MPA 5 mgs, or given continuously in combination with 2.5 mg MPA. Prempro™ might work, but *because she is only six months past her last period, she may have bothersome erratic spotting and bleeding for several months.* A transdermal patch, .05 mg with 2.5 mg of daily MPA, may work. Or she might try a progesterone-containing IUD with continuous oral or transdermal estrogen. A .0375 mg or .025 mg patch or Premarin® in 0.3 mg dose or a half-dose of Ogen® or Ortho-EST® or Estratab® could be selected, but the woman would have to be aware that both are a lower than normal dose. Some physicians use progesterone-like medication every second or third month to decrease the frequency of bleeding. The final decision really depends on her other risk factors. If there are no risk factors, no therapy should be a major consideration.

This third woman, in addition to not wanting monthly flow, also has bone loss: If so, it may be possible to combine a lower dose of estrogen, 0.3 mg for example, with a preventive 5 mg dose of Fosamax®. Studies on such combinations should be completed soon. However, at the time I am writing, results are still unknown. If osteoporosis is your main or only worry, try Fosamax® in full therapeutic dose (10 mg) or raloxifene and forgo the estrogen. No matter what you finally choose, sufficient calcium and exercise must be added to your daily routine. More nitty-gritty facts: If you decide to take Fosamax® or raloxifene, you need 1,500 mg of calcium daily between diet and supplements. If you take estrogen, which improves your ability to absorb calcium, you need to take only 1,000 mgs in your diet and in supplements. And don't forget that you also need 400 to 800 IUs of vitamin D. The need for the higher dose of vitamin D occurs as we get older. Actually, new information is that all adults, both male and female, over the age of sixty-five should have 1,500 mg of calcium and 600 to 800 IUs of vitamin D daily obtained usually in a combination of diet and supplements.

The fourth woman has migraines: This woman should get relief from transdermal estrogen. Patches provide constant levels of estrogen that relax the cerebral blood vessels and decrease the spasms that cause migraine. This woman should be given daily continuous MPA or micronized progesterone either cycled or in a low daily dose to best control her headaches. If the progesterone-type medication creates an increase in headache, this woman should consider a progesterone-containing IUD. She may also be a candidate for low-dose estrogen-only therapy, given without progesterone.

The fifth woman had a superficial thrombophlebitis in the past (not associated with estrogen use and not causing embolism): This woman's first choice should be a transdermal patch, rather than an oral, because patches have no effect on clotting factors that predispose her to thrombosis. Oral therapy can be tried at a lower dose first, if the patient cannot tolerate patches or is willing to assume a possible minimal increased risk of blood clots. Regardless of how her estrogen is given, she can be cycled with any of the progesterone-like medications. Or, again, depending on her risk factors, no therapy might be selected.

The sixth woman has hypertension: Her hypertension should be controlled first with antihypertensive medications. Then I would recommend a transdermal patch. Cycling with MPA or micronized progesterone would be best, or a progesterone-containing IUD could be used. An oral estrogen would also be a good choice. Because of a tiny subgroup of two or three patients in my practice who developed increased blood pressure on Premarin®, I usually prefer other orals.

The seventh woman has diabetes mellitus or has known coronary artery disease: This woman needs the best cardiovascular protection we can offer. Premarin® 0.625 mg or any oral would be good because of their beneficial effect on blood lipids. I would then give her the least possible dose of progesterone-type medications. So I would cycle her on micronized progesterone 200 mg at bedtime for twelve days, offer a progesterone-containing IUD, or MPA 5 mg for ten days (which comes out to *less* than the MPA dose of 2.5 mg given for thirty days, as used in Prempro™). I might also consider using MPA every second or third month rather than monthly because of MPA's potential ability to induce vascular spasm in women with preexisting vascular disease. Smokers probably fall into this same category as they have a high likelihood of preexisting vascular disease.

The eighth patient weighs 225 pounds: First, I would have to be very sure that this patient had documented low estrogen levels and symptoms that really required therapy. I would also want to know her lipid profile and any other risk factors she might have for cardiovascular disease. If I did treat her, I would likely choose a transdermal because overweight women are somewhat more prone to thrombophlebitis, but, if she had cardiovascular risk factors, I'd recommend an oral. I would also make sure that she received MPA in adequate doses for *twelve* days. I encourage women who are obviously overweight to have a biopsy of the lining of their uterus prior to therapy because they are at higher risk for uterine cancer. I then follow her with ultrasound and closely monitor any abnormal bleeding. This close observation is necessary because women who are heavy have increased production of estrone-type estrogen in their extra body fat. I feel that appropriate hormone replacement may actually help to *decrease* their risk of endometrial cancer because it provides progesterone to properly balance the hormonal milieu. Another fact: Women who weigh over 180 pounds are normally at low risk for osteoporosis. If her symptoms are not severe, and her lipids are good, therapy could be postponed, or perhaps local vaginal therapy could give relief until her next visit.

The ninth woman has loss of libido: Most women regain sexual appetite when replenished with estrogen. Estrogens contribute to desire and prime the sexual organs and the brain (the most important erotic organ). The physical aspects of sex often improve because vaginal dryness and pain diminish. However, if *after making sure that she is not depressed* or just in a bad or boring relationship I find that estrogen alone does not remedy the situation, then adding male hormone may improve her ability for sexual fantasy and intensify her sex drive. Estratest® H.S., an oral tablet containing a balance of male and female hormone, currently is the first choice. Injectable combinations of male and female hormone such as Depotestadiol® are available, but less frequently used, as are subcutaneous implants of male hormones. A transdermal patch containing estrogen and testosterone, and sublingual and gel forms will be available soon. (As an aside, hypothyroidism can also contribute to lack of libido.)

The tenth woman is on hormone replacement and still has flashes or feels "down." Remember, estrogen is absorbed best after or with meals. However, sometimes some women seem not to absorb oral estrogen well. This may be a time to measure blood levels of estrogen. This rare patient with persistent flashes may do better on a transdermal. Or she may simply need to have her oral estrogen increased or switched to another more potent oral or to Estratest® H.S., where an androgen is added to the estrogen.

Androgens may also help to improve mood and energy level. Rarely, injectable estrogen or estrogen/androgens need to be used.

ALL OF THE FOLLOWING WOMEN ARE IN THEIR SIXTIES

The first woman has symptoms: Obviously, this woman has not had menses for a long time. She could be started on almost any regimen and might never bleed. Or she might. Prempro™ 0.625/2.5 given daily might be all right. However, many women who are started on this preparation complain of breast tenderness and/or bloating. Her dosage can be cut by eliminating the Prempro™ on Sundays—it's my "never on Sundays" routine. Sometimes, it's "never on Sundays and Wednesdays" to keep patients comfortable. However, I would be more likely to choose other orals for this woman. Certainly, Estratab®, Ogen® or Ortho-EST® with cycled or continuous progesterone-type medication will give her excellent relief and cause less bloating. Some physicians use unopposed estrogen, using 0.3 mg of Estratab®, Ogen®, or Premarin®, or 0.5 mg of Estrace®, or a low-dose patch. Then they use ultrasound to monitor these women who are far past their last menstrual period. Exact choices and doses tend to depend on other factors, such as heart and bone risk factors. For cycling, MPA or micronized progesterone will do nicely. A progesterone-containing IUD probably would be difficult to insert into the uterus of a sixty-year-old.

The second woman has no symptoms: This woman is obviously considering estrogen for another reason, such as cardiovascular protection, bone protection, fear of Alzheimer's, etc. Depending on her personal risk factors, appropriate doses of raloxifene could be used. If there are no risk factors, no therapy should be considered as well.

The third woman only has complaints of vaginal dryness and atrophy: This woman has the choice of any oral or transdermal estrogen, or if she does not want systemic therapy, she has the choice of the Estring™ ring, or tiny doses of intravaginal estrogen-containing creams used along with an over-the-counter lubricant.

THE FOLLOWING WOMAN IS IN HER SEVENTIES

This woman, as is typical for a woman her age, takes estrogen because of its protective effect after she has been documented to have osteoporosis or cardiovascular disease. A low dose should be given initially because traditional doses may cause fluid retention or other discomfort, especially since many of these women are tiny. Ogen® or Ortho-EST® in 0.625 mg dose could be given, beginning with half a tablet. Estratab® 0.3, Estrace® 0.5, or Premarin® 0.3 could be tried and the dose titrated as her comfort and risk factors demand. Transdermals starting with .025 or .0375 doses are fine. Raloxifene would be another choice. Again, no therapy may be fine, depending on her individual health factors and wishes. "If it ain't broke, don't fix it" comes to mind. However, good diet, calcium and vitamin D supplementation, and activity must always be encouraged.

HRT FOR WOMEN WHO HAVE HAD A HYSTERECTOMY

These women fit into all of the above categories, except that they do *not* require progesterone-type medications added to their regimens. Women with no uterus and no ovaries should also, some experts feel, have their male-type hormones replaced to ensure libido and possibly their bone mass as well. The use of Estratest® and Estratest® H.S. as well as other means of taking androgen, i.e., transdermal, injectable, sublingual, are being investigated. Currently, however, most women who have had a complete hysterectomy take oral or transdermal estrogen alone. This may change in the future, or other proandrogen-type compounds, such as DHEA, may be added. (See page 120.)

Who Really Needs Hormones?

A woman must know what the reasons are for taking hormone replacement, or she will most likely never fill her prescription or will soon discontinue therapy. Understanding why HRT is important to her own body is of paramount importance. On the other hand, if symptoms are so bad that she has not slept in weeks and is about to "lose it," then relief of her symptoms is all important and little else may matter for the moment.

Some women come for help later, when hot flashes have already begun to dissipate. But they feel life isn't as good as it used to be. Sleep isn't as sound, vaginal dryness has begun to be bothersome, memory is playing tricks, skin isn't quite as luminescent as it used to be. These women can live with all of the above, but there are more basic questions they want answered. What about my risk of heart attack? Am I going to lose bone quickly, or do I already have bone loss? Suddenly, the decision whether or not to take HRT has become complex.

Whether to take HRT has always been a complex decision, but many doctors and patients didn't really think about all of the factors that go into tailoring HRT to the woman. And sometimes they ignored what was really right for her and her psyche and genetic and social background. To begin with, not every woman needs hormone replacement. Some don't because they are simply too uncomfortable and afraid of the idea. That has to be respected by both doctor and patient. Some don't need hormone replacement because they truly have few risk factors. For example, if a woman has few overt symptoms, has a good lipid profile, and has good bones, there may be precious few reasons to take hormones, at least for now.

The basic things to consider when thinking about starting HRT are the risk and benefits for *you*. If you have a strong family history of heart disease, if you have a poor lipid profile or you have already had a heart attack, this should be a powerful motivator to begin HRT. It is important to realize here that family history of early heart attack includes early heart attack in *male and female* family members. For example, if your brother, sister, mother, or father died at or before the age of fifty-five, you are in a higher-risk category and you might be wise to consider taking hormones. If you are at increased risk for fracture and bone loss because of a family history of osteoporosis in a mother or sister, or because of personal factors in your own life (see chapter 6 on osteoporosis), then I encourage you to take HRT or Fosamax® or raloxifene as well as to exercise and take calcium with vitamin D. Remember, women on HRT who take sufficient calcium in their diet or as supplements improve their bones more than women on HRT alone.

If your love life is suffering because of vaginal dryness and tenderness, or your bladder is beginning to show signs of weakness resulting in urinary incontinence, it may also be time to say yes. But instead of taking hormones by mouth or by patch, you may have another choice: treating the problem locally with a tiny dose of estrogen cream or the Estring™ vaginal ring. If the dose of vaginal cream is kept to one gram per week, it is enough to improve the vaginal tissues and bladder outlet without much systemic absorption. If you have had breast cancer and do not want to take any estrogen product, the Estring™ ring, because it does not get any measurable estrogen into the bloodstream, is probably safe, according to many experts.

For those of you who have had a hysterectomy and bilateral oophorectomy, the decision may be easier. Many of you had surgery prior to the age of menopause. The abrupt transition from normal hormone levels to zero hormone levels can be devastating, causing constant severe hot flashes and drenching sweats. And unless the surgery was for a hormone-dependent cancer, such as endometrial cancer, your doctor will usually quickly prescribe estrogen replacement. And because there is no uterus, there is no endometrium to protect, so no progesterone is needed. Surgery done postmenopausally when ovarian function is minimal will not likely result in major symptoms and you would have to weigh your risk factors in the same manner as other women in your age category.

Often, women are puzzled, and need to know a good, persuasive reason to take or continue taking hormones. When blood work, lipid profiles, and symptoms are not creating any urgent situation, a bone density test may help in making the decision. Finding out that your hip has major bone loss, putting you at high risk for fracture, can be a significant motivating factor in beginning hormone replacement. Or if your bone density is good, you may decide to wait and reevaluate your blood and bone parameters the next year. In fact, there is reassuring data that hormone replacement begun in your sixties may greatly improve your bone density, maybe not quite as much as taking HRT from the day you became menopausal, but very substantially. This, of course, would limit the number of years on hormone replacement and many women find that waiting is an attractive alternative. Women in their late sixties and seventies can also be assured that starting hormones now will actually build bone and give them protection against fracture.

No decision should be forever. That goes either way. You and your physician should engage in mental gymnastics at least once a year, reevaluating whether to start, continue, or discontinue your therapy. All decisions should be based on how you feel mentally and physically as well as on lab comparisons over the prior six to twelve months. I find that I often have to remind my patients that they are taking hormone replacement, not birth control pills. That they will not get pregnant if they miss one pill, and that we can modify their hormone regimen in many ways to assure their physical comfort. In fact, this is why there are so many ways to take hormone replacement. No one way is right, it just has to be right for you.

And so it is important to have a physician who has experience and interest in menopausal therapy and who will be willing to listen and alter therapy as needed. I have heard new patients say that their previous doctor told them they had to stick it out with Premarin® or discontinue therapy. If your doctor makes such a statement, perhaps you should bring him/her this book. Premarin® is the oldest and most popular estrogen in this country. It is an excellent drug and it works well for many women. However, there are now many other choices and so this "take it or leave it" attitude is intolerable. The ability to alter doses or change to a more compatible estrogen preparation is the art of therapy, an art that will give a woman the fine-tuned hormone replacement she deserves.

Ways to Take Hormone Replacement

ESTROGEN, ESTROGEN WITH PROGESTERONE

If you have had your uterus removed, estrogen replacement is easy: Estrogen is usually taken on a daily basis in continuous fashion. On the other hand, if you have breast tenderness or bloating, it is possible to decrease the dose a bit by either lowering the dose or decreasing the actual number of days they are taken per week.

If you have a uterus, you will take estrogen along with progesterone-like medication (PLM) to prevent an increased risk of uterine cancer. Therefore, you have two hormones to juggle, and you and your doctor can be very creative. The old standard was to take estrogen cyclically for twenty-five days, i.e., from the first of the calendar month to the twenty-fifth, adding PLM on day 14, 15, or 16, continuing up through the twenty-fifth, then stopping both hormones. Depending upon your age, hormonal dose, estrogen compound selected, prior amount of menstrual flow, and luck, you might or might not get a period. Women who are younger, women with a history of heavy menses, women who are started on cyclic HRT within weeks or a few months from their last menstrual period are more likely to get a withdrawal bleed when started on HRT. However, after time, which could be months or years, the endometrium gradually stops functioning and bleeding stops.

The next step was to take estrogen continuously, i.e., every day of the month, and take PLM as well during the first two weeks of the month. Because bleeding normally occurs one to two days after discontinuing progestins, patients would get a midmonth bleed. Or the progestin can be taken from days 16 through 25. Although many of my patients use the day 16 to 25 regimen, it has one distinct disadvantage—you wind up with a period on Christmas, New Year's, and almost every Thanksgiving. No matter when the PLM is added, I prefer a continuous estrogen schedule, because it prevents symptoms of hot flashes and night sweats from occurring as they sometimes do when both hormones are discontinued for five days at the end of the monthly cycle. Plus, it gives continuous uninterrupted daily protection to arteries that feed the brain and heart.

On the other hand, in order to not produce a menstrual flow (which most women don't want), several innovative schedules have been designed. One is to take a small daily dose of PLM along with *any* daily estrogen. Wyeth-Ayerst has introduced Prempro™, the first combination pill that contains both Premarin® and medroxyprogesterone acetate. It is available in the United States. This may *not* be the best way to start women who have recently stopped having periods because erratic breakthrough bleeding may be especially bothersome for the first six to eight months. However, after patients have already been on a cyclic regimen for six to eighteen months, changing to Prempro™ often stops further monthly bleeding. On the other hand, this continuous combined schedule can be used initially for women who are several years postmenopausal when they first start HRT and generally will not cause bleeding.

If you are good at math, it will be apparent to you that with a continuous combined regimen, you wind up getting a larger dose of PLM than with cyclic schedules that use 5 mg of MPA for ten days. This could be a disadvantage. Not only is the total dose important, but the continuous PLM may counteract on a daily—rather then on a limited cyclic—basis some of the cardiovascular benefits of the estrogen. In addition, there have not been long-term studies that can totally reassure us that good endometrial protection is achieved by this method. It seems common sense that it should, but I would like to see long-term study results. However, there may be a possible benefit to the use of low-dose continuous PLM with estrogen in the sense that continuous combined use may decrease cellular activity in breast tissue and (although this is unproven) might decrease the risk of breast cancer. In the future PLM may be added in a variety of different ways to continuous estrogen. Small studies show that when PLM doses are alternated—a few days on and a few days off—it may be possible to turn off hormonal receptors in the endometrium and possibly in breast tissue also. Other regimens call for PLM to be used only every second or third month for those women who find it hard to tolerate menses or progesterone-type side effects.

On the other hand, it may be possible to use lower doses of estrogen than we used in the past. Low-dose estrogen has recently been reported to prevent bone loss while causing little endometrial stimulation, even without the use of PLM. The compound used in this two-year study was Estratab® 0.3 mg. Low-dose .0375 and .025 mg patches are also now available. Or, by choosing less potent compounds such as 0.625 mg Ogen® or Ortho-EST®, there will be less growth of the lining of the uterus and often no flow, or only the scantiest of flow.

Natural and Synthetic Progesterone-like Medications

In the near future, micronized progesterone will play a more important role in hormone replacement. At this time, however, few large-scale studies have been done. One of the reasons is that progesterone is not patentable and will not generate large enough profits for a drug company that carries out the studies. Therefore, women may need to have close monitoring of their endometrium until we are more sure of how much progesterone is really the correct amount. This is because the rapid metabolism of this natural product may create variation in individual absorption and metabolism. Also, because it is rapidly metabolized, larger doses, e.g., 200 mg (versus 5 mg of MPA), are normally taken. And just because the hormone is "natural" does not mean it is without side effects. Several of my patients have had significant side effects, primarily sleepiness; one had her speech become slurred; and one lost coordination, perhaps because she felt so tired. Therefore, it is usually prescribed to be taken at bedtime.

Micronized progesterone received its first real boost when used in the Postmenopausal Estrogen-Progestin Intervention (PEPI) Trial. This study involved a total of 875 healthy postmenopausal women between the ages of forty-five and sixty-four. Prometrium®, the trade name of the progesterone product used in the PEPI trials, turned out to have less adverse effects on HDL cholesterol than medroxyprogesterone acetate. It has been available in Europe as Utrogestan® and in Canada from Schering-Plough for years. Sold in 100 mg capsules, the suggested dose from the PEPI trial for hormone replacement is two 100 mg capsules to be taken at bedtime for twelve days each month. Side effects such as fatigue and sleepiness should not be a problem as the medication is taken at bedtime. The other good news about micronized progesterone is that it doesn't cause PMS-like symptoms as do the synthetic progestins.

Some women buy natural progesterone creams that are rubbed on the skin. Please *don't* unless and until one is FDA approved for use in HRT. See page 109 so that you will understand: Natural progesterone creams that are presently available have not been proven to balance the estrogen in hormone replacement.

The FDA has approved Crinone™ from Wyeth-Ayerst, a vaginal gel that contains micronized progesterone. It is used for infertile women who are undergoing assisted reproduction and have been found to be progesterone deficient. It has also been FDA approved to be used for treatment of irregular bleeding, but *not* yet for menopausal therapy. Studies by Dr. Mona Shangold indicate that micronized progesterone used vaginally causes less drowsiness and fewer side effects than when used orally. Her studies also showed that Crinone™ was able to protect against the development of endometrial abnormalities.

There is another thought on how to get your progesterone. The Progestasert® IUD contains natural progesterone. When inserted into the uterine cavity, it slowly releases a small amount of progesterone onto the endometrial lining of the uterus. This tiny amount of progesterone works locally, and does not get into the bloodstream, thereby avoiding any undesired side effects. Furthermore, this IUD tends to decrease menstrual flow and cramping. Though an ideal method (except for the fact that it needs to be changed once a year), it is rarely used. I have often suggested it to patients, but few seem willing to try it. IUDs that contain more potent PLMs and last much longer than the Progestasert® are available in Europe. When they make their way into the States, more women may select IUDs as an option.

Other PLMs are currently being used here and in Europe. All of these—norgestimate, levonorgestrel, gestodene, and desogestrel—are being studied for lipid effects, clotting, and other problems. A recent study involving different PLMs in birth control pills, cited in the British medical journal *Lancet,* showed a slightly increased incidence of venous thromboembolism when some compounds were used as compared with others. Much work is still to be done.

ANDROGENS

Androgens are male hormones. Men produce female hormones as well as male hormones, e.g., testosterone and androstenedione. Therefore, it shouldn't surprise you to find out that ovaries and women's adrenal glands secrete androgens. Androgen levels peak when a woman is twenty and begin to fall through the perimenopausal years. With the onset of menopause, androgen production by the ovary falls by approximately 50 percent and then continues slowly to fade over the next few years. On the other hand, if your ovaries are surgically removed, your ovarian source of androgen is immediately zero. The question then might arise, should androgens be replaced in women along with estrogen and progesterone? Or at least in women who have had their ovaries removed? There are many who feel that this is a neglected subject.

Androgen's effect on postmenopausal women has been studied over the past decade because male hormone is known to affect the sex drive. Androgen is always given to women in conjunction with estrogen. The most often prescribed oral tablet is Estratest® H.S. Many women report that the addition of androgen makes them feel better, elevates their mood, and increases their energy level and their ability to concentrate. There is now evidence that androgens may offer bone protection as well. In fact, along with estrogen, androgens may help increase bone mass beyond the effects of estrogen alone. Women with vertebral crush fractures have been noted to have lower levels of testosterone than women who have not fractured.

On the downside, depending on dose, balance with estrogen, or individual sensitivity, androgens may increase appetite; cause weight gain, hair loss, acne, deepening of the voice, and growth of facial hair; and may decrease HDL cholesterol. However, with careful adjustment of doses, most unwanted side effects can be avoided. If non-oral forms of androgen are used, i.e., injectable or implanted pellets of androgen, the effect on blood lipids seems to be reduced. In Europe, transdermal gels are available for testosterone and androstenedione. Soon, combination patches containing estrogen and androgen will be sold in the U.S. If you are considering using androgens, it might be a good idea to get a testosterone test with your initial blood work to see if your male hormone levels are actually low. Also, remember, it will still be necessary to take a PLM along with the estrogen and testosterone, if you have a uterus.

New studies are beginning to show that DHEA* or DHEAS† and androstenedione also play a part in the quality of sexual life in women. Androstenedione is a weak androgen. Unlike testosterone, it is only weakly attached to proteins in the blood, so that it can easily leave the bloodstream and enter the tissues. Furthermore, DHEAS and androstenedione are present in large amounts. They are becoming a source of great interest in studies of arousal and sexuality (see page 120).

---

*DHEA—dehydroepiandrosterone—an adrenal hormone with male-type effects.

†DHEAS—dehydroepiandrosterone sulfate—a prohormone of DHEA. DHEAS becomes biologically active after the sulfate has been removed.

THE NUTS AND BOLTS OF TAKING HORMONE REPLACEMENT

Starting HRT

Whether a woman will use HRT for a few months, or for several years, before starting on hormones, a baseline evaluation must be completed. The initial history, physical exam, and lab data will be the basis for determining whether or not she will benefit from therapy. *The key we need to aim for is individualization of therapy.* The evaluation should include:

1. Complete physical examination including a breast and pelvic exam. Blood pressure, height, weight, thyroid, heart, lungs, and abdomen as well as extremities should be checked.

2. Complete blood work, including a complete blood count, and chemistry profile that includes cholesterol, triglycerides, HDL, liver function tests, blood sugar, body salts, kidney function, and if indicated, or for screening purposes, a TSH to evaluate thyroid function. Ideally, this should be done fasting, i.e., prior to breakfast, after a twelve-hour fast, for the most accurate cholesterol/lipid profile.

3. Pap smear.

4. Mammography, unless it was done within the preceding twelve months.

5. If any abnormal bleeding pattern has occurred within the last several months, if there is an abnormal finding on pelvic exam, or if significant fibroids are present, or if there is any question about the pelvic examination, then a pelvic ultrasound and/or an endometrial biopsy should be ordered.

6. Bone density test to evaluate the spine and hip for any bone loss may be indicated.

7. If there is any question about whether a woman is truly menopausal or has stopped menstruating for other reasons, then blood tests known as FSH (follicle-stimulating hormone), and estradiol or prolactin may be obtained.

Once her physical exam, mammography, and blood labs are evaluated, it is time to decide whether or not to begin HRT.

Six-Week Checkup

I feel that a woman who begins HRT needs to be seen for a short visit after six weeks, because there are usually so many questions that come up, plus she already has a very good idea of whether or not she is comfortable with her therapy. This is the time to make sure that hot flashes have decreased and to reassure her that some symptoms such as breast tenderness are to be expected. It is also the time to make sure she is happy with her therapy and generally feeling well. If she has a uterus, this is the time to review whether or not she had a withdrawal bleed, and if so, whether it was light or heavy. Hormonal adjustments can be made if needed.

The visit involves a blood pressure, a breast examination, and a pelvic exam to check the vaginal mucosa visually. In just six weeks, it is possible to see dramatic change in the vagina. Thick, pink, moist, healthy folds of tissue indicate that there has been good absorption of estrogen. A vaginal estrogen level test can be quickly and inexpensively performed. Cells wiped from the lateral wall of the vagina are placed in a drop of saline solution and looked at with a microscope. One can easily tell by viewing the cells whether or not estrogen is present, and whether or not levels are sufficient.

There are rare times when women continue to have complaints of flushing while taking usual doses of oral estrogen. This may be the time to measure estrogen blood levels (see below).

After her six-week visit, my patients on hormone replacement therapy are seen every six months. I encourage *all* patients who are over forty to return at six months for their breast and pelvic exam. I think that this interval is best, so that I can be aware of new complaints my patient may have or discover abnormal physical findings early.

When to Measure Estrogen Levels

By this time you're almost a doctor! If symptoms persist in the face of what should be adequate doses of estrogen, or if side effects persist even if doses are standard or low, estrogen levels should be measured. In these cases, doing a blood or urine estrogen test may be a way to get a handle on what is happening. If you are on Estrace® or a patch, you are taking pure 17 beta-estradiol, the exact molecule that your ovaries used to make, and blood estradiol measurements are easily done by standard tests. Estradiol levels should be at least 50 pg/ml to protect you, but the levels may be anywhere between 50 to 120 pg/ml. Anything over that level is unnecessary, and may cause heavy bleeding or breast tenderness due to excess estrogen.

However, if you are on Premarin®, you cannot simply measure an estradiol level because Premarin® is a mixture of several estrogens. Therefore, we normally order a blood test for total estrogens. This test measures three different estrogens: estrone, estradiol, and estriol. However, this is still not the total amount of estrogen, for Premarin® also contains equilins, or horse estrogens, which we are unable to measure. Therefore, any woman on Premarin® should know that her total estrogen level is actually somewhat higher than reported on her blood test, due to the equilin component. Nonetheless, the 50 to 120 pg/ml range still holds.

Basically, doctors want to make sure that patients are on *adequate* doses that will protect their bones and cardiovascular systems. So it is probably best to measure hormone levels when they are at their lowest ebb. Therefore, if you take your Premarin® in the morning, have your levels measured before your morning dose. If you take your pills at bedtime, measure the levels in the afternoon.

Abnormal Bleeding Problems on HRT

If you have been on hormones and you have a uterus, it is possible that at some time you might have bleeding. As has already been discussed, irregular bleeding can often happen when you begin continuous combined estrogen/progesterone therapy with a product such as Prempro™. It is possible to bleed for part of a day, a day, three days, or five days at a time with little or no pattern. With time, however, bleeding should become lighter and the bleeds will become wider spaced. Then, one hopes, the bleeding should disappear. While some women on this schedule will never get even one bleed, others may and finally get frustrated and need to change to a different brand of hormones or different method of taking them.

Women on cyclic regimens (i.e., where a PLM is taken days 16 through 25 of each month) may also never have even one bleed; those who do should bleed one, two, or three days after the PLM has been stopped. Others bleed on the last or next to the last day while still taking progesterone. That's okay too. However, bleeding earlier than that may indicate that a patient is not taking a sufficient dose of progesterone. Bleeding that occurs on any other day, for example, midcycle, is considered abnormal. A sometimes overlooked common cause of bleeding is often simply that the woman forgot to take one or two pills.

In all of the above regimens, what is *not* okay is to have progressively heavier bleeding that lasts longer and longer. Whether continuous combined or cyclic schedules are followed, periods should be light to moderate in amount of flow, and last no more than four to five days. And although most women do not have major problems with abnormal bleeding, it may occur and needs to be fully checked out so that both patient and doctor are sure that no ominous changes are occurring.

The workup is somewhat cookbook. It usually involves a pelvic ultrasound exam and/or an endometrial biopsy done in the office. While either one of the exams may provide sufficient information, it is sometimes best to have both procedures done. Normally, a transvaginal ultrasound is done. A slender vaginal probe is gently inserted into the vagina. The woman is encouraged to guide it in herself. And because the vaginal probe is so close to the uterus and ovaries, great detail can be seen. With ultrasound it is easy to find an ovarian cyst that may be producing hormone, or to measure the thickness of the lining of the uterus. If a woman is not on hormone replacement, and is postmenopausal, her uterine lining should be no thicker than 3 to 5 millimeters. On the other hand, if the woman is premenopausal or cycling on hormone therapy, the lining will be thicker. Just how thick is normal for her depends on where she is in her hormonal cycle. Abnormal findings will need to be followed by an in-office biopsy of the uterine lining.

Sometimes the measurements reported on ultrasound and the final tissue diagnosis just don't seem to agree. Therefore, your doctor needs to have good clinical judgment. Also, if a woman is easy to examine—she can relax well, and is not obese, etc.—an endometrial biopsy may be the only exam needed. In my original book, few methods then existed to accomplish a biopsy; now there are several. All of them basically do the same thing: They suction off a tiny amount of the lining of the uterus, and the specimen is analyzed by a lab. The whole procedure takes no more than a minute or two. There is a cramp-like sensation as the probe enters the uterine cavity and suction is applied, but it is fleeting. Afterward, I always watch my patients carefully for a few minutes and then offer them hot tea or juice. A beverage and time to talk are always appreciated.

If the lab report comes back normal, then it is possible that no change in hormone therapy will be made. On the other hand, if the diagnosis shows an overgrowth of cells indicating an early hyperplasia, she needs more progesterone. Therefore, the progesterone dose can be increased, the total length of time the progesterone is taken can be increased, or another progesterone can be substituted for the original. Norethindrone acetate is often a better choice than medroxyprogesterone acetate for women with breakthrough bleeding. A little time and patience on the part of physician and patient will usually be rewarded with a normalization of the bleeding pattern, or no further bleeding.

Contraindications to HRT

You should know the conditions when HRT should *not* be used:

1. Current cancer of the breast
2. Current endometrial cancer
3. Known or suspected pregnancy
4. Undiagnosed vaginal bleeding
5. Active deep venous thrombosis
6. Thromboembolic disorders, especially when associated with previous estrogen use
7. Acute liver disease

Under these conditions, estrogen therapy should *probably not* be used:

1. History of breast cancer
2. History of endometrial cancer
3. Chronic liver disease
4. History of deep vein thrombosis
5. Large fibroids
6. Hepatic porphyria
7. Pancreatic disease

The following conditions may be associated with increased risks from hormonal therapy; *treatment with transdermal estrogen would be preferable:*

1. *Gallbladder disease.* Women on estrogen have been thought to have a slight increase in the formation of gallstones. If you are having symptoms, you should have an ultrasound of your gallbladder *before* starting HRT. If there is any question about your gallbladder or its function, use a transdermal estrogen, or no estrogen.
2. *Mild liver disease or a history of jaundice associated with taking oral contraceptives.*
3. *Epilepsy.* Because estrogen may cause fluid retention, it might make this condition worse.
4. *Hypertension.* If the hypertension is well controlled on medication, there should be no problem with taking HRT. On the other hand, it might be wiser to select a transdermal patch when considering estrogen.

5. *Migraine headache.* Women who suffer from migraine who are treated with continuous transdermal estrogen usually note that their headaches occur less often or are less severe. If needed, care must be used in selecting the progesterone. Aygestin® in 2.5 mg cycled dose should be a good choice, micronized progesterone either cycled or continuous might be better.

6. *High triglycerides.*

7. *History of thrombophlebitis.*

Other situations in which use of estrogen has changed:

1. *Diabetes.* Diabetes used to be thought of as a contraindication for HRT. It is clear now that diabetic women, because they suffer from early vascular disease, may experience *greater benefits* from HRT than nondiabetic women.

2. *Fibrocystic breast disease.* If this results from abnormal hormonal ratios, then providing a correct balance of estrogen and PLM may be beneficial. No such studies are yet available.

3. *Uterine fibroids.* It is known that estrogen may increase the size of fibroids. However, if a woman waits until she is at least three to six months postmenopausal and if her fibroids are no more than ten- to twelve-week size, I feel that she can take estrogen. Fibroids rarely grow on the small dose of estrogen used in HRT, but should be monitored by ultrasound at appropriate intervals until the uterus has shrunk to near normal size (see chapter 13).

4. *History of stroke or heart attack.* Women who have had a stroke or heart attack may have the most to gain by beginning HRT as *second episodes can be decreased by nearly 80 percent.* However, recent heart attacks or strokes must be fully evaluated before a woman begins hormonal therapy.

Let Us Try to Reiterate:

The postmenopausal time is a new evolutionary gift. In the 1940s when Robert Wilson wrote *Feminine Forever,* the first book on estrogen therapy, he talked about regaining your youth—your skin tone, your vaginal moisture—and getting rid of bothersome hot flashes. He only knew that women who suffered felt better after beginning to take estrogen. He had no idea, nor did anyone else at the time, that estrogen would one day be shown to protect bone and the cardiovascular system as well as the brain.

We know that more and more women make it to their hundredth

birthday. We hear their names on the *Today Show* on NBC every day. But for each of us who make it in relatively good shape, many more are frail and dependent.

What we are experiencing is medicine's first attempts to overcome what was thought to be inevitable. Now we are on a new mission, to try to prevent the early onset of chronic diseases. These attempts will become more sophisticated over the next one to two decades, so that when we look back, our experience with estrogen will all seem so primitive, similar to the time when the only antibiotics were penicillin and sulfa. Nevertheless, these two antibiotics saved many lives and limbs that would otherwise have been lost.

I believe that estrogen is good for us. Something that makes you feel so good again can't be wrong. I have treated too many women for too long who look good, feel good, and are good. One day we will not only try to extend our life's span, but will also try to make our lives robust well into our eighties. Using cocktails of complementary hormonal and nonhormonal substances will become the norm. Using smaller doses of each will decrease side effects. We must not close our eyes and minds. We must always search for better solutions to help us live better.

Now that you know about the available prescription therapies, let's go on to talk about alternatives, designer estrogens, and complementary choices. Please read the next chapter, whether or not you take hormone replacement. It will complete your education and give you some commonsense advice for those times when you still have symptoms even though you take hormones.

Financial help:

One last note: Many older women have overwhelming financial problems. More times than we would like to acknowledge, such women cannot even afford vital medication. There is help—and you should be aware that it exists. Free medication is available for those in financial distress.

PhRMA, or the Pharmaceutical Research and Manufacturers of America, publishes a directory *for physicians*. It contains names of member companies who provide prescription medicines free of charge to physicians whose patients might not otherwise have access to necessary medicines. Each company determines the eligibility for its program of free drugs. Eligibility criteria and application processes vary. If you are having financial difficulties that leave little or no money for medication, contact your physician and have him or her call 1-800-762-4636 for a directory. Then your doctor will be able to look up specific pharmaceutical company addresses and telephone numbers to get eligibility applications. I hope that this information is helpful to you or a loved one.

Notes

1. D.T. Felson and M.C. Nevitt, "Effects of Estrogen on Osteoarthritis," *Menopausal Medicine* 4, no. 4 (winter 1996).

2. *CA, A Cancer Journal for Physicians* (January 1996).

3. Kim Bennicke, M.D., "Study of 4,240 Danish Women," *British Medical Journal* 310 (1995): 1431–33.

References

Berger, Sarah, ed. "Brain, Behavior and Reproductive Function." *Seminars in Reproductive Endocrinology* 15, no. 1 (February 1997) (New York: Thieme Medical and Scientific Journals).

"Infertility and Reproductive Medicine." Clinics of North America, ed. Esther Eisenberg, *Menopause* 6, no. 4 (October 1995).

Lobo, Roger A., ed. *Treatment of the Postmenopausal Woman: Basic and Clinical Aspects.* New York: Raven Press, 1994.

Chapter 3

ALTERNATIVES, DESIGNER ESTROGENS, AND COMPLEMENTARY THERAPIES—THERE'S EVEN MORE GOOD NEWS

Women are tremendously interested in over-the-counter products. They read about them in magazines and are presented with hundreds of items in health food and grocery stores. Women can buy them on their own, without a prescription and without ever consulting their doctors. They hope that these substances will somehow keep them forever healthy. Manufacturers specifically target the large market of female customers with promises of "natural" ingredients—natural somehow interpreted by consumers as safe and without side effects. Women use these products when estrogen is contraindicated, they try them first before ever using estrogen, or use them when estrogen is too frightening. They also use them at the same time they are taking estrogen. Doctors at least should begin to understand what their patients are doing because so many women are turning to herbs and other alternatives.

Before we go on, it is critical that you be aware that currently, no single alternative, i.e, prescription or over-the-counter, drug or herb can replace estrogen. It alone has the ability to improve the myriad symptoms and problems that may accompany menopause. Estrogen protects you in so many areas—from your brain, heart, and bones to your bladder and vaginal tissue. However, looking back at the original list of menopausal symptoms on page 43 the key may be that not all of these problems are yours. You may be able to make changes in lifestyle and diet, or take other medications or products that will meet your needs. Will alternative therapy be as good as estrogen? Perhaps the question that many women should ask is, "Will it be good enough?" Not everyone has a compelling reason to take hormone replacement therapy. For many women, fear of breast cancer, warranted or not, will never let them begin.

Let us go through symptoms and problems one by one and talk about alternatives and just plain common sense. The good news is that more and more alternatives, including designer estrogens, are or soon will be available. Furthermore, they are going to offer new benefits and give women real choice.

Dealing with Hot Flashes

Hot flashes are the problem that brings most women to their doctors or to the local pharmacy or health food store. Remember, hot flashes are caused by abnormal functioning of the heat-regulating area in the brain, which is triggered by the withdrawal of estrogen and other substances. The following list contains suggestions that all women may find helpful.

LIFESTYLE CHANGES THAT HELP

1. Avoid alcohol. Many women know that alcohol, which dilates blood vessels, can precipitate major hot flashes. Drink nonalcoholic substitutes, or water down your wine and drink it as a spritzer. You'll save lots of calories this way too.

2. Avoid hot drinks. This includes coffee, tea, etc. Hot drinks make you hot and tend to bring on hot flashes. Caffeine is probably another culprit here.

3. Avoid hot weather. This is not always so easy, but women have more hot flashes in warm weather.

4. Cool your body in a cool room for two hours prior to sleep. This has been shown by Robert Freedman, Ph.D., of Wayne State University School of Medicine, to decrease night sweats. Engage in quiet activities, reading, TV watching, sitting at your computer, etc., in a cool place, wearing minimal amounts of clothing to enhance your body's cooling. In the winter lower the heat prior to bedtime and keep it down during the night. In the summer, run your air conditioner to cool the room.

5. Dr. Freedman also suggests that when you do feel a hot flash coming on, try to immediately relax and begin *slow,* steady, deep *abdominal* breathing. Concentrating on your abdominal breathing—counting to five

as you inhale and five as you exhale—will help blunt the flash and speed its end. Purse your lips as you blow out. You should take only six to eight breaths per minute. Practice abdominal breathing while lying down. Inhale slowly, letting your belly rise while your chest remains motionless. Exhale by contracting and pushing in slowly with your abdominal muscles.

6. Dress in layers. This way, you can take off and put on clothes as quickly as you need.

7. Avoid spicy foods. They may cause a reaction similar to alcohol.

8. Buy an extra air conditioner if you do not have central air-conditioning. Place it where you spend most of your time or in the bedroom.

9. Exercise moderately. Walk when and where it's cool. I personally like treadmills. If you own one, you never have an excuse for not exercising. Also, there are no neighbors' dogs to contend with, no potholes to twist an unsuspecting ankle, and no proper dress required except for good sneakers. I walk outside for social reasons, to talk with friends and to enjoy the breeze. On the other hand, if you will only do your daily walk with your neighbor, do it. Do whatever ensures that you will do it!

10. Stop smoking. Smokers tend to have the most intense hot flashes. Smoking also increases your risk of breast cancer, causes facial wrinkles, brings on menopause two or more years earlier than it normally would occur, and further lowers any remaining estrogen levels. It also contributes to bladder and cervical cancer, plus causes our number one cancer killer for all Americans, lung cancer!

11. Lose weight. Postmenopausal obesity is associated with an increase in breast cancer and the feeling of always being warm. On the other hand, many overweight women have fewer and less intense flashes due to increased estrone production in their excess fat.

12. Try not to engage in intense mental "exercises" for two hours prior to sleep. No calculations, preparations of tax returns, etc. Besides helping your flashes, it will help you get to sleep.

Herbs and Such

When it comes to herbal treatments for menopause, nearly everything is hearsay. Friends will tell you this, salespeople that, and advertisements tout all. Remember, there is little data, little to no scientific research, but lots of anecdotal stories. "But how can I go wrong?" you say. "Everything 'natural' is safe!" Wrong! Scientists are not even positive how much to take of some herbs. Will you believe the high school–educated health food store employee? Herbs usually do not even have warnings on the label. We need to proceed with caution before we take them and certainly should think twice about ever giving them to our children. Remember that herbs are not regulated by strict FDA control as are drugs, but are sold as food supplements. Therefore, there is no law that requires efficacy to be proven and safety documentation is not standardized.

In some respects, I see what is happening today as a return to the thirties when the only therapies we had were plants and herbs. Patients with heart failure were given foxglove because there was evidence that it helped. But it killed almost as many as it cured, because the plant contains multiple substances. In addition, the amount of active ingredient, digitalis, varied from plant to plant, from field to field, and depended on when it was picked and how long it remained on the shelves. Worse, the therapeutic dose and the lethal dose were quite close. In other words, to get the desired effect, you had to take a dose that was almost at a toxic level. You had to be very careful and very lucky to get a dose that was correct. When the digitalis molecule was finally replicated, patients with heart failure were able to get exact doses that we could adjust up or down, until the patient was better. We no longer had to guess, and patients were safer.

Doses of herbal substances vary from brand to brand, by whether an extract or a powder is used, and whether the original plant products were of good quality. Where plants are grown, what they are combined with, and the manufacturing processes used all impact on the final product.

Ground-up Cow Brain Swept off the Slaughterhouse Floor

Women now go out and buy menopausal remedies with ground-up mammary gland, ovary, and brain from cows. These substances are heavily advertised and make millions for the companies that manufacture and sell them. Is that really what you want to take? Nothing scares me more. We have all heard about Mad Cow disease (bovine spongiform encephalopathy). It is impossible to know whether the cow glands in a particular product came from Europe, England, or the United States. Prions (living particles) that cause the illness can survive filtration and heat processing and can theoretically be passed on in brain, and possibly in other powdered animal parts. Animal feed is now controlled in many areas to make sure it does not contain these substances. In fact, the United States government and the FDA have proposed a ban on using tissue from animals that chew their cud in animal feed. This complete list now includes cows, sheep, goats, deer, and elk, and more recently hogs and mink have been added to the list. In England, this has already been done. There is a possibility that a link exists between Mad Cow disease and Creutzfeldt-Jakob disease, a degenerative brain disease of adults, which is always fatal. I advise that you *not* buy any products containing powdered animal glands. Better to stick to manufactured exact copies of the hormonal substances they contain or forgo all of it.

Melatonin from the pineal gland in the brain likewise poses a risk, but why take any risk at all? I never recommended melatonin until there was a good synthetic. I felt that there were potential problems, and I had to be responsible for my recommendations. I am not alone: Experts in the field and veterinarians admit that the possibility of disease transmission to humans theoretically exists.

ADVERSE REACTIONS

Minor side effects such as rash, nausea, and diarrhea are fairly common with various herbal preparations. Licorice can cause diarrhea and, rarely, hypertension. Excess amounts of ginseng can cause hypertension, insomnia, and nervousness. Common chamomile tea can even cause rare cases of severe allergic reactions. Echinacea, often used for boosting the immune system to shorten colds, is a stimulant and has occasionally been known to cause rash and allergic reactions. Aloe taken internally can cause diarrhea, nausea, and vomiting. Black cohosh can also cause nausea and vomiting, uterine contractions, and slow heart rate if taken in large doses. One of my patients wound up in intensive care with a cardiac arrhythmia after using it for two weeks. Kava Kava, used for its sedative effects, can cause hallucinations, dermatitis, and shortness of breath. Valerian, often used as a sedative, has been known to cause liver damage and odd neurological movements. Comfrey and sassafras both contain carcinogenic compounds according to Dr. Catherine Crone, a psychiatrist in Fairfax, Virginia. Comfrey, used for stomach ulcers and as a blood purifier, can also cause liver damage in patients who combine it with phenobarbital and phenytoin (antiseizure medications). She also has noted that "excessive sedation can result when prescribed sedatives or sleeping pills are combined with valerian, hops or passion flower."

Herbal medicines may interfere with prescribed drugs and cause unwanted drug interactions. Many women use many different products and combine them with prescribed medications and never tell their doctors. One of my patients developed abnormal liver function on her blood tests. I was aware that she took over-the-counter products, but upon questioning her in depth I was amazed that this tiny woman was taking literally basketfuls of pills that she had never before admitted to me. I simply stopped all of her pills and her blood tests became normal. Then she began slowly to add back each one by one so we could see which one was causing her liver problems. We may be checking her liver function tests for the next year unless I can convince her to save her money and my time. Another patient, a dentist, developed fever and abnormal liver functions after taking powdered liver and adrenal. When she tried the capsules again at a later date, her blood tests became abnormal again.

Another patient came into my office and stated that she had stopped her Synthroid®, a thyroid medication. When I questioned why she had made that decision, she read from the flyer from her local health food store: "Thyroid medication causes bone loss and osteoporosis." The flyer recommended sea kelp instead. I sat back on my stool and explained that patients who have an overactive thyroid or who take excess amounts of thyroid hormone can lose bone. This is exactly why doctors carefully monitor patients on thyroid replacement with blood tests for T4 and TSH. These tests, done at least annually, verify that patients are on the correct dose and that their medication will not cause bone loss. The patient, who was already feeling fatigued, was relieved and glad to restart her needed medication.

HERBS FOR MENOPAUSAL RELIEF

Ginseng is used in capsules or as a tea. Ginseng has true estrogenic properties and attaches to our estrogen receptors. It is best used for women who are not on estrogen and have no contraindications.

Licorice root can be tried, black cohash actually has a fair amount of data on menopausal relief from German trials, fenugreek is sometimes mentioned. Recently a well-thought-out placebo-controlled trial by Dr. Bruce Ettinger showed that Dong Quai used alone was no better than placebo. Whether it would have activity when combined with other Chinese herbs, as is typical in Chinese medicine, is still unproven.

Follow the directions and never overdose! Because there are few good scientific studies of herbal menopause treatments, you are on your own. The bottom line is that we really don't know for sure whether women are wasting their money and possibly jeopardizing their health. Does the woman with breast cancer increase her risks by taking estrogenic herbs? On the other hand in soy may give some of the benefits of estrogen replacement therapy without the risks. The National Institutes of Health is already funding alternative medicine research, albeit on a small scale. One team of researchers has come together to study the effects of an ancient Chinese herbal formula on hot flashes. The research team consists of Fredi Kronenberg, Ph.D., of Columbia University in New York City, Cristina Matera, M.D., Mr. Jing-Nuan Wu of the Taoist Health Institute, and James Simon, M.D., from the Women's Health Research Center, Laurel, Maryland. These investigators will study a group of herbs that have been used in Chinese medicine for menopausal complaints. This study will be scientifically conducted with placebo pills that look and taste like the herbs they mimic. Study subjects will keep a regular diary of hot flashes and will have blood chemistries, blood pressure, temperature, and body weight monitored. In addition, their heart rate, skin temperature, sweating, and hot flashes will be documented. With studies such as this, we will get to know more about the role of herbs and whether they are helpful or not.[1]

Getting Rid of Flashes with Progesterone-like Substances

Prescription progesterone-like medications: Not really alternative medicine, progesterone-type prescription medications can be used as an alternative to estrogen for some women with contraindications to estrogen. They work by lowering FSH and LH levels. We know that Depo-Provera®, Provera®, and Megace® are all effective for decreasing hot flashes. For specific women, these medications can be a boon. But given in larger doses than usual, and without estrogen, as they are normally used in HRT, they tend to have adverse effects on the cardiovascular system, lipid profiles, and mood, and tend to increase weight and vaginal dryness. Depo-Provera® may cause significant depression in 10 percent of women. However, Depo-Provera® may be as effective at getting rid of hot flashes as estrogen. Medroxyprogesterone acetate (Provera®) and Megace® have been shown to decrease symptoms in 75 to 85 percent of women when compared to placebo.

Over-the-counter "natural" progesterone-like substances: "Natural progesterone creams" are often advertised. Women often erroneously believe that "natural progesterone" is structurally identical to the progesterone that is produced by our bodies. Micronized progesterone (USP grade) *is* identical to your body's own progesterone and is laboratory made. Natural progesterone creams from Mexican wild yam root are advertised as a rich source of diosgenin, a precursor to progesterone. In truth, *diosgenin produces little to no progestational activity because it cannot be converted to progesterone by the human body.* This conversion, whereby diosgenin is broken down to obtain progesterone, is only able to be done synthetically in a laboratory. Mexican wild yam root cream is therefore usually sold mixed together with laboratory-made micronized progesterone, or the diosgenin is converted to progesterone in a laboratory before adding it to the cream. Thus, when products claim that plain wild yam extract can be absorbed through the skin, it does not mean that it will result in a significantly increased level of progesterone in your body.

While these over-the-counter "progesterone-containing" creams are probably not harmful, they *should not be expected to cure osteoporosis or to balance prescribed estrogen replacement therapy. Therefore, these products should not be taken in place of your prescribed progesterone.* Even micronized progesterone creams that are standardized and available in Europe cannot provide high enough doses of progesterone to prevent endometrial hyperplasia because absorption through the skin is too slow. However, more potent progesterone-type compounds such as norethindrone acetate can achieve the needed levels and are used in transdermal patches, e.g., CombiPatch®. (On the other hand, because the vaginal route improves absorption, vaginal micronized progesterone, e.g., crinone, is able to achieve proper dose.)

Some women use progesterone creams in the hope that they will decrease hot flashes. It is important that you know that *progesterone is not a precursor of estrogen in humans,* even though it is in rats. In humans, the chemical pathways are different: We are missing an enzyme sequence that is present in rodents. So if the label on the progesterone cream states that it will produce significant amounts of estrogen in your body, that is an error. One more fact: In almost all studies on hot flashes, hot flashes are reduced by placebo nearly 30 percent. That means that without carefully controlled studies where a large matched group of women are studied, real data are hard to pinpoint.

Androgens: Androgens have been used alone and may be effective in decreasing hot flashes, but many androgens, especially in larger doses, convert to estrogens once in the body. Again, used alone, without estrogen, they tend to cause weight gain, hair loss, acne, and facial hair. Androgens combined with estrogens—such as in Estratest® H.S. or Estratest®, an oral Solvay product—may aid those women who continue to flash even on estrogen therapy. It appears that one of the main mechanisms by which oral androgens exert this effect is by freeing up the body's own estrogen. For some women, changing to this product may also improve their general sense of well-being, energy level, as well as their libido. A low-dose estrogen/androgen combination patch is in development. Subcutaneous androgen implants and injections, usually combined with estrogen, have been in use for years by physicians around the world.

SERMs (Selective Estrogen-Receptor Modulators)— Designer Estrogens

This is the "hot news" for menopausal women. Most women tend to limit their use of estrogen because of annoying bleeding problems or because they fear that it will increase their risk of breast cancer. Actually, only a small percent of women continue their hormone replacement beyond one year. Therefore, there have been tremendous efforts to research estrogen-like compounds that will help our symptoms, bones, and heart, but not hurt our breasts or uterine tissue. Estrogens that are currently used in hormone replacement are non-selective. That means they effect our estrogen receptors exactly like our own body's estrogen always did.

SERMs are a new class of compound. They were created in a laboratory, originally designed as antiestrogens to be used in the treatment of breast cancer. By attaching to breast cell estrogen receptors, these compounds can block the body's own estrogen and starve breast cancer tissue of natural estrogen. Unexpectedly, tamoxifen, one of the early SERMs was found to have a weak estrogen-like activity on the skeleton and cholesterol. This was confusing initially because this meant that tamoxifen acts like an estrogen in some tissues, and like an antiestrogen in others. And so the term SERM, or selective estrogen-receptor modulator, came into being. Interestingly, SERMs are *nonsteroidal* compounds and look different from our own estrogen which is a *steroid* (see diagram), but they have properties that may one day approach those of an ideal postmenopausal hormone.

TAMOXIFEN (NOLVADEX®)

Tamoxifen's estrogen blocking effects reduce the recurrence of breast cancer in pre- and postmenopausal women with hormonally dependent breast cancer by 50 percent. (See page 305.) Furthermore, the Breast Cancer Prevention Trial (BCPT) showed that tamoxifen can decrease the risk of developing breast cancer in women who do not yet have breast cancer but are at high risk. This was the first study to ever demonstrate that spontaneously occuring breast cancer can be prevented! Over 13,000 women participated in the trial for more than six years. Those taking tamoxifen had a 45 percent lower incidence of invasive breast cancers and a 47 percent lower rate of noninvasive breast cancers compared to those

Human estrogen

Synthetic estrogen used in most birth control pills

Horse estrogen

First generation SERM
tamoxifen

Second generation SERM
raloxifene

taking placebo. On the downside, tamoxifen caused an increased risk of uterine cancer in participants over the age of fifty. There were thirty-three cases of uterine cancer in the treated group versus fourteen cases on placebo, as well as an increased incidence of pulmonary embolism and deep vein thrombosis in those women on tamoxifen. Because of the increased risk of uterine cancer, women who take tamoxifen and have an intact uterus are followed at regular intervals with ultrasound of the endometrium and/or biopsy by some gynecologists.

Nonetheless, tamoxifen remains an important drug. Tamoxifen's estrogen-like effects improve bone and lipid profiles. These are important pluses for women with breast cancer who are not candidates for hormone therapy and may be helpful for women at high risk of developing breast cancer. In the meantime, the search continues for compounds that will only have beneficial effects.

RALOXIFENE (EVISTA®)

Raloxifene was also developed as an antiestrogen for the treatment of breast cancer. Unlike tamoxifen, this new SERM was found to block the effect of estrogen in the breast *and* in the uterus. Therefore, progesterone-like medications are unnecessary, bleeding is avoided, and there is apparently little or no increased risk of developing uterine cancer. This is a welcome advantage. Studies on over 12,000 women around the world have shown that raloxifene's estrogen-like activity helps protect against bone loss in a manner similar to low dose estrogen. The drug has been approved by the FDA for prevention of osteoporosis. In a two-year study published in the December 4, 1997, *New England Journal of Medicine,* raloxifene plus calcium was shown to prevent bone loss (approximately half as effectively as estrogen) while women on no therapy (placebo), continued to lose bone. The good news is that there are now three choices for preventing bone loss, hormone replacement, raloxifene (Evista®) and alendronate (Fosamax®).

There are also very encouraging and exciting reports that raloxifene decreases the risk of developing breast cancer. Dr. Steve Cummings from the University of California, San Francisco, and other medical centers studied 7,704 postmenopausal women to determine the effect of raloxifene on bone. In addition to preventing bone loss at the end of two years, the women on raloxifene had a 50% decrease in breast cancer and a significant decrease in uterine cancer compared to the placebo group.

Additionally, a review of raloxifene studies by Dr. J. E. Glusman, (12,000 women) showed a 58 percent reduction in the risk of developing breast cancer. The drug was also found to markedly decrease the incidence of uterine (endometrial) cancer.

Raloxifene has also been shown in many studies to improve the cholesterol profile. In a study by B. W. Walsh et al., in the May 13, 1998, *JAMA,* raloxifene was compared to estrogen *plus* progesterone. Although both regimens improved (lowered) cholesterol and LDL cholesterol, improvement in HDL cholesterol only occurred in women on estrogen. Drs. Rifkind and Rossouw, who commented on the study in the same issue of *JAMA,* felt that while both regimens produced similar effects on LDL cholesterol, raloxifene's "effects on other blood lipids were less likely to be cardioprotective." They cautioned that raloxifene's lesser effects on blood lipids might not be sufficient to create a future decrease in cardiovascular disease. They likened raloxifene's effect on lipids to that of tamoxifen where only one in three studies have shown a decrease in cardiovascular problems.

Most of this is very good news. However, to date, no medication is a panacea or without any side effects. Because raloxifene does not alleviate hot flashes, there is a question whether or not raloxifene will benefit the brain as estrogen appears to do, improving mental function and decreasing the risk for Alzheimer's disease. To date, we know nothing about its ability to alter mood. It also has no documented beneficial effect of vaginal tissues. Raloxifene may increase the incidence of venous blood clots slightly more than estrogen therapy. Side effects also include a small increase in leg cramps. Raloxifene is contraindicated in pregnancy or in women with active or a history of deep vein thrombosis, pulmonary embolism and retinal vein thrombosis. Safety has not been established in women with severe liver disease. Other information shows that cancer studies in mice given large doses of raloxifene showed an increase in both benign and malignant ovarian tumors. Whether this would ever have any human significance is unknown, and to date ovarian growths have not been reported in raloxifene users.

Finally, it is wise to remember that raloxifene is a new drug and only short term studies (several weeks to a few years) have been completed. In contrast, estrogen (Premarin®) has a fifty-six-year history. Therefore, it will take many more years before we know all of the facts about this promising SERM. Before it becomes a viable alternative to hormone replacement, longer trials will have to be done that establish its actual benefit/risk ratio. Furthermore, although raloxifene improves bone density, the proof that raloxifen will actually prevent future fractures is still pending further study.

Since most hip fractures occur twenty-five or more years after menopause, any preventive therapy including raloxifene must be safe and have minimum side effects over a very long period of time. One day we will hopefully have compounds that will be able to *increase* bone formation and quickly add bone mass in women who already have osteoporosis. Then, long term preventive medication will be unnecessary. Unfortunately, these agents will probably not be available for years to come.

In the future, women suffering with hot flashes and night sweats, may use estrogen as a transition therapy—for several months or a few years—until symptoms have passed. Then, raloxifene or another designer estrogen might be prescribed long term to protect the bones and the cardiovascular system. Postmenopausal therapy will change as new compounds come along and more and more novel therapeutic choices evolve. And with that evolution, there should be better compliance as fears about breast and uterine cancer diminish. Because protecting the postmenopausal woman is so important, it is necessary to continue the research for new and better alternatives.

TIBOLONE

Tibolone is currently being studied in the U.S. It is not a SERM, but rather a medication with weak estrogenic, progestational and androgenic effects. It has been used in Europe for several years as a substitute for hormone replacement. Problems such as bleeding, progesterone-type symptoms, and a decrease in HDL cholesterol levels make this only a second choice drug. On the other hand, it does not seem to affect endometrial growth and therefore may become another alternative for some women.

OLDER NONHORMONAL PRESCRIPTION DRUGS

Nonhormonal prescription medications go back decades to Bellergal®. It is used to stabilize the vascular system, but there is only a little controlled data that say it works. It does, however, contain phenobarbital, a well-known sedative, which may account for its long run in the marketplace. Contraindications are more often due to the other components, belladonna-like substances and ergotamine tartrate, which affect the autonomic nervous system. Women with peripheral vascular disease, hypertension, coronary artery disease, liver or kidney problems, or glaucoma should not use this drug, nor should patients taking dopamine for Parkinson's disease.

Clonidine (the trade name is Catapres®), given orally or by patch, has also been used and is generally thought to be modestly effective. It is an antihypertensive drug. For patients with normal blood pressure, there seems to be little effect on blood pressure. Side effects include dry mouth, sedation, and, less frequently, constipation, dizziness, headache, and fatigue. The drug can also enhance the sedative effects of alcohol and sedative medications.

There are European drugs that are not yet available; perhaps eventually they will make this list more inviting.

DEALING WITH VAGINAL DRYNESS RELATED TO MENOPAUSE

It has been documented that "use it or lose it" really has a basis in fact. Women who continue to have intercourse (more than three times per month) have a thicker vaginal lining, compared with women who abstain. This could be the result of mechanical friction that serves to increase blood flow to the area. Now we have added "more sex" to the list of alternatives to estrogen!

PREVENTION OF HEART DISEASE

You've heard much of this before and much is just plain common sense. Indeed, whether you take estrogen or not, all of these suggestions should be followed, for doing them all is good for you.

Stop Smoking!

One-half of all heart attacks can be attributed to cigarette smoking. Even one to four cigarettes per day doubles the risk of a heart attack. More than a pack quadruples the risk. There is no safe number of cigarettes that you can smoke. Furthermore, levels of fibrinogen, the stuff that invites blood clotting, are increased by smoking. It is important to remember that there is a thirtyfold increase in the risk of heart attack in women over thirty-five who take birth control pills *and* smoke. These two substances synergize each other and multiply risk. However, the cigarettes are the real culprits, for birth control pills used alone in nonsmoking women, even up to the age of menopause, cause little or no increased risk of heart attack. As for cigarettes and men, not only does smoking ruin the arteries to their heart, but it also makes them impotent (unable to have an erection). By prematurely clogging the arteries that bring blood to the penis, men lose the ability to enjoy a normal sex life at an earlier age than normal. Tell that to the next male smoker you see. Smoking likewise destroys a woman's ovarian hormonal production, bringing on menopause two or more years earlier than normal for her. Smoking is a risk factor for osteoporosis and has a direct toxic effect on bone cells.

Walk!

Walking will help reduce your risk of cardiovascular disease by more than 50 percent. That is, of course, only if you do it and do it on a regular basis, four to five times a week. It will also help raise your endorphin levels that raise your spirits. Put on your walking shoes, grab your spouse, a friend, your overweight and underexercised dog, or just go by yourself and commune with nature. Or if you prefer, use a treadmill. The important thing is do it and start today!

Eat a Low-Fat Diet!

A 1 percent decrease in cholesterol will decrease the risk of heart attack by 2 to 3 percent. It's worth doing. Simply make better food choices. This information is everywhere. We're just lazy for the most part; we tend not to cook and instead grab the nearest fatty sweet thing when we're hungry. I know, I do it too, but I never grab more than one! Okay—two.

Lose Weight

Just being overweight increases your risk of heart attack. I'm going to give you two hints. First, resign your membership in the clean plate club. And if your mother's advice is too well ingrained in you, then put your dinner on a salad plate and clean that off. Too many of my patients never take time for breakfast and lunch, then are starved and eat all night. Second, try my diet (see page 23), which I use for patients with premenstrual syndrome, and to help patients lose weight. By eating every three hours, you'll be much less likely to have food binges, for you'll never be that hungry. Also, researchers at Tufts found that older adults burn fat from smaller meals as easily as younger adults. However, as meals become larger, this ability diminishes. This could make fifty- and sixty-year-olds much more likely to gain weight unless they eat smaller meals three to four times a day.

And if you're angry at your husband because he nags and says you're too fat, don't continue to eat and eat because you're depressed. Remember, the best revenge is to live and look great. So stick it to him and get even by losing the weight. Then you'll decide whether or not you want to continue to stick with him.

Control Your Blood Pressure

This will be necessary with or without hormone replacement. A normal blood pressure helps protect you against stroke, heart attack, and other cardiac problems. Being overweight increases your risk of high blood pressure. When I start overweight patients on antihypertensive drugs, I tell them if they could just lose some weight, they probably would not need medication.

Take Antioxidant Vitamins

They may play an important role in prevention of heart disease. Hard scientific evidence is beginning to accumulate.

Vitamin E is the most important and has been said to decrease the risk of heart attack by 40 percent. By preventing the oxidation of LDL, vitamin E (like estrogen, which is also a powerful antioxidant) reduces the ability of LDL cholesterol to damage blood vessel walls. Vitamin C helps vitamin E work. Folate, or folic acid, one of the B-complex vitamins, is also a very important substance in decreasing the risk of heart attack. I think *all women should take vitamins and antioxidants.* I do not consider this alternative medicine, but just plain common sense. (See chapter 7 on vitamins and minerals for women.)

Take Cholesterol-Lowering Drugs

These medications can have a major effect on your heart's health by lowering your total and LDL cholesterol. They have been shown to decrease the risk of a first or second heart attack. Talk to your doctor if your cholesterol or LDL is too high and dieting and weight loss have not lowered your blood fats to safe levels.

Take Aspirin

Low-dose aspirin (one baby aspirin or one 80 mg aspirin) is thought to decrease the incidence of heart attack by 25 percent for both men and women. Please confer with your own physician before beginning low-dose therapy, as aspirin can cause bleeding and other problems.

Remember, half of the strokes in the U.S. occur in women and the risk of stroke increases after menopause and with each successive decade. The haunting statistics are that one out of five to one out of six women in this country will have some cerebral vascular disease in her lifetime. Aspirin therapy will decrease the risk of stroke by 20 percent.

Drink a Controlled Amount of Alcohol

One ounce of alcohol, one glass of wine (preferably red), or one twelve-ounce beer a day can decrease the risk of cardiovascular disease by raising HDL levels and lowering LDL levels. Red wine can also decrease platelet stickiness and has some antioxidant activity. However, alcoholic drinks have calories. And to their detriment, they increase the risk of breast cancer and liver disease, and increase blood pressure when consumed at the rate of more than two drinks daily. All this makes for tough decisions.

Drink Purple Grape Juice

Another alternative that even teetotalers can enjoy is plain purple grape juice. Like red wine, it can decrease platelet stickiness, thereby slowing the formation of artery-clogging clots. John Folts of the University of Wisconsin Medical School studied seventeen healthy volunteers who drank three glasses of grape juice daily. He found their platelet stickiness decreased by 65 percent. (Aspirin cuts platelet activity by 45 percent.) A second experiment had study subjects drink ten ounces of grape juice daily for a week. Two days after they discontinued the juice, their platelets remained less sticky. White grape juice, orange juice, and grapefruit juice and pure alcohol do *not* have antiplatelet activity.

New Hormonal Medications

The following hormones, some of which are available over the counter, may have rejuvenating effects. Along with estrogen, more youthful levels of these substances may be part of the reason why some seventy-year-olds look fifty. All of these hormones decrease as we age. Does this decline contribute to frailty? Can we bypass disability and illness by supplementing with these substances and make our extended lives more vital? We have fifty years of experience with estrogen and still do not understand everything about it, while research on these newer hormones has just begun. Remember that before you go off to the store.

Melatonin: Melatonin decreases as we age, with a steep decline at puberty and then a slower decline. Melatonin sets the clock for many of the body's activities: eating, sleeping, and for secretion of other hormones. Although used primarily to induce sleep, melatonin has been touted as an antiaging product. Healthy older people tend to have circadian rhythms more like those of younger people, and their melatonin levels tend to be closer to those of younger people as well. On the other hand, there is no evidence that giving melatonin will give better health to older people—at least for now.

This hormone is produced in the pineal gland of the brain. Light, acting on the brain, sets the secretion rate of melatonin, which in turn regulates our body's clock and temperature rhythm. Melatonin is synthesized from tryptophan in the body. Therefore, high tryptophan (milk products) in your diet may influence the amount of melatonin actually made. That may be why a glass of warm milk at bedtime with a cookie or cracker helps you sleep. Melatonin secretion can also be influenced by how "nervous" we are or by other medications that we take.

Decrease in melatonin secretion with age has been associated with sleep disturbances in the elderly. One study found significantly lower melatonin levels in elderly insomniacs than in the elderly without sleep problems. Two milligrams of melatonin shortened the time it took to fall asleep and decreased nocturnal awakening without causing an increase in the amount of time actually asleep.[2] In other words, it increased the efficiency of sleep without affecting REM (rapid eye movement) sleep, as happens with other sleeping pills.

Melatonin may become a promising alternative to the commonly used sleep preparations because these tend to cause rebound insomnia when discontinued or sometimes have to be used in increasing doses that cause increasing side effects. Melatonin, however, has been reported to cause headache, upset stomach, and depression. In the future, we may better know and understand how to use melatonin to our advantage.

DHEA (Dehydroepiandrosterone) and DHEAS (Dehydroepiandrosterone sulfate)

Diabetes, loss of immunity (known as immune senescence), and cancer all seem to occur as we age. In addition, aging is associated with a reduction in protein synthesis with the result that there is less bone, less muscle, and more fat in our bodies. These phenomena are paralleled by declines in DHEA and growth hormone.

DHEAS is simply the sulfated prohormone (earlier form of the DHEA molecule) that has a sulfate attached. DHEAS has been proven to progressively decline after it peaks at age twenty-five to thirty. At seventy, levels are only 10 to 20 percent of what they were. We cannot know for certain whether this is a deficiency or just secondary to aging. Does the loss of DHEA help to accelerate other aging processes? In rats, mice, and dogs, DHEA decreases obesity and diabetes, promotes learning, improves the immune system, and prevents cancer. But rodents make very little DHEA during their lives, so is its effect physiology, pharmacology, or something else?

In mice, DHEA decreases the risk of cancer. To date there is no data on DHEA and cancer risk in humans, although decreased DHEA levels have been found to be associated with breast and lung cancer. However, this finding may be due to stress of the disease, rather than a causal factor, because our adrenal glands *react to stress by increasing cortisol and decreasing DHEAS secretion.*

Dr. Samuel S. C. Yen, a renowned researcher at the University of California in San Diego, has researched DHEA for years. In one small study of older patients given DHEA or placebo for a year, there was increased feeling of well-being, better ability to sleep, and more energy. In addition, men experienced a 5 percent decrease in fat and an increase in muscle and bone. Although this did not occur in women, a mild antidiabetic effect was seen in postmenopausal women. Although the immune system usually declines as we age, he showed that postmenopausal women and elderly men given DHEA had an increase in the number of a type of white blood cells called natural killer cells. This would be expected to protect the body from infection and cancer. Other researchers have had similar findings; for example, a single dose of DHEA prior to receiving a booster dose of tetanus toxoid injection or flu vaccine was shown to enhance antibody formation in older patients. Also, a dose of DHEA prior to bedtime enhances REM sleep, which is thought to be important for memory. Though certainly interesting, all of these studies are preliminary and need to be confirmed by larger clinical trials.

With the use of small 25 mg doses, it may be possible to reproduce the DHEA levels found in premenopausal women. One of the basic rules that all people forget is that when we take a drug such as DHEA, we want to attain the normal blood and tissue *levels that we had when we were younger.* These are known as physiological levels. *More is NOT better!* High doses can overwhelm the system or cause it to shunt metabolism in other than the normal direction. For example, using high doses of DHEA in women can produce unwanted and unhealthy androgenic (male-like) effects, such as adverse effects on lipids or abnormal liver function. That is why it is important, when taking DHEA, to follow directions and not to think that more is better. For women the recommended dose of DHEA is 25 mg; men normally take 50 mg. (Again, you should confer with your physician if you are taking over-the-counter medication.)

DHEA may turn out to be a possible adjunct used in a complementary fashion to HRT or other therapies. Physiological levels of estrogen actually impair secretion of androgen in cell culture. *DHEAS levels are reduced, as are androstenedione levels and free testosterone levels, in women on oral hormone replacement.* According to Elizabeth Barrett-Conner's Rancho Bernado Cohort study, there is a 50 percent decrease of these substances in estrogen users versus women on placebo. Dr. Peter Casson's studies from the Baylor College of Medicine and other studies also showed similar trends.

DHEA, when given orally, is a prohormone. It is actually a precursor for estrogen, testosterone, and many other hormones. Much of its conversion to these hormones goes on in the tissue where it has its effect. Therefore, if you make a decision to take DHEA and you are already on estrogen, it may be necessary to consider decreasing your estrogen dose. And because the conversion goes on within the cells themselves, serum levels may not really reflect correct hormonal levels. And so, you see, we really don't have enough information yet to recommend its use.

Is DHEA the fountain of youth? Perhaps there is a kernel of truth here, but there has been a lot of premature hype; and with the substance already on drugstore and health food store shelves, many women are taking it before definitive research is completed. If you take DHEA, you should have your doctor follow your liver function tests as well as levels of DHEAS. If you can wait, however, data should be coming in the next two or three years.

GROWTH HORMONE

Human growth hormone replacement therapy is another "replacement" on the horizon. Like the other hormones, growth hormone levels decline as we age, starting at age thirty to forty. At the University of Wisconsin Medical School, 900 study participants were treated with growth hormone for an average of 191 days. They experienced a decrease in total cholesterol, triglycerides, and a significant decrease in body fat, especially belly fat! More than 80 percent of the patients reported increase in muscle size and strength, exercise endurance, energy levels, and sexual potency. Sixty-four percent felt that their memory had improved. There seem to be no data that growth hormone increases the risk of tumor formation, but it can increase the size of various body organs, and cause fluid retention, joint pain, worsening of diabetes, and heart failure. Some of these side effects can be reduced by decreasing the dose used.

Growth hormone is normally secreted at night during slow-wave (deep) sleep. This phase of sleep can be disrupted by medications or possibly by melatonin abnormalities. With loss of this sleep pattern, there may be additional loss of growth hormone. In addition, as we become more and more sedentary with aging, less growth hormone is produced. Exercise increases growth hormone production.

Currently the National Institute on Aging is conducting several studies on the effect of growth hormone on older men and women. The results of these studies will be available in the next year or two. Growth hormone is given as an injection daily or nearly daily. Although synthetically made, growth hormone costs run nearly $15,000 a year for treatment of an older patient. Transdermal and oral methods are currently being researched.

PHYTOESTROGENS

Some of the original interest in these substances began when it was first realized that postmenopausal Japanese women living in Japan had few complaints of hot flashes and had less breast cancer than Western women. It was apparent that Japanese women eat large amounts of soy products on a daily basis. These soy products contain phytoestrogens, which have estrogenic effects. This may partially explain why postmenopausal Japanese women have so few menopausal complaints. Proof of this estrogenic activity can be seen by noting that vaginal cells mature as if the woman were taking estrogen therapy. Since Asian communities have lots of soy in their diets and have lower rates of breast, ovarian, endometrial, colon, and prostate cancer, it seems that these plant estrogens may have anticarcinogenic qualities. As Westernization of the diet occurs or when these women move to Western countries, cancer rates increase and these advantages seem to disappear.

Before discussing soy and related products, I believe it is important to realize that this is only one possible reason among many others why Japanese women have fewer menopausal symptoms. And although they may have fewer menopausal symptoms, they also refer to them and perceive them differently. There is no word for hot flash in Japanese; instead, the Japanese refer to it as "blush." Furthermore, in Japan, the elderly are honored, so that attaining a menopausal status means increasing prestige within the family. In the United States, youth is honored, and older women always yearn to look younger whether or not they really wish to be younger! In addition, Japanese women have smaller breasts and therefore less breast tissue in which to develop breast cancer. Moreover, there are other physical differences. For example, their pelvis has better and thicker muscles than Caucasians.

In addition, Japanese women have almost never been exposed to birth control pills and rarely smoke. They have also rarely consumed milk or milk products. They eat lots of fish rich in omega-3 oils, and a low-fat diet, and have always exercised. Although they are at high risk for spine fracture, they have one-third fewer hip fractures, although their hip density is low. This could be for a variety of reasons. One is that Japanese women are shorter. In general, shorter women have fewer hip fractures because of the shorter length of the femoral neck (the top of the thighbone that angles to fit into the hip socket). Shorter women have less distance to fall than tall women. Also, Japanese women spend more time in squatting positions, which may add more muscle and protect this area. In addition, older Japanese women generally don't wear high heels, and may be more likely to limit their activities to their homes and protected immediate surroundings rather than jogging down streets and roads. All this is to say that soy is not the whole story and that we have much to learn. Now let us go on to talk about soy and phytoestrogens.

Phytoestrogens are basically estrogenic substances produced by plants. That plants could contain estrogen-like substances was discovered nearly fifty years ago when sheep feeding on clover became infertile and were found to have increased estrogen levels. (This was known as Clover disease and could be thought of as giving the sheep a clover-based birth control pill.) As time went on, research efforts proved that these substances competed with estrogen for binding sites on cells that are known as estrogen receptors. Once either estrogen or phytoestrogen binds to the receptor, the cells show an estrogen-like response.

Phytoestrogens are found in fruits, vegetables, beans, and soy, probably the best-known source. Actually, soy contains a botanical mix of many different substances. It is possible that the mixture itself may benefit us more than any single extracted portion. Soy contains isoflavones, the most potent class of phytoestrogens. Isoflavones are found in highest concentration in soybeans and soy products. Another type of phytoestrogens, lignins, are found in almost all cereals and vegetables, with the highest concentrations in linseed (flaxseed). There are many different phytoestrogens, each with a different structure. There are also a number of classes of phytoestrogens, including lignins, isoflavones, coumestans, and resorcylic acid lactones.

Soy made it into the mainstream of medical literature when a major study was published by Anderson et al. in the *New England Journal of Medicine* in August 1995. It was a retrospective meta-analysis of thirty-eight studies involving more than 740 subjects. The study showed decreases in serum cholesterol by nearly 10 percent, LDL 13 percent, and triglycerides 10 percent, as well as a small increase in HDL when soy, a vegetable protein, was substituted for animal protein in the diet. An average of 47 grams per day was consumed. The researchers found that soy was more effective in reducing cholesterol in those people with higher than normal cholesterol levels. They speculated that the beneficial action of soy is due in large part to its estrogen-like activity because of the similar lipid changes that occur with both substances. In addition, phytoestrogens' vasodilation effect on blood vessels is similar to that seen with estrogen. Therefore, phytoestrogens seem to protect the cardiovascular system in many ways, as does estrogen.

The Japanese have the highest dietary intake of soy products, consuming some 200 mg per day. On the other hand, in the U.S. we consume less than 5 mg per day. Whether phytoestrogens protect bone density as well as estrogens is still not known. However, Asian women do suffer from osteoporosis, even though they consume large amounts of phytoestrogens. Another intriguing aspect of these plant proteins is that they may decrease the risk of breast cancer. There is some evidence that these substances may decrease blood vessel growth to tumors, depriving the tumor of its blood supply.

On the other hand, American lifestyles, environment, and backgrounds are different from that of the Japanese. If research continues to give good news about soy, much more effort will be needed to educate the American public. New ways to incorporate soy into our foods and recipes will have to be learned. Soy milk gives 9 grams of soy protein in an 8-

ounce glass. A cup of soy flour contains about 30 grams, tofu has 1 gram per ounce, and textured protein (like veggie burgers) is the most concentrated source at 16 to 23 grams per ounce.

Commercial soy products may be different in composition from those used in the Far East; in addition, they may be produced by different processes, and no laws require manufacturers to list the isoflavone, genestein, and daidzien content in their botanical mixture. In addition, there are differences in manufacture, with some companies using ethyl alcohol extraction for preparation of soy concentrates. This process removes a major portion of the isoflavones and saponins, could reduce the benefits of the final product. Also, because soy is low in zinc, iron, and calcium, you should take a well-rounded diet in addition to the soy or add a vitamin and mineral supplement.

After eating an average amount of soy, extremely high levels of isoflavones can be found in our blood, in the range of 100 to 800 ng/ml. In contrast, levels of plasma estradiol are often 50 to 70 pg/ml in the postmenopausal woman on hormone replacement. Therefore, it is not surprising that these high phytoestrogen levels create an estrogen-like response.

Soy products have been a staple for centuries in Asia, so we hope that there are no major surprises as we Westerners increase our consumption of them. Most Americans know soy only through soy formulas given to infants who are allergic to cow's milk. Whether we know all there is to know about its safety is not clear. Major changes in diet or eating more potent compounds could create a hormonal imbalance. Studies have shown that adverse effects are possible with a prolongation of the length of the menstrual cycle and suppression of the usual mid-cycle surge of LH (Cassidy et al., 1994). Also, cases of uterine bleeding have been seen with high intake of soy products. We simply don't have all the answers yet.

Summary

Ongoing studies in many parts of the world are looking at nonhormonal therapy for menopausal women. Some are using traditional Chinese herbs, others are using specific plants and extracts, and still others are researching different forms of phytoestrogens. In the not too distant future, we will have many options for the menopausal woman. I think that it will soon be clear that aging per se is caused by a deficiency of many substances, and not just by the loss of estrogen alone. Frailty, cancer, and our body's resistance to disease can be improved with research effort. This research will save billions of dollars in medical care and give senior citizens more of the vitality they had in their youth.

Hormonal therapies are likewise being developed with new compounds that are tailor-made for specific effects. Designer estrogens are on the horizon that will have powerful antioxidant effects to protect our cardiovascular system, and anti-inflammatory effects to protect us from arthritic disease. They will be designed to have little or no effect on the endometrium so that bleeding will not occur, and to not affect breast tissue. In the future, we may take our daily vitamins with a cocktail containing small amounts of estrogen or designer estrogens, plus some bisphosphonates for our bones and phytoestrogens in addition to a nighttime dose of melatonin, DHEA, calcium, growth hormone, and vitamin E. All this will have to be tailored in amount to each woman's personal needs.

Physicians and researchers are trying hard to find the right answer for postmenopausal women. As the next century approaches, we will also be trying hard to do equally well for men. Remember that for the time being, estrogen is still the gold standard, having been studied and used by millions of women since 1942. Actually, estrogen was the first alternative to just plain having hot flashes. Not only do we know more about it than any other therapy, but also we know that it has the ability to benefit more different aging problems than any other single known compound.

After you have digested all of this information, try to take care of yourself by doing all the commonsense things your mother would have advised. Then, consider your own individual risks and make the decision that makes the most sense, at least at this time. Remember, I'm in the same boat with you. Good luck to all of us!

Notes

1. If you are interested in participating in this or other related studies, please contact The Columbia University Center for Complementary and Alternative Medicine, New York, New York, tel. (212) 543-9550, or The Women's Health Research Center, 14201 Laurel Park Drive, Suite 104, Laurel, Maryland 20707, tel. (301) 953-9677.

2. D. Garfunkel et al., "Improvement of Sleep Quality in Elderly People by Melatonin," *Lancet* 346 (1995): 541–44.

Chapter 4

ESTROGEN AND THE BRAIN—KEEPING YOUR MIND

WITH HOWARD FILLIT, M.D.

I tried to hire Howard Fillit, M.D., as a geriatrician many years ago for my women's center, but the Mount Sinai Medical Center in Manhattan had more pull. Dr. Fillit is an internationally recognized expert in geriatric medicine. He has been actively involved in research on aging and in 1985 was the first to report that estrogen replacement therapy improves cognitive function in postmenopausal women with Alzheimer's disease.

In 1980, in a chapter in *No More Menstrual Cramps and Other Good News*, I wrote that estrogen had a profound impact on the brain:

> My first acquaintance with estrogen replacement therapy came when I, as a new doctor just out of medical school, was making house calls with Florence, my senior associate. We were let into a thoroughly messy apartment by a disheveled, middle-aged woman in a bathrobe. She told us that she couldn't cope any longer. She was extremely depressed, and her whole life seemed to be made worse by her constant hot flashes. Florence gave her an injection and a few pills. When we got back into the car, I asked, "What did you give her?"
>
> "A shot of estrogen and some estrogen pills."
>
> That was my first experience with estrogen therapy. It had never been taught in medical school.
>
> Some ten days later, I was working in the office when I noticed a patient I had never seen before sitting in the wait-

ing room. She was pretty, neatly dressed, and made up; she sat there smiling with her gloved hands calmly folded in her lap.

"Who is that?" I asked Florence.

"Don't you recognize her? That's the woman we gave the estrogen to on our house call." I was flabbergasted. Seeing the remarkable transformation in that woman made an indelible impression on me, and in 1964, I began to use hormone replacement therapy rather freely for patients with hot flashes and night sweats, who also had depression.

In 1983 in *No More Hot Flashes and Other Good News,* I wrote about a patient who "was on handfuls of tranquilizers and antidepressants. I suggested that we add estrogen. Soon after, she was able to cut her drug intake to small bedtime doses and was much more functional than when she was so heavily sedated."

Scientific data now have proved that estrogen has a direct effect on the brain, and when added to antidepressant medication, enhances the antidepressant effect in postmenopausal women. Read on, for there is good news for your most precious body part, your brain.

• • •

How could estrogen, a sex hormone, be useful in the treatment of postpartum depression, perimenopausal and postmenopausal memory, attention and mood problems, and senility in late life? To find the answer to this question, we need to first understand the basic and important role that sex hormones, including the female hormone estrogen and the male hormone testosterone, play in the development and function of the brain and in human behavior.

John Gray's best-selling book *Men Are from Mars, Women Are from Venus* (New York: HarperCollins, 1992) delineates and discusses the differences between men and women in the way that we think, feel, speak, and behave. Gray uses an approach that is probably necessary for us to get some perspective on ourselves and recognize the differences in how men and women think. He asks us to view our differences from outer space. He contends that it is difficult for us to really see and understand our differences because we are too close and involved with them.

We tend to take these differences for granted. And yet, every day, we live these differences in our marriages, our relationships with friends (which are usually of the same sex because only friends of the same sex really "understand" us), and in the workplace.

Women and men differ in their appearance, hair distribution, bone and muscular structure, breast development, and sexual organs. The female hormone estrogen and the male hormone testosterone are responsible for these differences. Just as our bodies are different, or "differentiated" according to gender, so are our brains. What could be the evolutionary basis for this?

Reproduction and survival of the species. Sex is vital to life. It is responsible for carrying on the species. Without sex there is no life. No wonder that gonadal hormones play a fundamental and important role in behavior. Reproduction involves not only the physical aspects of procreation but also, perhaps even more importantly, the behavioral aspects of getting the male and the female together in the first place for the purpose of procreation. As we all know, the female needs to be able to signal to her mate that she is receptive, and the male needs to be able to tell the female that he is interested and capable. Furthermore, both sexes need to be able to choose the strongest and most capable mate they can find; this is good for both the species and for the ultimate survival of the individual child. For example, even among humans, the best predictor of longevity is having parents who lived to be old; having good genes and finding mates with good genes is crucial to the mating process.

Animals do this primarily based on physical strength. Males fight for dominance and the winner gets the chance to mate with a receptive female. But in humans, this is obviously much more complicated and involves all of the aspects of mind and emotion that make us human. Underlying John Gray's fundamental point is the fact that sexual behavior in humans underlies much of what we are all about as humans. In fact, research has shown that sex hormones play a role in many human behaviors, such as flirting (receptivity), jealousy (keeping the mate monogamous), imagination (sexual fantasies), and being able to evaluate the physical (i.e., aggressive), intellectual, emotional, and social strengths and weaknesses of a potential mate.

In fact, until relatively recently, adult roles in human life were much more sexually differentiated than they are today. Sexually differentiated roles for men and women were true for cavemen; men went hunting and women were food gatherers and responsible for child raising. These social roles may have had a biological basis. Men were bigger, and had better visuospatial skills for hunting, while women had better social skills and verbal skills necessary for attending to the communal needs of the children and the family and promoting communal child rearing and related social networks. Not much has really fundamentally changed. In fact, sexual differentiation of the brain and behavior is a fact of life for all species, not just humans.

The Neurobiology of Sex Hormones

What is the biological basis for the effect of sex hormones on the brain? Scientific research has clearly shown that sex hormones, estrogen and testosterone, play a crucial role in brain development and function.

Many years ago, gonadal hormones such as estrogen were found to play a vital role in the *behavior* of animals. In animals, scientists discovered that gonadal hormones are essential for brain cell growth and function, much as they are responsible for the development and function of the body.[1]

Sex hormones do this in two ways.

ORGANIZATIONAL AND ACTIVATIONAL EFFECTS

Organizational Effects

Hormones are responsible for the development and growth of the brain in the fetus. They "organize" the brain according to gender. Think of this as the "hardware" of the brain. In essence, during prenatal development, these hormones cause brain cells and circuits to develop and organize according to gender, making a male brain and a female brain. In fact, all humans, and most animals for that matter, begin with a "female" brain; subsequently, in males, development is altered in utero by testosterone to create the male brain.

At a cellular level, scientists have found that there are "estrogen receptors" in certain cells in crucial circuits in the brain that are responsible for a number of important behaviors, including memory, learning, and emotions. These estrogen receptors are similar to the estrogen receptors that are seen in breast cells and are active primarily during brain growth development. In males, specific brain cells recognize testosterone (male hormone). However, within the cell, testosterone is converted to estrogen, which is ultimately the active hormone in males as well.

These "organizational" effects are "trophic," which means that the way estrogen causes the brain to become a "female" brain is through its effects on specific "estrogen-responsive" cells, making them grow into "female" circuits. These are the effects that may account for as the following: that early in life, little girls (on average) clearly have better verbal skills, and obtain them earlier (in general) than little boys. On the other hand, on average, little boys are much more likely to participate in "rough-and-tumble" play.

EFFECTS OF ESTROGEN ON THE BRAIN

Organizational Effects
occur primarily during development
directly affect the growth of brain cells (trophic effects)
result in permanent changes in the brain
differentiate the brain according to gender

Activational Effects
occur primarily during adult life
affect the function of brain cells
alter the neurochemistry of the brain
support gender-related behavior in adult life

Activational effects

Once the brain is "organized" as a female brain, estrogen continues to have an effect on brain function after birth, and throughout life. The estrogen-responsive circuits seem to remain estrogen responsive, and may require the continuing "trophic" effects of estrogen to survive. In addition, estrogen modulates the function of these cells and circuits. These effects during postnatal and adult life are called "activational" effects. Think of these effects as the "software" of the brain. Estrogen "activates" these circuits and modulates the production of important neurotransmitters that are crucial to normal brain function in adult life.

For example, the monoaminergic (MAO) neurotransmitters system plays an important role in emotion; abnormalities in this system are thought to be a cause of depression. MAO inhibitors are used in the treatment of depression. They re-equilibrate the monoaminergic system back to normal in depressed individuals. Another important neurotransmitter system in the brain is the cholinergic system. This system plays an important role in memory and in learning. Drugs that cause amnesia block the cholinergic system; drugs that enhance learning increase the activity of the cholinergic system.

To prove that estrogen and testosterone can affect brain function in adult life, scientists have done thousands of experiments over the last fifty years. For example, in the early 1970s, investigators at The Rockefeller University in New York showed that ovariectomy of rats (removing the ovaries, an event that produces effects similar to the menopause, when women lose the function of their ovaries) resulted in a decrease in the activity of the cholinergic system (associated with memory loss and an inability to learn) and an increase in the activity of the monoaminergic system (associated with depression).[2] Giving these ovariectomized animals estrogen replacement reversed and normalized the levels. These findings have obvious clinical implications.

Other experiments looked into how the growth effects of estrogen may play a role in adult life. Dr. Bruce McEwen, also at The Rockefeller University, studied the number of possible connections that brain cells can make in the hippocampus, the area of the brain responsible for memory and learning in female rats both after ovariectomy and also through the phases of rat menopause.[3] His group found that after ovariectomy (the "menopause" equivalent), or during the nonfertile part of the menstrual cycle, the actual structure of the brain cells was altered. The dendrites (parts of the brain cells that is the equivalent to the "wires" connecting the cells that carries the signals) actually lost spines ("connectors"). This would indicate that during menopause, or during the nonfertile phases of the menstrual cycle that are associated with low estrogen levels, the number of potential connections that could be made by the brain cells in this area of the brain decreased. Of even more interest, when the animals that had had ovariectomies were given estrogen replacement, the number of spines increased. In addition, during the fertile phase of the menstrual cycle (a period associated with high estrogen levels), the number of spines also increased.

Could these changes have effects on memory and learning? In recent work, other scientists have shown that after ovariectomy, rats have a decreased learning capacity. However, after being given estrogen replacement, these rats increased their learning capacity, bringing it back to a normal level.[4]

SEX HORMONES AND THE HUMAN BRAIN

What does all of this have to do with human conditions? A great deal. Periods of alterations in estrogen levels in women are frequently associated with changes in mood and cognitive ability (including memory and learning) in several important phases of the life cycle. For example, we often say that adolescents are "hormonal." This change in behavior, often associated with sexual maturity, but involving a variety of complex human cognitive and emotional changes, must have a biological basis. Similarly, recent evidence shows that postpartum depression, a period of rapid and large decreases in estrogen levels, can be treated with estrogen replacement.

SEX HORMONES AND THE HUMAN BRAIN AT THE MENOPAUSE

One of the most important periods of change in estrogen levels in the life cycle is at the menopause when, after a lifetime of estrogen availability, estrogen drops to very low levels. This is often associated with changes in mood and cognition, which women frequently acknowledge as occurring in varying degrees. Although these symptoms are generally "subclinical," and for the majority of women do not significantly affect function in either the workplace or at home, many menopausal women experience anxiety, irritability, depressed mood, forgetfulness, and difficulty concentrating. The changes in mood and cognition are often noticeable to family and other loved ones and may affect quality of life.

The problem with attributing these symptoms to the abrupt menopausal loss of estrogen is that menopause is a complex psychosocial and physiological event. For example, women may view the loss of reproductive fertility either as a negative sign of aging or as a positive liberation from menstrual periods and potential pregnancies. These psychological variables might affect whether a menopausal woman going through this phase of life will have depressive symptoms or not.

In addition, the menopause is associated with hot flashes and sleep disorders, which are generally considered systemic effects of the menopause. Of course, one could make the argument that anyone not sleeping well and experiencing hot flashes throughout the day and night would be irritable and anxious, and might therefore be distracted enough to complain of memory loss and difficulty concentrating. However, it is of interest, and not generally recognized, that sleep disorders and hot flashes (which are real physiological disorders associated with menopause) are, in fact, the result of the abrupt loss of estrogen on the brain. Hot flashes are the result of blood vessel dilations, which are mediated by a disturbance of the hypothalamus of the brain. Sleep disorders represent a disorder of the biological clock located in the brain.

In the face of these confounding factors, how can we know whether menopausal women's irritability, anxiety, memory loss, or difficulty paying attention are attributable to an adjustment reaction, hot flashes, and sleep disorders, or are real effects of abrupt estrogen loss on the function of brain cells (neurons) and circuits responsible for memory and mood?

A number of previous studies by physicians have investigated this question during the past twenty years.[5] These studies have shown that estrogen replacement therapy during the menopause clearly reduces irritability and anxiety, and improves memory and attention. In one study, the influences of hot flashes and sleep disorders were distinguished from the possible "central" effects of estrogen directly on memory and mood. Improved mood and memory were found even in women who were not suffering sleep disorders or hot flashes. We may also conclude from these studies, in addition, that regardless of whether menopausal women are suffering hot flashes and sleep disorders or not, estrogen replacement therapy at this time improves mood and memory.

From a scientific perspective, none of the studies on memory and mood during the menopause was performed according to strict standards employing appropriate controls, leaving the interpretation of the results in question as far as the scientific establishment is concerned, and preventing these concepts from entering the clinical mainstream. However, recent studies by psychologist Barbara Sherwin have, at least in part, addressed this problem.[6] Sherwin chose an interesting model: the surgical menopause. In these studies, women who had a bilateral ovariectomy experienced a surgical menopause. In essence, these women experienced the same operation the scientists performed or laboratory animals as described above. Before and after the surgical procedure, the psychological profiles of the women were characterized extensively with regard to their mood and memory and other cognitive functions. Then, after the surgery, some of the women were given estrogen (and in some experiments testosterone as well) while others were given a placebo. Neither the scientists measuring the women's psychological function nor the women themselves knew whether they were getting the placebo or the hormone treatment.

These experiments clearly showed that the surgical menopause resulted in depressed mood and in memory and learning impairments. The experiments also demonstrated that hormone replacement either improved mood and cognition, or at least prevented it from worsening as a result of the operation. For example, in studies of the learning ability of women experiencing a surgical menopause, Sherwin's group showed that women who received placebo had impaired learning ability, while women who took estrogen did not. In this context, then, we may conclude that estrogen prevented the decline of cognitive function in these women. This concept has important implications for our understanding of aging and estrogen replacement. Sherwin's studies further demonstrated that the effect of estrogen replacement on memory and mood in these women was not the result of improvements in sleep disorders or hot flashes but was more likely due to direct effects of estrogens on estrogen-responsive neurons and circuits.

Sherwin's studies also showed that testosterone replacement improved mood and libido in surgically menopausal women. These studies point out the interesting fact that the female brain is also responsive to testosterone. In fact, both male and female brains are responsive to testosterone in the same way. Testosterone-responsive neurons have an enzyme called an aromatase that converts testosterone to estrogen inside the cell. Ultimately, estrogen is the hormone that alters neuron function in both males and females. In women, most testosterone is derived from the adrenal glands. Some women may develop lower levels. What was important in Sherwin's studies, and others, is that testosterone influenced the level of the women's sexual libido. After the surgical menopause, women sometimes suffer lower libidos. Since this can be measured by asking women about the number and types of sexual fantasies they have throughout the day and night, one can roughly measure the activity of the libido. Postmenopausal women who received testosterone had significantly improved libido. This is interesting for two reasons: One, it showed that the female brain responded to testosterone after the menopause with improved function. But the experiments also show that sex hormones affect one of the most fundamental activities of the mind that make us human, namely imagination!

Other studies have investigated the efficacy of estrogen in the treatment of depression in women. Dr. E. L. Klaiber demonstrated that estrogen may be useful in the treatment of depression in some women.[7] Others have confirmed these findings, also suggesting that dosage was important. When estrogen blood levels were brought to premenopausal blood levels, women improved; subtherapeutic levels did not improve mood, and high blood levels were associated with excessive side effects.

The Long-Term Effects of Estrogen Loss and Aging of the Brain

Most women today can expect to live about thirty years beyond the menopause. As other parts of this book describe, this has important implications for the aging women. Osteoporosis primarily results from estrogen loss at the menopause. But the real effects of osteoporosis do not occur until thirty years later. The average age at which women experience a hip fracture is seventy-nine years, even though women begin losing bone density at the onset of the menopause.

What are the long-term effects of estrogen loss on the brain? From the time of brain development to the menopause, brain structure and function are influenced by estrogen levels. However, after the menopause estrogen levels drop to very low levels, contributing to a number of chronic illnesses associated with aging, such as osteoporosis and heart disease. This is a result of the loss of the trophic effects of estrogens on these tissues. The loss of trophic effects on estrogen-responsive neurons may also lead to their degeneration, contributing to cognitive aging and even senility. Could senility be likened to "osteoporosis of the brain"? It is of interest that the average age of onset of senile dementia is also seventy-nine years, the same as the average age of hip fracture from osteoporosis in elderly women.

Though the terms "senility," "senile dementia," "dementia," and "Alzheimer's disease" are used frequently in this chapter, these terms are not all interchangeable. As I have said earlier, "dementia" is a medical term for what we commonly call senility. The best way to understand Alzheimer's disease and why it is not interchangeable with dementia is to think of it this way: The *most common cause of dementia is Alzheimer's disease*. However, *dementia can also be caused by many other things,* such as minor or major strokes, and a number of other causes that are very uncommon. There are also other reversible causes of cognitive impairments in the elderly such as the use of certain medications, depression, and thyroid disorders.

Could estrogen replacement therapy be an effective treatment for cognitive decline in late life?[8] In fact, this is not a new idea. In the early 1950s, Barbara Caldwell, a gerontologist at Washington University in St. Louis, performed elegant studies of estrogen replacement therapy in elderly women. In these studies a group of about fifty women with an average age of seventy-six years were given hormone replacement therapy over a period of eighteen months. Using very sophisticated mental tests, including the standardized Wechsler-Bellevue IQ test, Caldwell showed that hormone replacement therapy in these elderly women significantly improved cognitive function. In fact, Caldwell showed that hormone replacement increased memory, comprehension, and verbal IQ in women receiving estrogen compared with controls who received only a placebo.

The problem with Caldwell's studies for our modern understanding is that, until recently, senility was considered a normal part of aging. We do not know the condition of the women that Caldwell studied, other than that they were old. We now have a much better understanding of cognitive aging and recognize that senility is not a normal part of aging. While some memory loss occurs with age, generally cognitive decline associated with normal aging does not result in loss of daily function. When it does, a diagnosis of senility, or dementia, may be made. Now-classic autopsy studies performed by Tomlinson, Blessed, and Roth in 1970[9] were the first to recognize that Alzheimer's disease, previously known as a cause of presenile dementia or dementia in younger persons, also caused senility (the medical term is dementia) in elderly individuals. They finally confirmed that senility is not a normal part of aging.

About the same time, Michael and Kantor[10] employed estrogen replacement therapy with conjugated estrogens to treat women living in a nursing home. While they also did not have a diagnosis of Alzheimer's disease in modern terms, they knew the women had cognitive and functional impairment. Over a period of thirty-six months, women who received estrogen improved significantly, while those who did not receive estrogen showed progressive cognitive and functional decline.

Estrogens, Alzheimer's Disease, and Related Dementias

In the early 1980s, a group of neurobiologists studying the effects of sex hormones on animals' brains joined a group of physicians studying Alzheimer's disease on clinical rounds at The Rockefeller University Hospital. Headed by Dr. Howard Fillit, the clinical group was trying to discover new treatments for Alzheimer's disease. In this era, most scientists thought that Alzheimer's disease was the result of a loss of cholinergic system activity in the brain (the neurochemical system that plays an important role in memory and learning). Scientists Luine and McEwen had shown that estrogen improves cholinergic function in the brains of ovariectomized rats. They suggested that, from a basic neuroscientific perspective, it might make sense to give women with Alzheimer's disease estrogen as a means of improving their cholinergic function. Fillit, a geriatrician, was familiar with the use of estrogen for the treatment of osteo-porosis in elderly women as a form of prevention. The stage was set.

Over the next three years, studies were conducted that demonstrated, for the first time, that estrogen replacement therapy was effective in improving cognitive function in some elderly women with Alzheimer's disease.[11] Estrogen treatment improved both mood and memory in a small group of women, average age seventy-six years, who were treated. In some women who had completely lost their learning ability, estrogen restored this capacity.

Over the next ten years, slowly other investigators read the studies by Fil-lit and repeated them, finding the same thing: Estrogen replacement ther-apy improved cognitive function and mood in women with well-documented Alzheimer's disease.[12] For example, Ohkura found that same effect of estro-gen on improving cognitive function in elderly postmenopausal women in Japan. Of interest, in these studies, Ohkura found that estrogen also improved cerebral blood flow in these women. In 1996, the National Insti-tutes of Health finally recognized these important findings by initiating a clinical trial that will be conducted at over twenty-four sites throughout the United States with over 120 women to be entered and studied using sophis-ticated cognitive and emotional testing. It is hoped that this large multicen-tered and well-controlled study will definitively demonstrate whether or not estrogen is effective in the treatment of Alzheimer's disease.

However, another potentially even more important question is whether estrogen can prevent Alzheimer's disease. As with osteoporosis, it may be possible that if women take estrogen from the time of the menopause until old age, they will be protected from neuronal degenera-tion by the continued presence of the growth-promoting effects of estro-gen. Some tantalizing data have appeared in the past two years to indicate that this possibility is quite real.

Paganini-Hill and V.W. Henderson[13] studied a group of over eight thousand people who were part of the Leisure World Study. This is one of several longitudinal studies of aging currently being conducted in the world. In this epidemiological study, older people who live in an adult community have agreed to participate in long-term research, primarily involving questionnaires, so we can learn about what factors contribute to their longevity. In the early 1990s, Paganini-Hill and her group rean-alyzed the data from the study according to whether women stated they have ever used a variety of medications, such as thyroid replacement, estrogen, and a variety of other drugs, and then identified individuals who had died and looked at their death certificates to determine whether they had died of Alzheimer's disease or any related dementias.

Incredibly, of all the medications studied, only the use of estrogen correlated with a reduction in the incidence of Alzheimer's disease and related dementias. In fact, use of estrogen decreased the incidence from Alzheimer's disease by about 30 percent, a very significant reduction. Furthermore, reduction in rates of dementias was correlated with both the dose and the duration of use of estrogen.

More recent studies[14] conducted at the Columbia-Presbyterian Medical Center in New York by Richard Mayeux and his group investigated the relationship between estrogen use and the incidence of dementia. In this population-based study, women who reported they used estrogen also had a reduction in the incidence of Alzheimer's disease. Again, these investigators found that this reduction correlated with the dose and duration of estrogen use. In fact, for women who used estrogen for more than one year, the incidence of Alzheimer's disease was reduced by almost 90 percent!

These epidemiological studies need even further confirmation before we can conclude for certain that estrogen can prevent Alzheimer's disease, much as it has been demonstrated to prevent osteoporosis and hip fractures, and probably heart disease. As a result of these epidemiological studies, a new and major study is being undertaken as part of the Women's Health Initiative (WHI), a study of one hundred thousand American women funded by the National Institutes of Health. It will seek to determine if estrogen can prevent Alzheimer's disease. This study will take at least six years.

Alzheimer's disease is not the only form of dementia. Multiple small and/or large strokes are also a common cause of dementia, especially in women over the age of eighty-five years. We do know that estrogen can protect against heart disease, and has significant effects on the vasculature. This is likely to be true for the brain as well. In fact, as mentioned previously, estrogen improves cerebral blood flow in postmenopausal women. Some early studies have also shown that estrogen improves cognitive function in elderly postmenopausal women with cerebrovascular disease. Improvements in cerebral blood flow may also be one of several mechanisms by which estrogen can prevent and treat Alzheimer's disease.

Other Factors in Preventing Cognitive Decline in Late Life

There are a number of other factors that may contribute to robust cognitive health in our later years.[15] These factors are important for all men and women, including those women who may be unable (or who choose not) to take estrogen replacement therapy.

Considering that one of the important causes of cognitive decline in our later years is related to vascular disease (previously thought of as "hardening of the arteries"), control of risk factors for vascular disease may also prevent cognitive decline and senile dementia. In general, these are the same risk factors that are important in the prevention of heart disease. Controlling hypertension, if you have it, is very important in preventing stroke and deterioration of brain function in late life. Often we think of strokes as those events that lead to paralysis of the body. However, small strokes that do not cause paralysis can cause loss of memory and reasoning, difficulty with speech, and changes in our personality. Other risk factors for vascular disease in general, such as smoking, high cholesterol, diabetes, and certain forms of heart disease, are probably also risk factors for vascular disease of the brain and contribute to cognitive decline in late life. In general, then, the healthy lifestyle that we adopted in middle age to prevent heart disease becomes increasingly important in old age to prevent cognitive decline.

Exercise is also very important in maintaining brain function in late life, although we do not know exactly how exercise does this. It may be that exercise improves blood flow to the brain and keeps brain cells healthy. Exercise appears to improve brain function, at least in part, by improving how "sharp" we are. The brain, like a computer, operates on "processing speed" called reaction time. This is centrally a fundamental process of brain function. Exercise clearly improves brain processing speed. In addition, exercise is known to play a role in the prevention of vascular disease, and this may also be an important factor in the ability of exercise to maintain brain function in late life.

The brain is "like a muscle." Perhaps we have all heard this before, but it is true. As with our muscles, we must keep our brains "in shape." The expression "use it or lose it" definitely applies to the brain. In fact, like muscles, which can be seen to physically increase in response to exercise, the brain also "grows" in response to use. More connections or synapses are made, greater redundancy is created, and the brain becomes less at risk for decline. Amazingly, some of the most important risk factors for cognitive decline in late life are related to intellectual stimulation. Having a high level of education and continuing participation in a complex social or occupational environment protects the brain against decline in late life. Another crucial factor associated with high levels of intellectual functioning in late life is a spouse who is also of high intellectual capacity. Apparently, being married to a "smart" spouse is crucial to maintaining cognitive health in late life. Finally, maintaining vision and hearing is important in maintaining a healthy brain in late life.

Conclusions

Beginning in early infancy, estrogens have profound effects on human behavior, the way we act, think, feel, and interact with others. These effects are real, and have a biological basis. The menopause is now considered by many to be a hormone-deficiency state. We are in the relatively early, but very exciting, stages of understanding how this estrogen deficiency state in the postmenopausal woman affects the brain, both short term during the menopause, and long term during aging. If estrogen can prevent Alzheimer's disease and other dementias, particularly vascular dementia, this would be a great improvement in women's lives. Many women question whether the benefits of long-term estrogen replacement therapy are worth the risks, and are especially concerned about breast cancer. There are also the bothersome aspects of compliance with taking a pill every day and of possibly reinstated menstrual periods. If the benefits are limited to possibly preventing a hip fracture at age seventy-nine, thirty years of estrogen replacement treatment may not seem worth it. But the thought of losing one's mind at age seventy-nine is far more fearsome. Dementia is probably the most tragic outcome in old age. Preventing cognitive decline is crucial to quality of life in old age.

There are also many other things we can do to prevent cognitive decline in late life. Continuing many of the healthy habits we adopted in middle age to prevent heart disease can prevent cognitive decline in old age. A healthy lifestyle is crucial not just for the heart but also for the brain. In addition, our remaining connected to our families, our communities, and our occupations can provide continuing stimulation and growth for our intellectual capacities, and prevent cognitive decline due to disuse. In the absence of serious physical disease, old age can be a time of growing wisdom, intellectual and social contribution to the community, and satisfaction in living.

Notes

1. D. Toran-Allerand, R. C. Miranda, W.D.L. Bentham, F. Sohrabji, T. J. Brown, and B.S. McEwen, "Steroid Hormones: Effect on Brain Development and Function," *Hormone Research* 37, suppl. 3 (1992): 1–10.

2. V. N. Luine, A. I. Khylchevskaya, and B. S. McEwen, "Effect of Gonadal Steroids on Activities of Monoamine Oxidase and Choline Acetyltransferase in Rat Brain," *Brain Research* 86 (1975): 293–306.

3. C. S. Woolley and B. S. McEwen, "Estradiol Mediates Fluctuations in Hippocampal Synapse Density during the Estrous Cycle in the Adult Rat," *Journal of Neuroscience* 12 (1992): 2549–54.

4. M. Singh, E. M. Meyer, W. J. Millard, and J.W. Simpkins, "Ovarian Steroid Deprivations Results in a Reversible Learning Impairment and Compromised Cholinergic Function in Female Sprague-Dawlay Rats," *Brain Research* 644 (1994): 305–12.

5. H. Fillit, H. Weinreb, I. Cholst, V. Luine, R. Amador, J. Zabriskie, and B. S. McEwen, "Hormonal Therapy for Alzheimer's Disease," in *Treatment Development Strategies for Alzheimer's Disease,* edited by T. Crook, R. Bartus, S. Ferris, and S. Gershon (Madison, CT: Mark Powley Associates, 1986), 311–36.

6. B. B. Sherwin, "Hormones, Mood, and Cognitive Functioning in Postmenopausal Women," *Obstetrics and Gynecology* 87 (1996): 20s–26s.

7. E. L. Klaiber, D. M. Broverman, W. Vogel, and Y. Kobayashi, "Estrogen Therapy for Severe Persistent Depression in Women," *Archives of General Psychiatry* 36 (1979): 550–54.

8. See for review: H. Fillit, "Future Therapeutic Developments of Estrogen Use," *Journal of Clinical Pharmacology* 35 (1995): 225–28.

9. B. E. Tomlinson, S. Blessed, and M. Roth, "Observations on the Brains of Demented Old People," *Journal of Neurological Science* 11 (1970): 205–42.

10. C. M. Michael, H. I. Kantor, and H. Shore, "Further Psychometric Evaluation of Older Women—the Effect of Estrogen Administration," *Journal of Gerontology* 25 (1970): 337–41.

11. H. Fillit, H. Weinreb, I. Cholst, V. Luine, B. McEwen, R. Amador, and J. Zabriskie, "Observations in a Preliminary Open Trial of Estradiol Therapy for Senile Dementia–Alzheimer's Type," *Psychoneuroendocrinology* 11 (1986): 337–45.

12. See for review: H. Fillit, "Estrogens in the Pathogenesis and Treatment of Alzheimer's Disease in Postmenopausal Women," *Annals of the New York Academy of the Sciences* 743 (1994): 233–40.

13. A. Paganini-Hill and V. W. Henderson, "Estrogen Deficiency and Risk of Alzheimer's Disease in Women," *American Journal of Epidemiology* 140 (1994): 256–261.

14. M. X. Tang, D. Jacobs, Y. Stern, K. Marder, P. Schofield, B. Gurland, H. Andrews, and R. Mayeux, "Effect of Oestrogen during Menopause on Risk and Age at Onset of Alzheimer's Disease," *Lancet* 348 (1996): 428–32.

15. H. M. Fillit and R. N. Butler, eds., *Cognitive Decline: Strategies for Prevention (Greenwich Medical Media)* (London: Oxford University Press, 1997).

Chapter 5

ACHES AND PAINS—KEEPING YOUR MUSCULOSKELETAL SYSTEM STRONG

BY JEFFREY E. BUDOFF, M.D., WITH ROBERT P. NIRSCHL, M.D.

In 1983, in No More Hot Flashes and Other Good News *I complained to my then teenaged son about upper body fatigue from sitting for hours and typing. With his guidance I decided to try weight lifting using the bench-press set up in his bedroom. He looked at my skinny arms and set up the bar (25 pounds) with no weight on it. After two months I was still lifting only the bar, but got up to three sets of ten repetitions. I finally added five pounds of weight, and felt that that was an accomplishment for me.*

Over the years I have had mixed emotions seeing my son Jeff play football, wrestle, swim, play rugby and only after the fact found out that he boxed with the Harvard boxing club and bungee-jumped while on a visit to Australia. He made up his mind to be a physician, and chose a field that would combine his love for sports and give him the ability to help those with joint and muscular problems. He remains dedicated to exercise and practices daily what he preaches. He firmly believes that all of us should do the same.

I have not been a star pupil. I try in spurts, but find that I'm like most women who are over fifty; exercise was not part of our world, and learning new tricks takes effort. I know, however, that it's worth it. Nothing gets rid of aches and pains like exercise activity. Nothing makes me feel better and more energized than walking on the treadmill and doing my newly learned Tai Chi exercises.

Jeff's chapter contains the basics of preventive medicine. His mentor, Dr. Robert P. Nirschl, a well-known expert on sports medicine problems of the elbow and shoulder, contributed many of the ideas presented here, and most of the analogies are "Nirschlisms." Follow their instructions, and you will live a longer, more active life. With a mother's pride.

The musculoskeletal system can be a major source of pain and disability as we age. Overuse, tissue degeneration, and especially deconditioning (allowing ourselves and our muscles to get out of shape) contribute to many of the musculoskeletal problems experienced by the middle-aged and older.

With the current focus on fitness (every other magazine article and daytime television show seems to be dedicated to this), we are all trying to remain active longer. While this unquestionably benefits the cardiovascular system and overall health, and is certainly to be encouraged, it often takes its toll on overworked tendons and joints. However, the other end of the spectrum, allowing ourselves to become inactive and out of shape, also predisposes us to a multitude of nagging aches and pains. A balance between our activity level and overall fitness is desirable in order to allow us to maximize function and minimize discomfort. Therefore, as we get older it is prudent to become more careful, and more knowledgeable, in order to avoid injury. This chapter is dedicated to giving you the knowledge that will allow you to remain active and injury-free, as well as to understand more about any injuries that you may suffer. We hope you will find this to be important reading on a practical level.

The musculoskeletal system is made up of the body's muscles, tendons, ligaments, bones, and joints. Practically speaking, it encompasses the arms, legs, back, and neck. The musculoskeletal system is unisex, of course, even though I will often use the pronoun "she" in this chapter—however, the information applies to both men and women.

All of our muscles need regular exercise to maintain strength and tone. If you don't routinely exercise to stay in shape, then you allow your muscles to weaken. As we age, this predisposes us to aches, pains, and injuries in two ways: (1) The muscle itself becomes more easily injured, and (2) the rest of your musculoskeletal system (your tendons, ligaments, and joints) becomes more vulnerable to injury.

Let's talk about muscle first. I'd like to introduce the concept of stress tolerance. There is a certain amount of stress (externally applied force, such as a lifted weight) that each of us can absorb without injury. When we experience stress above that amount, injury occurs.

Muscles are like the shock absorbers of our body. They absorb energy, and disperse the stresses that we're subjected to. The better shape our muscles are in, the more shock they can absorb. When we become "deconditioned" (i.e., out of muscular shape), stresses that our muscles would normally absorb without difficulty can hurt us. A bumpy car ride, a roller coaster, a boat ride, etc., that a person with good muscle tone wouldn't think twice about, can leave you—if you're a deconditioned person—sore for days. That's because your muscles aren't in shape to absorb the shock. The stress tolerance of your muscles has decreased, rendering them more vulnerable to injury.

Not only that, deconditioned muscles also leave the rest of the musculoskeletal system more vulnerable to injury. The bones that make up the skeleton of our bodies are supported by both muscles and ligaments (strong rope-like structures that connect your bones to each other). For example, in order to pull a turkey drumstick off its body you have to break through both muscles (the meat that you eat) and ligaments (the strong white structures deep to the meat that hold the bones together). The same arrangement occurs in the human body. Your muscles help your ligaments to support your skeleton, from your spinal column to the arch of your foot. If your muscles are weak, the shock absorber fails, and now all the stresses that you experience are passed on to the tendons (which attach muscle to bone) and ligaments. This predisposes them to injury.

This is why athletes are most likely to be injured when they're tired. When muscles are well rested and strong, they absorb most of the forces the body is subjected to, protecting the tendons and ligaments. When muscles fatigue, or are weak, they cannot contract strongly, and are therefore less able to help absorb energy. And deconditioned muscles, which are out of shape from inactivity and disuse, lack both strength and endurance. They are therefore less able to absorb energy, subjecting your tendons and ligaments to more stress. This leads to "stress overload" (an abnormally high concentration of forces in a vulnerable area).

Stress overload may lead to tissue damage. This often occurs in the tendon that attaches an overworked muscle to the bone. (By definition, tendons attach muscles to bone, ligaments attach bones to other bones.) This breakdown may be acute (related to a specific traumatic event), but more often it is chronic in nature. Rather than being injured by one single massive event, the tendon is injured by thousands of little stresses. This is called repetitive overload, and is a major cause of tendon breakdown and injury. Usually, no specific cause can be remembered—"It's been hurting for months." Tennis elbow, rotator cuff problems, and heel pain commonly present this way.

Many of the injuries that occur as we age are related to tendon breakdown, usually from accumulated trauma. This degenerative process is called tendinosis. It used to be called (and unfortunately still is by many) tendinitis. But this is a misnomer. The suffix "-itis" means that inflammation is present. However, several pathologic studies (where the tissue is removed from the body and looked at under the microscope) have failed to show any evidence of inflammation. Tendinitis is simply the process of tissue degeneration and the body's attempt to repair it.

It is important to understand that not all exercise is beneficial to your body. In fact, overly intense exercise may contribute to tissue degeneration and overuse injuries. To understand that exercise may either be helpful or harmful to your body, you must first realize that there are three types of exercise.

The first type is rehabilitative exercise. Rehabilitative exercise is designed to take injured tissue, help your body to repair it and get it back to normal, or as close to normal as possible. Rehabilitative exercise strengthens a particular muscle, or muscle group, that is weak, injured, or deconditioned. In addition to restoring strength, flexibility, and endurance, your exercising of a specific damaged muscle within the limits of pain also helps to bring more blood supply into the damaged region so that the injured tissue can heal itself. Rehabilitative exercise targets *specific* muscles with low weights and high repetitions. An example of rehabilitative exercise would be a physical therapy program prescribed by a knowledgeable physician.

The second type of exercise is fitness exercise. Fitness exercise presumes that everything—the muscles, tendons, etc.—is *healthy to start with*. Fitness exercise is performed *in moderation* in order to tone up the body, stay in shape, and improve cardiovascular conditioning. Working out in a gym, jogging, or doing aerobics are all examples of fitness exercise.

The third type of exercise is performance exercise. Performance exercise is concerned with meeting a specific goal (such as winning the local tennis tournament, scoring a touchdown, beating your friend in golf, or bench-pressing three hundred pounds). This experience, however, is not necessarily beneficial to your musculoskeletal system's condition. In fact, it may often be *detrimental* to the body's good health. A quick survey of the injury report in the sports section of any newspaper should confirm this. Any competitive sport should be considered performance exercise, even your weekly tennis matches (which are, after all, the "civilized equivalent of war"). Performance exercise (which often includes fitness exercise that is overdone) doesn't get you into shape; it subjects you to stresses that are potentially injurious. Appropriate rehabilitative and fitness exercises are what get you into shape.

And you need to make sure that your *entire* body is strong enough to withstand the stresses you plan to put it through, *before* you begin your activity. You wouldn't tell your sixteen-year-old child, "Play baseball to get into shape." You'd tell him or her, "Maybe you'd better get into shape to play baseball."

You say, "But doctor, I've been playing tennis for thirty-five years. I play three times a week. Of course I'm in shape." You may be in shape as far as the heart and lungs are concerned, but this may not be true of your muscles, tendons, and joints. In fact, it may be the performance (competitive) nature of tennis that caused the overuse injury to your deconditioned musculoskeletal system in the first place. What you need to do to heal your injuries, and avoid future ones, is rehabilitative exercises to strengthen *specific* muscle groups so that they can absorb the stresses they're subjected to.

Even though you've been active for a long time, and have good cardiovascular conditioning, it may be that not all of your muscles are in shape. In fact, some of your smaller muscles may be weak, deconditioned, and vulnerable to overuse. The reason this happens is that when we perform a certain activity (run, play golf, play tennis), we rely mainly on our big muscles. Our smaller muscles may not be used as much, and may therefore be relatively weak. Consequently, they may be vulnerable to injury from repetitive overload. By *specifically* strengthening these smaller muscles we may avoid or treat these nagging injuries.

As aging proceeds, the body's recovery from injury slows. Just because you were able to play three sets of tennis, four days a week when you were twenty years old, that doesn't mean you can do it when you're sixty. Your body needs more time to recover. And even if you do take it slow and steady, it is still possible to become injured from accumulated wear and tear.

Take the example of weight lifting. Common sense dictates that the longer you work out, the stronger you get. You may plateau at times, but overall, over time, you get stronger. Well then, why don't seventy-year-old men bench-press 500 pounds? Why don't seventy-year-old women bench-press 150 pounds? The answer is because most weight lifters who constantly push themselves accumulate injuries. They hurt their shoulders, for example, and have to take time off. I've often heard middle-aged ex-athletes explain, "I used to lift 300 pounds, but I got injured, and just can't do it anymore." That injury was due to a training error, the same training error that people playing tennis, golf, or other recreational sports frequently make: They train too intensely with not enough rest between. And as you age, the amount of rest your body needs between exertions increases. If you fail to appropriately decrease the frequency and intensity of your activities as you age, you may be predisposing yourself to injury, especially if you don't maintain good overall muscular fitness.

Overuse injuries may also occur while participating in recreational sports, while working around the house, or occasionally from nothing apparent at all. Even if you're just doing your spring cleaning, or merely living out your sedentary existence, your body experiences more stresses than you may give it credit for. Professional musicians, construction workers, and many other "occupational athletes" routinely, if not daily, stress their bodies to meet a performance goal. The culprit behind the injury is frequently a combination of overuse and "selective deconditioning."

If you're like most people, you'll push yourself to succeed. You may not realize that in order to attain your goals you are subjecting your body to strains that, as you age, it is less able to tolerate. The repetitive nature of the activity stresses your vulnerable tissues, often leading to pain, injury, and weakness.

So, after curing yourself with *rehabilitative* exercise, you prevent subsequent injury through *fitness* exercise, and avoidance of excessive *performance* exercise that overloads the body's *stress tolerance*.

You may protest, "But my sister is out of shape, and she never has pain." Understand that injury occurs when the forces experienced by the body exceed its ability to absorb them. By becoming deconditioned, and allowing your muscles and tendons to weaken, you predispose yourself to injury, like a bald tire looking for a piece of glass. If that bald tire never hits a piece of glass it may function well, and the driver may never know that one of her tires is dangerously worn out. Likewise, if the inciting event never occurs, you may never realize how weak a certain part of your body has become. Then when a seemingly trivial incident occurs, like catching yourself to avoid a fall, you wonder why you hurt.

There is a balance between tissue quality and applied stress. As long as the tissue quality is greater than or equal to the applied stress, you're okay. But once stresses exceed tissue quality, you experience pain and injury. Therefore, to get rid of your pain and avoid future injury you have two options: (1) improving the quality of your tissues (adding tread to your tire), or (2) reducing the stresses you subject yourself to.

Maybe golf isn't that important to you. You could give it up. But many would rather die of pain than give up golf. The alternative is to take a lesson with a pro, to make sure that there's no flaw in your swing that is unnecessarily increasing the stresses you experience and contributing to your injury. Now Lord knows, no readers of mine could possibly have a flaw in their golf swing. Still, some people may turn their trailing hand over too much. Not only does this cause you to hook the ball (which is far more important than your elbow pain, I understand that), but it also subjects the muscles that rotate your forearm (whose tendons are located at your elbow) to unnecessarily high stresses. By correcting this problem with your swing mechanics, not only will your elbow feel better, but also you may actually keep the ball on the fairway.

The same thing goes for the tennis swing. By correcting poor swing mechanics you may reduce the stresses on your shoulder, elbow, and wrist, and prevent injuries, or help to heal one that already exists.

The same thing goes for many people with chronic, nagging lower back pain. Not only are most of them deconditioned, but they also have poor lifting techniques, and repetitively subject themselves to unnecessarily high stresses, often on a daily basis. Then they get injured and wonder why.

Now for the vicious cycle: Because you hurt, you do less. This allows your muscles to become even weaker and more deconditioned. And because you are still employing the same poor mechanics that led to the injury in the first place, you keep on reaggravating the same muscle strain. Continuously.

Another important point to understand is that once an injury occurs to one part of your body, the rest of your body now becomes predisposed to injury. For example, if you hurt your right elbow you will use your right arm less. It's natural—everybody reacts to pain with inactivity and disuse. But this disuse affects the entire arm, not just the specific part injured. It causes all of the arm's muscles to become weak and deconditioned. And so, when your elbow finally feels better and you resume your normal activities, you hurt your shoulder. Bad luck? No—bad rehabilitation. In order to avoid future injury you must strengthen both the elbow and the shoulder.

The same applies to hips and knees. After finally healing a knee injury or a hamstring pull, after having done months of supervised physical therapy to strengthen an injured knee, after making that knee the best it's ever been, you go back to whatever activity you do and pull your groin muscle. Bad luck? No—bad rehabilitation. You never realized that by limiting your use of that leg as a whole you weakened your hip muscles, which were also not being utilized. While you did physical therapy exercises to specifically strengthen your injured knee, you neglected your hip muscles (which, incidentally, include the groin muscles). Then you went back to playing golf, or taking in the groceries, with your hip deconditioned and predisposed to injury—"a bald tire looking for a piece of glass."

You've got to think of the body, certainly each limb, as an interrelated whole. When one part of that limb becomes injured, you've got to recognize that it deconditions the rest of that limb, if not the entire body. So before you consider yourself healed, you'd better be sure that the *entire* limb is adequately strengthened.

This is why some people ache all over. They get deconditioned (lacking muscular fitness, i.e., strength, flexibility, and endurance) and injure something. This makes them even more deconditioned, so that they injure something else, and a vicious cycle occurs. They may even see a physician for their injuries. Unfortunately, many physicians have been taught to treat these aches and pains with pills and rest. The problem is that pills and rest do nothing to restore strength, endurance, and flexibility, which is what the injured patient really needs. In fact, reliance on pills and rest often results in a patient who is even more deconditioned at the "end" of treatment than at its start.

And here we must address the difference between comfort and cure. Pills and rest (and modalities such as heat, ultrasound, iontophoresis, or whatever else is in fashion this week) merely make a patient more comfortable. They do nothing to cure the problem. Now, there's nothing wrong with being more comfortable. It helps if you're comfortable while you're performing the curative exercises that restore strength, endurance, and flexibility. But please don't make the mistake that's all too often made: Don't confuse temporary comfort with long-term cure. Just because medication or modalities temporarily take away the pain, that doesn't mean the problem is solved. Too often, the physical therapy that the patient thinks is curative is merely concerned with comfort and modalities.

If the injury is minor your body may be able to heal itself with some rest, and a little time off. But if your muscles are weak and deconditioned, the predisposition for injury still remains. The tire is still bald. And the road of life is filled with many pieces of glass. So once you're comfortable, it will pay to recondition yourself, and add some tread to your tire.

Start slowly as you place new stresses on your body's tissues. Injury is especially common during times of "transition," that is, changes in the frequency or intensity of activity. Your muscles, tendons, and even your bones need time to adapt to new stresses. If you fail to give them that time, injury may occur. This is often obvious in retrospect. For example, say a well-conditioned teenager came to you with shin splints, and told you that she had just started jogging, and that she got shin pain after running ten miles. What would you tell her? That maybe she should start by jogging one mile a day, then slowly advance to two miles a day after a week or two, and so on until eventually maybe she could handle ten miles without pain. The same concept, if not the same distance, applies to all of us. By starting slowly, we give the muscles, tendons, and bones of our musculoskeletal system time to adapt.

As we place stress on a bone, over a period of time it gets stronger. If we don't load a bone it loses calcium, leaving the bone weaker. This is known as Wolff's law—bone is strengthened according to the stresses it experiences. The same thing happens in muscles and tendons as well (and is known as Roux's law). But load the tissue quickly, before it has a chance to adapt, and injury may result.

So start slow, and increase the frequency and intensity of the activity slowly. Don't try to do too much, too soon. Rapid transitions in the intensity, quality, or duration of your activities put you at risk for developing overuse injuries. All transitions should be performed slowly and smoothly.

We all know someone who bought a $400 jogging suit, started jogging, got shin splints, and never jogged again. The problem is that instead of this person honestly and accurately assessing her body's condition (pretty out of shape) and assessing realistic goals for activity progression (advancing speed and distance slowly and consistently), she jumped in and overdid it. This is a common source of problems for "weekend warriors" of all ages. They sit in front of a computer console all week, do nothing to stay in shape, then play basketball at 110 percent all weekend, and wonder why their knees hurt on Monday morning. Understand that performance activities associated with abrupt transitions lead to the greatest risk of injury.

A word about people who have pain in multiple joints, who hurt all over. Many of these people may have poor quality collagen. Collagen is the protein that makes up all of our connective tissues (bone, tendons, muscles, and ligaments). The quality of this collagen is determined genetically. And some people may simply have better collagen than others.

Those people with weaker collagen may be genetically predisposed to overuse injuries. This has been referred to as the "mesenchymal syndrome." These people have a lower stress tolerance, and consequently experience more injuries and aches and pains, often in multiple locations (both elbows, both shoulders, etc.). They don't have any disease that we can identify (such as rheumatoid arthritis, lupus, etc.) would also decrease the quality of the collagen. They are just put together with slightly weaker material. It's like buying thirty-thousand-mile tires for your car instead of sixty-thousand-mile tires. They wear out sooner. These people simply have a thinner tread on their tires. They may also have an increased susceptibility to tennis elbow, rotator cuff tendinosis, nerve entrapments (including carpal tunnel syndrome), trigger fingers, and overuse syndromes. This syndrome may have some overlap with fibromyalgia and other pain disorders. It may occur in up to 15 percent of patients with overuse syndromes. X rays and lab tests are characteristically normal.

Certain diseases, like rheumatoid arthritis, lupus, and other inflammatory diseases, will weaken what may have started out as normal collagen. Some people may have joints that are damaged by injury or arthritis, and are consequently less able to tolerate stress. This is like starting out with sixty-thousand-mile tires, but then somebody comes along with a knife and pares down your tread so that you only have thirty thousand miles left. Same idea.

People with these syndromes have a predisposition for overuse injuries and should be especially careful about maintaining the strength of any limbs that bother them. Staying in the best overall physical shape possible may help relieve present problems and help prevent future problems a lot more than you'd think. It may also dramatically decrease the amount of pain you feel. It certainly works a lot better over the long run than manipulations, massage therapy, and the like.

However, before you think, "Aha—that's my problem, I'm just put together poorly," you'd better be sure that your injuries and aches and pains aren't just due to deconditioning. In fact, because joint problems, systemic illness, and the mesenchymal syndrome lead to pain, they also lead to deconditioning, which must be corrected if their symptoms are to be minimized.

The message is this: (1) Educate yourself—the more you understand about your body and its maladies, the better you will be able to help correct present problems and avoid future injuries; (2) recondition yourself—use rehabilitative exercises and stretching to restore strength, endurance, and flexibility; and (3) reduce stresses by only engaging in activities appropriate for your level of fitness, and by correcting poor mechanics.

And now on to some *specific complaints*.

LOW BACK PAIN

First, a little perspective. You should know that the majority of the adult population, between 60 and 80 percent, will, over the course of their lifetime, experience low back pain severe enough to interfere with the performance of normal activities. Every year, 2 to 5 percent of Americans will get low back pain. It's almost to be expected. It's certainly not unusual.

Furthermore, the majority of low back pain goes away by itself. Fifty percent of people with low back pain recover in two weeks, and 90 percent have no pain by three months, regardless of treatment. The 4 percent of individuals who have back pain for over six months (defined as chronic low back pain) account for about *85 to 90 percent* of the *$50 billion cost* of low back pain in the United States every year. After one year only 2 percent still have pain, again, regardless of treatment.

The cause of low back pain in 80 to 90 percent of adults is unknown.

That means that no anatomical problem can be identified. What this usually represents is a combination of many factors, including muscle strain and spasm. These injuries are usually due to poor lifting mechanics and deconditioning, leading to stress overload.

So if low back pain is common, usually goes away by itself, and no certain diagnosis can be given in the vast majority of cases, what is important to know about it? Glad you asked.

While low back pain is commonly due to muscle and ligament strain, the differential diagnosis of low back pain (the list of things that can cause low back pain) is long. Back pain can be of three types: (1) mechanical, (2) nonmechanical, or (3) referred.

1. Mechanical means that the pain is increased by activity, and improves with rest. Frequently with mechanical back pain, certain positions, such as sitting or standing, cause it to be better or worse.

2. Nonmechanical means that the pain at rest is equal to or greater than that with activity. Nonmechanical back pain is much less common, and is caused by infection, tumor, metastatic disease, inflammatory diseases, or metabolic diseases of the bone itself.

3. Referred means that a pain originating from another place in the body, such as the organs of the abdomen, pelvis, or the kidneys, radiates to the back. Referred pain is the least common of the three types of low back pain.

Mechanical low back pain is by far the most common, and is the type we will focus on. While the cause of mechanical low back pain is almost always mechanical overload, the exact tissue (i.e., disk, ligament, muscle, or bone) that is actually damaged and symptomatic is often unknown. Besides muscle or ligament strains and sprains, other causes of mechanical low back pain include arthritis, stenosis (not having enough room for the spinal cord or one of its nerves), an acutely symptomatic herniated disk (uncommon in people over fifty), stress fracture, or severe spinal deformity or instability. Regardless of the causative event, the end result is usually muscle spasm and strain, which is quite painful in and of itself.

It should be noted that mechanical (activity-related) low back pain is *not* usually caused by infection or tumor. These diseases usually cause nonmechanical, or referred, low back pain.

Your physician will take a history and examine you. As most mechanical low back pain is benign in nature and resolves quickly, X rays are usually not indicated unless the pain has been present for over six weeks. Of course, there are certain exceptions. There are some "red flags" your doctor will be looking for, things that indicate that something dangerous (like a tumor, infection, fracture, significant neurological injury, or metabolic disease) may be going on. These are: recent unexplained weight loss, a history of cancer, pain that awakens you from sleep, pain worse at rest, fever above 100.4° F, acute loss of bowel or bladder control (such as incontinence, retention of urine, or frequent, small-volume urination), significant leg weakness, a history of major trauma, drug or alcohol abuse, steroid use, or a previous history of spinal column disease. The presence of any of these requires more tests.

In addition, pressure on the nerve roots may cause pain that radiates down the back of the leg *past* your knee. This leg pain may be associated with tingling or numbness that radiates into your feet or toes. This is known as a radiculopathy, or radicular pain. It has also, classically, been referred to as sciatica, but "sciatica" has become somewhat a lay term, and has been loosely used by some to refer to *any* leg pain.

Uncommonly, certain nerve roots that exit higher up in the spine become entrapped (by arthritis, a herniated disk, etc.), potentially leading to pain down the front of the leg to the knee. However, pain radiating to the buttocks or to the back of the thigh, but not past the knee, is usually not a radiculopathy (i.e., due to nerve root entrapment). Pain radiating to these regions is usually referred from the lower back without the benefit of compressed nerve roots, probably by the muscles crossing over the injured area. Therefore, most people developing back pain that radiates down to the buttocks and the back of the thighs, but not past the knee, should still think of this as low back pain, not leg pain (radiculopathy). I will refer to pain radiating down the back of the leg past the knee (radiculopathy) as "true sciatica."

And, just like most low back pain, most sciatica (true or otherwise) goes away by itself, although this leg pain may take a little longer to resolve than does the standard low back pain. Fifty percent of patients with true sciatica recover within a month, and 96 percent recover and function fully by six months. Most herniated disks, even large ones, will dry up and become nearly undetectable within one year.

People often want to see the doctor to make sure that nothing bad is happening. This is often an important, but usually unspoken, "agenda." Pain is a very subjective phenomenon. Pain is the *perception* of discomfort. If we are scared that our pain may signify that something terrible is wrong, then we focus on the pain, and it bothers us more. Once we know that it's just pain, and that nothing dangerous is causing it, we generally pay less attention to it and are able to relax. And most mechanical low back pain is just that: a "pain" issue, not a "harm" issue.

Unless you have one of the "red flags" mentioned above (fever, unexplained weight loss, etc.) low back pain is usually not dangerous. Your doctor will perform a physical examination to make sure that you don't have a neurological problem. If your physician is concerned, a blood test such as an erythrocyte sedimentation rate (ESR), complete blood count (CBC), or others may be ordered to detect a major infection, tumor, or systemic disease. After six weeks of pain, X rays may be taken.

You've doubtlessly heard about magnetic resonance imaging (MRI), the so-called wonder test that tells all. The suspicion that most patients have is that an MRI would clear up all doubts and questions as to diagnosis, but the doctor, HMO, or whoever, is just too cheap to order one. The hype is that the test is perfect—if something is going on it will show up, if nothing's going on then nothing will show up. "My brother told me not to leave the doctor's office until he ordered an MRI" is a comment not uncommonly heard.

Unfortunately, reality is another matter. The truth is that MRIs are far from perfect, and often further confuse the issues and obscure the real cause of pain. On more than one occasion, MRIs have even led to unnecessary surgery. The problem is that they're *too* sensitive. For example, if you took one hundred people who have never had back pain in their life and got lumbar spine MRIs on them, approximately thirty-three of them (one-third) will have a "positive" MRI (i.e., abnormal, degenerated, or bulging disks, often at more than one level). Therefore, just because you have low back pain, and you have a bulging disk on MRI, does *not* mean that the bulging disk is the cause of your back pain. One-third of people without any back pain will have that same bulging disk. So what did the MRI change? Nothing. You wind up having your back pain initially treated with physical therapy, reconditioning, and all the other things you were going to do before you got the MRI anyway. The test didn't change anything. And it cost you and the rest of the health care community time, effort, and money (about $1,000 to $1,500).

Worse, you now probably have an *in*correct idea of what's causing your pain. You might think, "I have bulging disks at L3-4, L4-5, and a degenerated disk at L5-S1. That's why I have back pain." But in many instances you would be wrong. Your pain may be largely due to deconditioning, poor body mechanics, and repetitively exceeding your back's ability to absorb punishment on an almost daily basis. By thinking that your pain is due to bad disks you deny yourself the chance to improve the situation yourself.

An MRI is best for answering a *specific* question your orthopaedic surgeon may have; for example, it may be used to check for a specific diagnosis that may cause him to treat you in a different way (i.e., the pain is so bad, and has been going on for so long, that you're actually considering surgery); or your orthopaedic surgeon may feel a need to exclude more dangerous problems. It does *not* help you to get an MRI "just to see what's going on." Again, if you're not going to narrowly interpret the results to answer a specific question, you're probably going to find lots of things "going on," few of which have any relation to your back pain, which is the reason you ordered the test in the first place. This often results in focusing on radiographic "red herrings" instead of the true symptom-causing problem.

A key issue to understand is that treating mechanical low back pain is different from treating pain in other parts of the body. In other parts of your body a correct diagnosis is essential to initiating appropriate therapy. However, with regard to mechanical low back pain, the exact diagnosis may be somewhat less important. Why? Because the initial treatment for most mechanical low back pain is similar (i.e., reconditioning, which we'll discuss later). In fact, the response of the pain to the initial treatment, as well as the passage of time, is often one of the most important factors in determining an accurate diagnosis.

Even a herniated disk causing true sciatica is initially treated the same as a mechanical low back pain. Less than 10 percent of people with true sciatica (pain radiating below the knee) due to a true herniated disk require surgery. I'll restate that: Over 90 percent of people with a herniated disk leading to true sciatica don't require surgery. And patients are selected for surgical intervention based on their *symptoms, not* their radiological studies.

A herniated disk is unlikely to cause paralysis, and urgent surgery is rarely necessary. Unless you're experiencing progressive leg weakness or the acute onset of bowel and bladder problems, you should probably wait at least three months before you consider surgery. The MRI should then be obtained close to the time of your surgery because, believe it or not, the MRI changes over time. Most herniated disks will shrink in size, without surgery, to the point of being almost undetectable by MRI within one year.

By the way, if you *are* having bowel or bladder trouble (acute-onset urinary incontinence, urinary retention, or frequent, small volume urination) or progressive leg weakness associated with severe back pain, *these are emergencies!* See your doctor as soon as possible, or go to the emergency room.

X rays are also often misinterpreted. Yes, arthritis in your back can hurt. But almost everybody gets "arthritic changes," detectable on X rays, as they age. So again, just because you have low back pain and you also have arthritic changes on your lumbar spine X ray, that *doesn't* mean that the arthritic changes are the major cause of your pain. Lots of people with arthritic changes on their spine X rays have no back pain at all, especially those who maintain good muscle strength and flexibility.

The effect of emotional issues on the intensity and longevity of low back pain cannot be overemphasized. Anxiety and emotional stress may increase tension in your back's muscles, so that less of a mechanical "trigger" is needed to initiate muscle spasm and pain. This increased resting tone (or tension) makes the muscles of the back more susceptible to overload and injury. The subsequent pain of the injury, and fear of what the pain may represent, leads to further anxiety. This anxiety causes the patient to refrain from any activity that leads to pain. This inactivity then leads to deconditioning, which results in weaker tissues and more pain. This cycle of pain and anxiety may then lead to depression, which makes the ultimate treatment of the low back pain much more difficult.

Now, there is a multitude of alleged cures for low back pain, almost none of which have been scientifically validated. How many *have* been scientifically validated? To my knowledge, only three: education, exercise, and in a small percentage of patients with specific indications—surgery. Let's focus on education and exercise.

The first thing we've got to realize is how we got here, why we're having mechanical low back pain in the first place. Again, after ruling out dangerous problems and emotional or tension-related causes, the exact diagnosis is less important. What is important is the fact that education and exercise can help the vast majority of people with mechanical low back pain, no matter what the cause.

What you've got to do is break the vicious cycle of stress overload: You start with a minor strain (usually due to poor body mechanics), decrease your activity level, become deconditioned, become more vulnerable to future injury, continue to use the same poor body mechanics that got you into trouble in the first place, reinjure yourself, decrease your activity level even further, become even more deconditioned, become even more vulnerable to injury, continue to use the same poor body mechanics, reinjure yourself, and so on. It's a vicious cycle, and it's up to you to break out of it.

Let's use an example. You're out walking, you slip, almost fall, but manage to catch yourself. However, while catching yourself you feel something "pop" in your lower back, and boy does it hurt. The pain is worst when you try to move, and it radiates down into your right buttock and halfway down the back of your right thigh. Although your right leg feels weak, due to the fact that it hurts like heck to use it (so it will probably become deconditioned as well), the weakness is not increasing at a significant rate. You haven't had any bowel or bladder problems lately. It is classic mechanical low back pain—intense pain, but not harmful. You get home, limp into bed, and call your physician. Let's discuss the initial things you can do to help.

First things first: You're in pain, and you won't be able to start reconditioning until the pain quiets down to at least a dull roar. Here are the facts as far as pills and rest go:

Two to five days of *relative* rest usually suffices. In most cases, longer periods of rest do not provide any greater benefit. Conversely, a prolonged decrease in activity risks further deconditioning. Please note that *relative* rest does *not* mean absence from all activity, or total bed rest. It merely means that you should avoid activities that cause major pain. The way to stay most comfortable may be by frequent changes in your position, from bed to chair to standing, then back again. It is also important to continue ordinary activities within the limits permitted by your pain if possible. This continuation of ordinary activities has been shown to lead to a quicker recovery.

Although narcotics may be helpful for relieving the initial intense pain, no drug, including narcotics, has ever been shown to be superior to aspirin for relief of long-term low back pain. And it's been looked at to death. The truth is that aspirin is actually a pretty potent drug, but is often overlooked because of its common availability. Remember that pain is subjective (i.e., controlled by perception and emotion). If you think something will ease your pain, it probably will. If you don't think something will ease your pain, it probably won't. Control of anxiety and emotional stress (through education, and understanding that your low back pain is a pain issue and not a harm issue) is therefore an important component of pain control. This reduction of anxiety in combination with the pain-relieving and anti-inflammatory properties of aspirin can be very effective. In addition, aspirin is not addictive, won't make you drowsy, and has fewer side effects than narcotics. People with sensitive stomachs or a history of ulcers should be sure to take aspirin with food (milk alone doesn't count) to protect their stomachs, or should use an enteric-coated form such as Bufferin®, Ecotrin®, or Ascriptin®.

Motrin®, Advil®, Naprosyn®, and all the other nonsteroidal anti-inflammatory medications are cousins of aspirin, and all work about the same. These medications have the advantage of being longer lasting, and on occasion may be somewhat better at pain relieving. As some of the initial pain may be due to inflammation, these nonsteroidal anti-inflammatory medications should initially be taken "around the clock" in order to build up their concentration in your blood, reduce inflammation, and maximize their pain-relieving effect. In some instances a short course of oral steroids (a medrol dose pack) may be appropriate in order to decrease the inflammation present in the early phases of injury.

Valium®, muscle relaxants, and narcotics—are all commonly prescribed for people with acute back pain. The major function of these medications is to sedate you. They may help your mental attitude, reduce anxiety, and make it easier for you to rest, but they're not specifically altering your back's condition. There is no additional benefit to using muscle relaxants in combination with nonsteroidal medications (or aspirin) over using nonsteroidal medications (or aspirin) alone. And Valium®, muscle relaxants, and narcotics may all lead to drowsiness or dependency (addiction).

A word about modalities (ultrasound, massage, heat, ice, iontophoresis, etc.): These may make you temporarily more comfortable by "distracting" your nervous system from incoming pain messages, but they do not specifically cure your back's condition. Again, remember the difference between temporary comfort and long-term cure. It's like drinking a couple of martinis; you'll feel better, but the problem is the morning after. It's just not a long-term cure. And while there is nothing wrong with being comfortable as you go through the rehabilitative process, please do not believe that temporary comfort will actually make a difference in the long run.

In addition, there is no evidence that the benefits of high-tech modalities exceed those of simple hot or cold compresses. And although traction may provide some benefit in the initial treatment of radiculopathy (true sciatica), neither traction nor biofeedback have been found to be effective in the treatment of patients with acute low back pain.

Many people mistake comfort for cure, walk into their physician's office, and inform him that they've *already* been through physical therapy and their back still hurts. Their implication is that further physical therapy is a waste of time. But many times, what they've unfortunately had during physical therapy has been the pure application of modalities, without any rehabilitative exercises (i.e., the failure to implement true rehabilitation).

Likewise, a chiropractor's manipulation has occasionally supplied temporary comfort. But long-term benefit is another issue. Manipulation may be helpful for acute low back pain *without* true sciatica during the first month of symptoms. At the time of this writing, there is no evidence that manipulation is beneficial for patients with true sciatica. It is also unclear as to whether manipulation leads to any long-term benefits or is, in the long run, any more useful than the other modalities (heat, ice, ultrasound, massage, etc.). In addition, manipulation may be harmful in certain circumstances, for example, if a true herniated disk is present. If you do elect to undergo manipulation, you should know that its efficacy is unproven in cases where symptoms have persisted for greater than one month.

Remember: 98 percent of people with low back pain are better by one year, *regardless of therapy*. If they do nothing, 98 percent will be better by one year. If they have ultrasound, 98 percent will be better by one year. If they get manipulated, 98 percent will be better by one year. And if they paint their toenails green and drink prune juice every morning, 98 percent will be better by one year. That doesn't mean that painting their toenails green and drinking prune juice *made* these people better. They would have gotten better anyway. Except that the people who sell green nail polish and prune juice want to take the credit for the improvement so they can sell more green nail polish and prune juice. Understand?

Once a few days have gone by and you're a little more comfortable, you can begin the real long-term cure: education and reconditioning. Please understand that physical therapy requires your participation in order to work. Nobody can make you better; we can only show you how to make yourself better. It's a team effort, and you must be a player, not a spectator. You can't sit up in the stands, eat hot dogs, drink beer, have somebody rub your back, and expect to get better. You've got to suit up, get in the game, and work up a sweat.

Many different treatment protocols have been designed for mechanical low back pain. All require specially trained physical therapists in order to realize maximum benefits. Most good exercise regimes focus on strengthening the spinal extensor muscles (with hyperextension exercises of the thoracic and lumbar spines), followed by strengthening of the abdominal muscles (with sit-ups and similar exercises). Strengthening of the spinal rotators (twisting muscles) may also be helpful in selected cases. Following your supervised program of training sessions, you should continue to perform your strengthening exercises on your own, either at home or in a gym.

In addition to the gradual strengthening of the muscles of your trunk, it is also important to learn how to avoid placing excessive stresses on your back, and to eliminate poor back posture. Improving your cardiovascular (aerobic) fitness is also very important. Time will cure you; exercise, conditioning, and good body mechanics will help to prevent reinjury.

The treatment protocols for leg pain due to radiculopathy (true sciatica) from a herniated disk are somewhat different than those for low back pain. The first priority is usually to get rid of the leg pain. In many cases, this may be accomplished using passive spinal hyperextension exercises (for example, lie facedown on the floor, then push up with your hands to arch your upper body off the floor, while leaving your hips still touching the floor). This exercise tends to compress the back of your disks, and may be combined with epidural steroids (steroids injected alongside the spinal cord). Your therapist may individualize your program based upon which exercises increase or decrease your leg pain, and which exercises "central-ize" your symptoms (move them out of your leg and back up into your lower spine). Once the leg pain has "centralized" (retreated back up the leg), spinal extensor strengthening exercises are begun. These may then be followed by flexion exercises, and occasionally by rotational exercises.

In addition, your legs should be evaluated for strength and flexibility. Those muscle groups that are weak should be strengthened, and those that are tight should be stretched, especially the hamstrings. Remember, the legs and the back usually function together as an interrelated unit. If your legs are weak or tight, you may be compensating for their deficien-cies by transferring stresses to your back. Thus, your back may be paying the price for what is really primarily a leg problem. Also remember that the back pain will recur if the same stressful activities are reinstituted and rehabilitation has not been undertaken.

Besides reconditioning, education is important, very important. You've got to learn how to avoid placing excessive stresses on your back. Simple things like not bending over at the waist to pick up objects on the floor; bend at the knees and keep your back straight. Lift from the legs, not the back. Keep lifted weights close to your body. Never lift and twist at the same time. When you wash your face, instead of keeping your knees straight and bending at the waist, you should put one leg on a step stool to keep that knee bent. This takes pressure off your back. Little things like that can be very important to your back, especially when repeated many times each day over many years. In addition, smoking has been associat-ed with low back pain, one more good reason to quit.

The philosophy of most good patient education regarding back pain is to change the patient's focus from being a passive recipient of health care to becoming an active guardian of her own health. This promotes self-sufficiency and helps the patient to regain a sense of control over her life. The patient should realize that, for the most part, whatever cure he or she will experience lies within him- or herself, not within medication, or the passive receiving of modalities or manipulation. Therapists and physicians should be viewed more as teachers, rather than administrants of pills or other comfort treatments.

And while most back pain resolves, in some people it may improve but never entirely go away. Accept this. Many people live their entire lives with minor aches and pains from sports injuries and the like. The trick is not to focus on them. Don't empower pain to ruin your life.

Psychological factors such as depression, anxiety, and emotional stress have been associated with low back pain, and clearly magnify its severity and duration. For those patients with these issues, psychological review may be very helpful. This approach may help because, even though the pain is real, all pain is still subjective. How we feel about ourselves and our lives as a whole greatly affects how disruptive the pain becomes.

And if you do develop chronic pain, don't think that surgery is always the answer: Whether or not you operate on a herniated disk for pain, after four years the results are the same—minor backache in a certain percentage of patients whether they were operated on or not.

So the message is this: Mechanical low back pain is so common that most will get it at some point in their life. It's usually due to excessive stresses placed on poorly conditioned muscles. Most of the time the immediate pain will resolve by itself. If it doesn't, the long-term cure is education and rehabilitation, not pills, rest, or modalities.

NECK PAIN

The concepts of neck pain are very similar to those of low back pain. Neck pain, which is often associated with pain radiating down the arm due to nerve entrapment, is quite common. It has been estimated that slightly more than half of adults will experience these symptoms during their lifetime. Like low back pain, most neck pain is mechanical in nature, is due to deconditioning, and will improve with reconditioning and education, even if it doesn't resolve entirely.

Let's discuss why you might have neck pain. The muscles of your neck are a lot smaller than the muscles of your back. These smaller muscles have to carry around a twelve-pound bowling ball (your head) all day long. And they get tired, especially if your shoulders slouch forward, because when your shoulders slouch forward your neck follows and leans forward as well. And now, instead of supporting a well-balanced load at the top of a straight column, your cervical (neck) muscles are trying to hold up a bowling ball on top of a column that is continually leaning forward. That takes a lot more effort, and over the course of the day your neck muscles are going to let you know about it. In addition, slouching forward means that your neck has to extend more to keep your head upright. This extra extension may close off the openings (vertebral foramina) from which your nerve roots exit the spine, leading to pinched nerves (nerve root compression).

Again, the cure is reconditioning. Start with isometric strengthening of your neck in flexion, extension, side bending, and rotation. This means applying steady force with your hands in those directions, and resisting with your neck muscles so that your head doesn't actually move. Place your hands on your forehead, not on your chin, which could aggravate your temporomandibular joint (the joint just in front of your ears, where the lower jaw hinges on the skull). You should also stretch your neck in these directions (bending to the right and left, rotating to the right and left, and flexing forward). You may want to avoid stretching back into extension, as this may aggravate any arthritis or stenosis (narrowing of the bone around the spinal cord or its roots) that you may have.

In addition, you should strengthen your scapular retractors (the muscles that pull back on your shoulder blades). It's very important that these muscles be strong so that they can help to keep your shoulders back. Rows or pull-downs (exercises performed in therapy or at the gym) are good for these, but you must be shown how to isolate these muscles or the exercises will probably be ineffective. In addition, some find that generalized shoulder strengthening helps. Any good physical therapist can teach you these exercises. Page 164 shows other suggested neck and scapular exercise programs, for which I thank Frank A. Pettrone, M.D., who permitted me to reprint them here.

In addition, you must learn proper posture. Keep your shoulders and neck back. And just as mother admonished you—don't slouch forward. If you spend a lot of time looking at a computer screen, make sure it's at eye level. If you have to look down at it you will spend the whole day slouching your neck and shoulder blades forward, placing a lot of unnecessary stress on your neck muscles. And at the end of the day, they're going to hurt. Simply elevating the computer screen (i.e., placing the monitor on a box) may help.

However, even though most neck pain is due to muscular strain, you should still pay at least one visit to your physician, preferably a specialist such as an orthopaedic surgeon, to make sure that nothing more serious is going on. The things you want to rule out as a cause of neck pain are radiculopathy (a trapped nerve root), myelopathy (compression of the spinal cord itself), arthritis, infection, and cancer. In addition, if the symptoms were due to an injury, a fracture must be ruled out.

A cervical radiculopathy (a pinched nerve in your neck) causes pain that radiates down your arm, or occasionally to the shoulder. This may be accompanied by numbness, tingling, or arm weakness. Pain may be

NECK EXERCISE PROGRAM

ISOMETRIC NECK EXERCISES—REPEAT TWICE EACH DAY. BEGIN WITH A TEN- TO FIFTEEN-MINUTE MOIST HEAT TREATMENT TO THE NECK, THEN DO THESE

EXERCISES:

1. Lie on back with head on a pillow. Try to push your head back through the pillow. Breathe normally, hold for three seconds. Relax.

   (a) Increase from one to three repetitions as tolerated.

   (b) Increase hold time until you are able to hold for six seconds.

2. Turn over so that you are lying on your right side. Place both hands under right cheek. Push head down as hard as you can. Relax. Repeat as indicated above.

3. Lie on your stomach with forehead on the pillow. Push head down as hard as you can. Relax. Repeat as above.

4. Lie on your left side with a pillow and both hands under your left cheek. Push head down as hard as you can. Relax. Repeat as above.

SHOULDER SHRUGGING:

Repeat frequently throughout the day.

1. Shrug shoulders toward ears. Repeat several times.

2. Shrug shoulders in a circular motion. Repeat several times.

ISOMETRIC RHOMBOID EXERCISES:

Repeat several times during the day.

Stand with arms down at sides, palms facing front. Pull arms behind your back and squeeze shoulder blades together. Hold for three seconds. Repeat several times and increase to ten repetitions as tolerated.

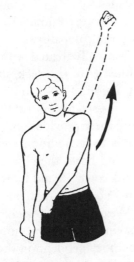

Rotate hand outward so that thumb leads motions. Now raise arm diagonally up and across body and beyond involved shoulder, thumb pointing back. Arm is halfway between shoulder and head. Turn slowly and return to starting position. (Picture yourself pulling a sword out of a sheath.)

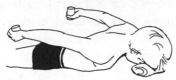

SHOULDER Progressive Resistive Exercises Extension (prone)
Raise arms off floor with weights, keeping elbow straight. Repeat.

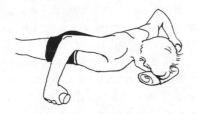

SHOULDER Scapular Exercises Prone Retraction
Keep arms out from sides and elbows bent as you pinch shoulder blades together. Hold. Repeat.

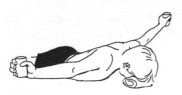

SHOULDER Scapular Exercises Stabilization in Prone
Raise both arms off floor with weights. Keep elbows straight. Hold. Repeat.

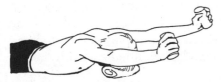

SHOULDER Scapular Exercises Flexion in Prone
Raise arms from floor with weights. Hold. Repeat.

referred to the area between the shoulder blades by either the overlying neck muscles or by an irritated nerve root. Therefore, pain radiating from the neck into this location is not necessarily a radiculopathy.

Like neck pain in general, radiculopathy is usually treated with a progressive exercise regimen to strengthen the muscles of the neck, shoulder blades, and shoulder. Modalities, cervical traction, TENS units (nerve stimulators), medications, or a soft collar may be used to comfort you during the initial period of pain and spasm. Again, these provide comfort, not cure. The best way to obtain long-term cure is to recondition your neck muscles so they can help support your neck and head, thereby relieving symptom-causing nerve compression. The soft collar should be worn on a continuous basis for only a few days, certainly no longer than one or two weeks. You should then wean yourself off it. Wearing it longer can lead to deconditioning of your cervical muscles, making the collar counterproductive. If your muscles weaken and you become dependent on the collar for support, it becomes difficult, if not impossible, to support your head and neck properly. Not a good idea. If no improvement occurs, or if progressive arm weakness or myelopathy (discussed in the next paragraph) occurs, then surgical intervention may be required. However, the majority of patients with neck pain and/or radiculopathy should be able to avoid surgery.

Myelopathy means that the spinal cord itself is being compressed (as opposed to a single nerve root). Herniated disks, arthritic spurs, thickened ligaments, and cervical spinal deformity may all contribute to this compression. Myelopathy is serious, and often requires surgical decompression to treat. The symptoms of myelopathy include arm weakness, lack of fine motor control of the hand (which may lead to difficulty buttoning your shirt, writing, handling change, or performing other intricate tasks), leg weakness or clumsiness (which causes difficulty balancing and walking normally), or pain in your arms or legs with neck motion. Hyperactive reflexes, spasticity (excessively increased muscle tone), sexual impotence, and bowel or bladder changes (incontinence, retention of urine, or frequent, small-volume urination) may also occur. The natural history of myelopathy (what happens without treatment) is one of exacerbations and remissions. That is, it gets better, then worse, then better. It may stay better for years. However, neurological function of the affected arms or legs will not return to normal without surgical decompression. Fortunately, myelopathy is relatively uncommon, and cervical radiculopathy rarely progresses to myelopathy.

Infection and cancer usually lead to severe, unrelenting pain that is unrelated to activity or position. Classically, this is pain that awakens you from a sound sleep. However, these conditions are very uncommon, and unless there is some reason to suspect them (a history of cancer, intravenous drug abuse, nonactivity-related pain over a long period of time that is unresponsive to therapy), it is unproductive to be unduly anxious that you might have them. If you don't have myelopathy, infection, or cancer then you probably don't need surgery.

Neck pain may lead to headaches in the back of the head if the upper nerve roots are compressed, or there is arthritis of the upper cervical spine. Injection of steroids around the nerve roots, or occasionally, surgical decompression, may help relieve this problem.

Again, as in the lumbar spine, X-ray changes in the cervical spine must be interpreted with caution. Degenerative (arthritic) changes are common in the neck after forty. Twenty-five percent of people aged forty to fifty, who have no neck pain, have degenerative changes on their cervical spine (neck) X rays. More than 70 percent of the population have degenerative changes on their cervical spine (neck) X rays by age seventy. These "arthritic" changes are often found in individuals without neck pain, and frequently do not correlate with neck symptoms. Again, just because you have neck pain, and you have X-ray changes (arthritis) in your neck, that doesn't mean the "arthritis" is causing your symptoms. Much of the pain may be coming from your muscles, and may respond well to stretching and strengthening exercises.

Whiplash injuries are a common complaint, affecting one million people in the United States every year. These are usually the result of a rear-end auto collision in which the head snaps backwards, then rebounds forward. This may stretch the structures in the front and/or the back of the neck, causing pain. The pain may come from the muscles, the ligaments, or the disks. The symptoms may begin immediately, or may be delayed for up to a week. The pain may radiate to the shoulders, the head, or to the area between the shoulder blades. Fifty percent of the time whiplash injuries are associated with low back pain. The presence of a radiculopathy (pain radiating to the arms) is associated with a worse long-term prognosis (i.e., a more severe injury that has a lesser chance of completely resolving).

The first step in treating the symptoms following a whiplash injury is the correct diagnosis. Your orthopaedic surgeon will make sure that there is not a specific etiology for the pain, such as an acutely herniated disk, broken bone, or a pinched nerve. Usually there is just generalized soreness, tenderness, and pain with motion, without a specifically identifiable injured structure, i.e., the whiplash syndrome.

There is no magic bullet for this injury. After a short initial period of rest, the basis of therapy is exercise, as you may have guessed. And the key is to realize that therapy requires helping yourself. Again, this is not a spectator sport. Avoid addictive medications (narcotics or muscle relaxants). You'll probably need a physical therapist to show you the exercises to do. But within a short period of time (a few weeks to a couple of months) you should progress to a home program or a gym program, where you continue the exercises on your own.

Unfortunately, on occasion, this injury tends to lead to long-term pain. The lingering of symptoms may be correlated with those patients who are more anxious, or who experience more stressful lives. Even long periods of treatment may not fully resolve the symptoms, especially without stress control. You may have to continue your exercises for a long time, possibly years. It may be helpful to consider them something you'll always need to do on a daily basis; you brush your teeth every day, you comb your hair every day, and you do your neck exercises every day. And while modalities (ultrasound, electrical stimulation, manipulation, etc.) may help to get you through the initial period of pain, they should probably only be used for a relatively short period of time (usually less than one month). Again, these are for comfort only, not cure. Don't confuse the two.

If a brace is given to you, it should be turned around and worn backward (putting the high part in the back). The reason for this is that these braces were designed to protect people with broken necks from flexing forward. Your neck is not broken (the X rays have already shown that), and what you want is to prevent your neck from extending backward, which is the direction that injured you in the first place. As previously noted, after two to three days start to reduce or eliminate brace use. Wearing it for longer periods of time may further decondition your neck muscles, which is precisely what you're trying to avoid. Prolonged disability (extended time off work, etc.) should be avoided, as this also leads to further deconditioning. Surgery is not helpful for the standard whiplash syndrome.

There may be a role for certain psychoactive medications, such as amitryptiline or other related drugs, in the treatment of chronic pain. A pain specialist—usually an anesthesiologist or a physiatrist (rehab doctor)—may be of value here.

Although you obviously need to be initially evaluated by a medical doctor (M.D.), once your physician has ruled out a specific injury, the initially intense pain has somewhat lessened, and you've begun an exercise program, there may be little reason to routinely follow up with a medical professional over a prolonged period of time. Again, taking responsibility for your own pain is a fundamental part of the treatment. Taking responsibility for your pain gives you some measure of control, and becoming independent of pain medications, physical therapists, chiropractors, and ultimately physicians is a worthwhile goal.

SHOULDER PAIN

The shoulder is a common source of complaints in the middle-aged and elderly. Two problems that commonly occur are rotator cuff disorders and the frozen shoulder.

Shoulder pain, especially rotator cuff pain, is usually felt on the outside of the upper arm. This is because pain is often "referred" from an injured area to another area farther down the arm, or leg, as the case may be. Pain originating in the shoulder may even radiate down to the elbow. It would be uncommon for shoulder pain to radiate down past the elbow, and any pain that does so is probably local in origin (actually originates below the elbow) or comes from irritation of the nerve roots in the neck.

Rotator Cuff Problems

Rotator cuff disease is an incredibly common source of pain as we age. First, an anatomy lesson. The shoulder is a ball-and-socket joint. The ball is called the humeral head; it is the head of the large bone of your upper arm, the humerus. The socket is called the glenoid. The shoulder is the most mobile joint in the body. This great mobility allows you to place your hand in space with a great degree of freedom. But the shoulder pays for this great mobility by having the least amount of bony stability of any joint in your body. The ball of the shoulder is like a golf ball precariously balanced on a tee (the glenoid, or socket). The shoulder is therefore highly dependent on soft tissue structures, such as ligaments and muscles, to maintain both its stability and its power. Younger athletes commonly have problems with instability due to ligament damage, but this is less common as we grow older.

Older people have problems with their muscles and tendons, especially the rotator cuff, which is the merging of four tendons over the humeral head (the ball of your shoulder). A tendon is the structure that attaches a muscle to its bone. As an analogy, let's imagine a horse pulling a cart with a rope. The horse is the muscle, the rope is the tendon, and the cart is the large bone of your arm, the humerus. No matter how hard the horse pulls, if the rope breaks, the cart is not going to move. And that's how it is with rotator cuff tears. The rope gets more and more frayed until it finally breaks. The fraying of the rope (degeneration of the rotator cuff) hurts, and an actual tear may hurt even more. A rotator cuff tear is also commonly associated with weakness.

The two muscles that allow you to lift your arm over your head are the deltoid, the big muscle that goes over the top of the shoulder, and the rotator cuff (actually a muscle-tendon unit). The deltoid originates from the acromion, the piece of bone that you feel on top of your shoulder, over your shoulder joint. If the deltoid acted alone, every time you raised your arm, the deltoid would pull the humeral head up into the acromion. It is the rotator cuff's job to stabilize the shoulder so that this doesn't happen. It prevents the humeral head from riding up and hitting the acromion every time you raise your arm. These two muscles, the rotator cuff and the deltoid, oppose each other so that the shoulder's ball remains centered in its socket as the arm is raised.

The problem is that the deltoid is a lot bigger and stronger than the rotator cuff. The rotator cuff is a smaller muscle-tendon unit that is in a critical area, with a critical function. We tend to preferentially use the big muscles of our body, and allow our smaller muscles to weaken. This is one of the reasons why the deltoid muscle maintains its strength better with aging. So if you don't take care of your rotator cuff, it degenerates and gets weaker more quickly than the deltoid does.

Rotator cuff degeneration, or tendinosis, is most commonly an overuse injury. Overuse occurs when repetitive activity leads to cumulative tissue damage that is greater than the body's ability to heal. In other words, you're damaging the tissue over time at a pace that exceeds the speed of repair. This repetitive "microtrauma" eventually leads to tissue breakdown. This should be contrasted with "macrotrauma," in which you injure yourself quickly in a single catastrophic event, like tearing a knee ligament during a fall.

Another factor contributing to rotator cuff degeneration is that the rotator cuff has a relatively poor blood supply and doesn't get enough oxygen for the amount of work it's required to do. The degenerative tendinosis tissue is in and of itself painful, just as any other ischemic (lacking adequate blood supply) tissue is painful: heart attack tissue, the uterus during dysmenorrhea (menstrual cramps), etc. In addition, any tears that occur in the rotator cuff may also cause pain.

As the rotator cuff gets damaged it also gets weaker and is less able to hold the humeral head down on the glenoid (socket) where it belongs. So when you raise your arm up the humeral head gets pulled abnormally higher by the large deltoid muscle. And as the humeral head rides higher, the rotator cuff on top of it bangs into the acromion (bone) above it.

This further damages the rotator cuff, which further weakens it, and so on in a vicious cycle. If the wear and tear goes on long enough the tissue can actually tear all the way through. This is called a rotator cuff tear, and usually indicates a more advanced and chronic problem.

Rotator cuff tendinosis and rotator cuff tears tend to hurt when you lift your arm over your head, and at night when you roll over onto that shoulder. They don't usually hurt with the arm hanging down at the side, or at night when you're lying on your back. Night pain that occurs while you're just resting, and not lying on your shoulder, is a more ominous symptom, and should definitely be mentioned to your treating physician. It may be due to a tumor or infection.

So now we know how the problem came about and why it bothers us. But how do we treat it? Again, we must understand the difference between comfort and cure.

As previously stated, pain occurs when your tissue is subjected to stresses too high for it to handle. Therefore, to get rid of pain you have two options: (1) limit your activity, and (2) improve the quality of your tissue.

If your shoulder hurts every time you raise up your arm, you can avoid pain by not raising your arm up. If you do this for long enough your shoulder may quiet down and not hurt so much. You might actually think that you're getting better. But you're not. In fact, the shoulder has a distinct "use it or lose it" character to it. If you don't use your shoulder's full range of motion you will eventually develop a (secondary) "frozen shoulder," where you have limited motion and are consequently unable to elevate it even if you want to. In addition, a frozen shoulder can hurt in and of itself. Not something you want to develop.

Again, pills, rest, or injections (or hot packs, ultrasound, or other modalities) may buy you comfort, but won't cure you in the long run. They may, however, enable you to better tolerate the cure.

And the cure? It starts with rehabilitative exercises to increase the blood supply to the tendon, strengthen the tendon, and, one hopes, promote the formation of healthy scar tissue. In many cases exercise is all that is necessary, especially if you catch it early. Again, rehabilitation is not a spectator sport; to be successful you've got to be an active participant in your own cure.

If exercise doesn't work, and the pain is bothersome enough, you may need surgery. If there is no complete rotator cuff tear then arthroscopic surgery (with two to three small, almost invisible, incisions) on an outpatient basis (come in that morning, go home that afternoon) is all that is needed.

The procedure involves the removal of the unhealthy rotator cuff tissue. This is analogous to cutting out dead, gangrenous tissue, while leaving the normal tissues alone. In selective cases, a portion of the bone above the rotator cuff, the acromion, that may be impinging against the rotator cuff, is also removed.

If there is a rotator cuff tear, then open surgery, with an incision, is required. (Actually, some surgeons are performing arthroscopic repairs of selected tears, but these repairs are, as yet, not quite as strong as the open repairs.)

Adhesive Capsulitis (Primary Frozen Shoulder)

Another shoulder problem that commonly occurs in the middle-aged is adhesive capsulitis, or primary frozen shoulder. This is especially prevalent in diabetics. Primary adhesive capsulitis should be differentiated from a (secondary) frozen shoulder due to a rotator cuff tear or a shoulder fracture. Both of those latter entities are tougher to treat.

What happens with a primary frozen shoulder is that the lining on the inside of your shoulder gets irritated and sticks together, for no apparent reason. This causes you to slowly lose motion, little by little—again, without any apparent causative event. And one day you notice that you don't have the range of motion you used to. But the process was actually going on for a while before you noticed it. In advanced cases, it can cause pain.

The cure is to stretch out the shoulder. After your orthopaedic surgeon makes sure that nothing else is wrong (such as other shoulder problems that might complicate treatment) you will be started on various stretches to attain motion. This usually works. If it doesn't, and your shoulder bothers you enough that you want it taken care of, the treatment involves putting you to sleep under general anesthesia (so you don't feel anything), manipulating your shoulder (i.e., stretching it out for you), and then arthroscopically cleaning out the inflamed lining of your shoulder. This last step greatly facilitates your rehabilitation, making it easier and less painful for you to resume your stretching exercises, saving you months of therapy. But you still need to do the therapy to *maintain* what your surgeon has *attained* for you. But again, surgery is only performed for those who *can't* attain good motion themselves.

Tennis Elbow

Tennis elbow is a degeneration of the "origin" of the tendons of your wrist and forearm muscles (remember that tendons attach muscles to bones).

The origin of a tendon is its starting point, at its attachment to the bone. The origins of these forearm tendons happen to be located by your elbow, but they aren't really elbow muscles. Even though the way the elbow is used may predispose them to injury (because they cross both the elbow and the wrist), they're really wrist and forearm muscles. It is necessary to understand this to know how to avoid and treat tennis elbow.

Tennis elbow is another example of tendon overuse, or degenerative tendinosis (breakdown of the tendon's tissue from overuse). It occurs most commonly on the outer side of your elbow, but may also occur on the inner side, and occasionally even in the back of the elbow. When it occurs on the inner side of the elbow it's called "golfer's elbow," but it's really the same problem. Either golf or tennis, or any other repetitive activity that stresses these tendons, can lead to tennis elbow, on either the inner or outer side. In fact, up to 95 percent of cases of "tennis elbow" occur in non-tennis players. Musicians, carpenters, assembly line workers, and many others who subject themselves to repetitive activities may develop tennis elbow. In fact, these "industrial" cases of tennis elbow are often the most resistant to treatment. In the industrial setting, the activities most likely to lead to "tennis elbow" involve forearm rotation or lifting with the hands in the "palm-down" position.

The ulnar nerve (funny bone) lies on the inner side of your elbow, fairly close to the tendons. Inflammation or degeneration of the tissue on the inner side of your elbow may irritate this nerve, leading to pain, tingling, or numbness radiating down to the small finger. This will usually resolve when the tendon problem does.

The most important risk factors for developing tennis elbow are age and activity level. That is, it's not the years, it's the mileage. If cumulative trauma occurs at a rate that is too rapid for your body to heal, tendon degeneration, or tendinosis, occurs.

Again, the balance of tissue stresses versus tissue quality comes into play. You don't want to load the tissue too much too soon. Avoid training errors. Start slow, and increase the frequency and intensity of activity slowly. Rapid transitions in the intensity, quality, or duration of your athletics put you at risk for developing overuse injuries.

Proper technique is also important to minimize the stresses placed on the arm. In tennis, swing from the shoulder and step into the ball to generate proper forward body weight transfer. This uses the big muscles of your shoulder, trunk, and legs to generate swing power. This minimizes the work your smaller forearm and wrist muscles have to do; they should only be used to hold the wrist straight. Not stepping into the ball, and trying to swing the racket with your elbow and wrist, places a tremendous amount of stress on these tendons, which can rapidly lead to injury. Inexperienced players often hit the ball late, when it is at their side or even behind them, resulting in little if any forward body weight transfer.

Using a two-handed backhand reduces the stress on your tendons. Make sure that your backhand stroke doesn't allow the elbow ahead of the racket. Players who hit their backhands with a "leading elbow" may be at increased risk of developing tennis elbow. It also helps to play with others who hit the ball at a velocity that is comfortable for you.

The tennis ball should be hit at the center of the racket's percussion (the "sweet spot" in the racket's center). Off-center hits increase stresses in the forearm.

Players should avoid solid-core or wet tennis balls, which increase the forces required to hit them. Windy days also require more force to control the ball.

Don't hit against a brick wall; this requires the elbow to function six times as fast as when hitting to another person on a court. It also requires you to cope with the irregular bounces and angles associated with playing against an irregular surface.

You can greatly reduce the amount of stress your forearm tendons are subjected to, and reduce your chance of injury, or speed your recovery, simply by improving your swing mechanics. It might pay to see your local sports pro for an evaluation. In addition, if you have tennis elbow and you have to do some lifting, keep your hands in the "palm-up" position.

Using the proper tennis equipment will also help to avoid injury. The size and weight of the racket should match the strength of the player. If anything, it is preferable to use a racket that is slightly lighter, to ensure proper positioning of the racket head at the time of ball impact. While there is no absolute scientific proof concerning the best racket to use, a valuable clinical observation is that a midsized (ninety to one hundred square inches of hitting zone) graphite composite lightweight racket offers the best protection.

Oversized rackets have positives as well as negatives. While they tend to absorb vibrations better because of their larger sweet spot, they produce greater stresses with off-center hits, especially if the ball hits the metal frame. That is, oversized rackets reduce stresses as long as the ball is struck in the racket's center. Once the ball is struck off-center, stresses are increased as compared with regular-sized rackets.

Good quality synthetic string at the manufacturer's low-range recommendation for string tension (looser stringing) seems to work the best as well. Strings of smaller size (1.3 mm or smaller) have more "give" than thicker strings and may be helpful.

Using an appropriate grip size is also important. The proper grip handle size should be the same as the working length of your hand. Note that there are two transverse palmar creases. The working length of your hand is measured from the tip of your ring finger to the proximal palmar crease (the transverse palmar crease closest to your wrist, excluding the closest diagonal crease).

However, the evidence is very mixed as to whether a larger or smaller grip is better. Some investigators have found that switching grip size either way, from either large to small *or* from small to large, may improve the symptoms of tennis elbow.

Counterforce bracing has also been shown to be extremely effective in reducing the stresses to your forearm muscles. The counterforce brace is a strap that encircles your forearm muscles just below your elbow. The best braces are wide, have a longer side (which goes up top) and a shorter side (which goes on the bottom), because the top of your forearm is wider than the bottom. Braces that use two straps also seem to work better. The brace for inner tennis elbow should also have a little extension from its top edge to cover the inner side of your elbow.

Counterforce bracing reduces the tendon's load by: (1) preventing full contraction of your muscles (in this way maximal force cannot be generated, and the tendon will not be injured), and (2) by absorbing some of the stresses so that the tendon doesn't have to.

The counterforce brace should be put on as follows: The top part of the brace should sit about two fingers below the elbow crease. Make a tight fist to flex the muscles of your forearm and pull the brace fairly tight. It should be a little loose with your fist (and forearm muscles) relaxed, and should tighten up again when you make a fist. You may want to make some minor adjustments with respect to its location or tightness.

Activity limitation, proper technique, proper equipment, and counterforce bracing will help to decrease the stress load on the origins of your forearm muscles. The other side of the coin is to increase the quality of those tissues. This is done through rehabilitative exercises. The muscle groups worked are the wrist entensors, wrist flexors, and the forearm rotators. In addition, a generalized shoulder-strengthening program should be done to avoid shoulder-deconditioning and future problems.

Weights used should *not* cause pain. Pain means you're further injuring the already damaged tissue. The idea is to strengthen the weakened muscles, not to add to the overuse injury. Wear your counterforce brace while exercising to further reduce the stresses on the origin of the tendons, as you're strengthening the muscles. Start with one-pound dumbbells or a one-pound can of soup. If that causes pain, then just raise your closed fist without holding any weight in it.

Rehabilitative exercises, combined with appropriate bracing, successfully manage about 95 percent of patients with tennis elbow. The other 5 percent continue to have pain that limits their activities. This occurs because the amount of tissue damage is too great for their body to repair. If you're in this situation, then you have a choice to make. Either (1) accept your condition and limit your activities accordingly, or (2) undertake a surgical solution.

The surgical solution involves a small incision, only about two inches long, through which the damaged, abnormal, unhealthy tendon is removed. The body then fills in the resulting defect with abnormal but healthy tissue called scar. The difference is that the tissue removed is pain*ful,* while the scar is pain*less*. It's like a scar on your skin—the scar is abnormal, in that it's different from your normal skin, but it works well enough, and it doesn't hurt. The same thing happens in your tendon. The rate of surgical success is 97 percent.

However, it should be stressed that this is a newer surgical concept. Older surgeries tried to "release" the origin of the tendons from the bone. Not only does this not work well, but it also weakens the forearm muscles, while leaving all of the unhealthy tissue behind. In addition, the release may damage the elbow ligaments located directly beneath the tendons, which may lead to further pain, as well as elbow instability. And once you've had an unsuccessful surgery, the chances that an appropriate surgery can help you decrease to about 84 percent.

HEEL PAIN

Heel pain is an incredibly common problem. The majority of it is due to plantar fascitis (another misnomer, because there is no inflammation, or "-itis," present). This is a degenerative tearing at the origin of the plantar fascia, much like the degenerative tendinosis found in tennis elbow or rotator cuff problems.

The foot's arch is supported by muscles, ligaments, and the plantar fascia. The plantar fascia runs from the heel bone (specifically, the medial tubercle of the calcaneus) to insert into all five toes. It functions as a tie bar: It holds the bottom of the two sides of the arch together, which prevents the arch from collapsing.

If overstressed from repetitive overuse, it suffers a degenerative tearing at its attachment to the heel bone. This leads to pain on the inside of the bottom of the heel. The pain is usually worse during the first few steps in the morning, or the first few steps after prolonged sitting. It generally gets better with a little activity, but may then get worse after prolonged weight-bearing. The pain may be so disabling that you can hardly walk.

On X ray a heel spur is often present. It was previously thought that this was the cause of the pain, and many people have had their heel spurs (unnecessarily) removed. I want to emphasize something right now. The heel spur is a *reaction* to the degeneration of the plantar fascia, *not* the cause of the pain. The spur is not even in the plantar fascia. It's in a muscle that is beneath the plantar fascia (the flexor digitorum brevis). If you take X rays of the opposite foot, which has no pain, you will often find a heel spur as well (63 percent of the time). Many people without heel spurs have very painful plantar fasciitis and many people (over 50 percent) with heel spurs have no heel pain whatsoever. Fifty percent of people with plantar fasciitis don't even have heel spurs. If you have a heel spur you do *not* need it taken out. Excision of the spur may actually make the pain *worse*, by altering the mechanics of the heel pad that cushions that area.

The way to cure plantar fasciitis and get rid of the pain is to take the stress off the plantar fascia. And the number one culprit putting stress on the plantar fascia is a tight heel cord (Achilles tendon and calf muscles). A tight heel cord makes you keep your foot more plantarflexed (ball of the foot down). A tight heel cord doesn't allow your ankle to dorsiflex (allow the ball of the foot to come up). Therefore, at the end of your stride, you tend to go up on the ball of your foot more. This puts more pressure on your arch and on the plantar fascia, which is trying to support it (keep it from getting stretched out).

With your knee straight you should be able to dorsiflex your ankle (bend your ankle so that the forefoot points up toward your head) ten to fifteen degrees from the horizontal. If you can't, there's no need to wonder why you have heel pain. Your tight heel cord is the answer.

And there's no quick fix. Even if you have surgery to correct the problem, if your Achilles tendon is still tight, the pain will probably come back.

So in order to relieve your heel pain you must stretch out your Achilles tendon. One of the best ways to stretch your heel cord is to stand on a step, with the edge of the step directly under the ball of your foot. Only the front of your foot should actually be on the step; the back of your foot should hang off it. Stand on one leg only (the leg that hurts). Hold onto the banister so you don't fall. Then lower your body down. This dorsiflexes your heel (allows your heel to sink down below the level of your forefoot). You should feel a pull in your calf muscles. Always stretch slowly, and in a controlled fashion. Do *not* bounce up and down—that's a good way to injure yourself. Hold the stretch for five to ten seconds, then repeat it. Do this ten times in a row, for at least four or five sessions a day.

Another way to stretch your heel cord is to loop a towel under the ball of your foot and pull up. You might want to stretch out when you get up in the morning, before you take that first (oh so painful) step. It'll help.

The other thing you can do to relieve forces on the plantar fascia, and reduce your pain, is to wear a counterforce brace. This is small, comfortable, cheap (about $18), fits in your shoe, and you'll never know it's there, except that you'll feel better. It works on the same principles that the counterforce brace for tennis elbow does. The important thing is that it works.

Arch supports (about $5 at any shoe store) may also take some stress off the plantar fascia, and make you feel better. However, our experience has been that the counterforce brace works a little better.

You don't need expensive orthotics. You don't need expensive orthotics. You don't need expensive orthotics.

Heel cups don't help plantar fasciitis that much. Heel cups merely gather the fat pad together under the heel to provide more cushioning. This works well for another, less common, cause of heel pain that is found in older patients—atrophy (thinning) of the heel's fat pad. These people have heel pain and tenderness right in the center of the heel, not on the inside of the heel. This is a cushioning problem, and is helped by heel cups and cushioned insoles, anything that increases padding around the heel. Your orthopaedic surgeon or podiatrist should be able to make the appropriate diagnosis for you. They will also make sure that your heel pain is not due to an entrapped nerve or part of a more generalized, systemic inflammatory condition like rheumatoid arthritis, gout, or related diseases.

You may also want to consider limiting your activities until your heel cord is fully stretched out. Cutting down on activities that involve more toeing off (quick walking or jogging) will help. You may also want to walk with shorter strides, as this tends to lessen the intensity of toe-off.

The reason that plantar fasciitis hurts so much in the morning is that we sleep with our feet plantarflexed (forefoot down). This allows our heel cords to get nice and stiff. This causes the plantar fascia, which has also stiffened overnight, to take a lot of load during the first few steps of the morning. The pain continues until we're up and around, which limbers us up. If you're having trouble stretching out the heel cords, it may be because you regress every night when you sleep. Consider night splints, which will keep your ankles at 90° so the heel cord doesn't tighten up. This may help.

If you need immediate comfort you may try some nonsteroidal medication like Advil®, Motrin®, Naprosyn®, or the like. Again, they buy comfort, not cure. You still need to take charge, get in the game, and stretch out those heel cords.

Similarly, a steroid injection or two (three should be considered an absolute maximum) may quiet things down and relieve some pain. But don't have too many—they may dissolve the fat pad, which will give you another reason to have heel pain, which is tougher to treat.

Surgery should only be considered after nine to twelve months of serious stretching, in patients who continue to have heel pain despite having limber heel cords. The injured part of the plantar fascia is released off the heel bone or excised (cut out). Fortunately, if you follow the advice given here, the vast majority of those of you with heel pain will not require surgery.

HIP FRACTURES

Hip fractures are a different sort of entity than the other aches and pains discussed in this chapter. They're not due to overuse or deconditioning. They don't get better with exercise. And they don't allow you the luxury of elective decision making.

They are a very serious, often life-threatening injury, and most often occur in a fairly elderly and debilitated individual. Almost all hip fractures require surgery, usually as soon as the physicians determine that it is safe for the patient to undergo anesthesia. This is usually within twenty-four to forty-eight hours.

Although young people can break their hips in car accidents, and other high-energy situations where there is significant trauma, the vast majority of hip fractures occur in the elderly. In fact, the incidence of hip fractures increases with increasing age, doubling for each decade beyond fifty years. Females are affected two to three times as much as males. The incidence in white women is two to three times that of black and Hispanic women. This is probably due to the increased incidence of osteoporosis (decreased bone density) in elderly white women (see chapter 6).

Hip fractures are serious injuries. Unfortunately, they usually occur in people who don't have the ability to handle a serious injury. The risk of death in the year following a hip fracture is between 14 and 36 percent (up to one in three). After one year, the mortality rate drops back down to normal.

Most (90 percent) of the hip fractures in the elderly result from simple falls, many in the home. So to decrease your risk of getting a hip fracture, you should try to decrease your risk of falling. The risk of falling increases with age due to decreased coordination, slower reaction times, and the prevalence of other diseases that may increase the risk of falling (Parkinson's disease, heart disease, etc.).

However, there are some things that you can do to decrease your risk of falling. Most of the following is probably common sense, but common sense may not be as common as we'd like to think.

First, you need to be honest with yourself. If your balance and coordination aren't what they used to be, then use a cane for support. True, this may be a blow to your dignity and your sense of independence, but it may help you to avoid falls and a subsequent hip fracture that could rob you of your independence even more.

Wear rubber-soled shoes. Many women's shoes have soles made of wood, plastic, or other slippery materials that even a young athlete would have trouble walking in without breaking her neck, especially on waxed or tiled surfaces. If you walk over a wet spot on the kitchen floor while wearing these types of shoes you could be in real trouble. Rubber-soled shoes provide the traction that could be the difference in whether or not you fall.

Wear flats or low-heeled shoes. It helps if the soles aren't too thick, because very thick soles may cause you to lose your sense of surefootedness, especially on uneven ground. Terry slippers are good for walking around the house.

Use the bannister whenever you go up or down the stairs, even if there are only two or three of them. And go up one step at a time if you need to. Try to avoid the stairs when you're tired.

Don't use a sleeping pill at night. As we age, we metabolize medications more slowly, meaning that they stay in our system longer. This can lead to confusion, especially in the dark. Many falls have been related to this. You may also be groggy the next morning, when you try to walk down the stairs to breakfast.

Night-lights are a good idea, and are useful to illuminate your path to the bathroom. If you don't like night-lights then consider having your remote control near at hand. Before you get out of bed, click it on and use the TV to illuminate your path. You can have the volume turned down to avoid disturbing your spouse. Make sure that all small objects are picked up off the floor. Throw away scatter rugs, as these frequently lead to falls, or put a rubber nonslip backing on them.

Maintain good eating habits and good nutrition. This won't help you to avoid hip fractures, but if you do break your hip, or develop another injury, it will go a long way toward helping you heal without ill effects.

If you do get a hip fracture, it probably means surgery. Depending on where the fracture is, and whether or not the two fragments of bone have displaced (moved apart from each other), your orthopaedic surgeon will either fix your hip (put metal into the fragments of bone to hold them together while they heal) or replace the broken part of your hip (with a metal prothesis). The reason we operate on hip fractures is to mobilize the patient (get him or her out of bed) as rapidly as possible. Immobilization may lead to life-threatening complications, such as blood clots in your legs that may break off and go to your lungs, or pneumonia. Therefore, you will be expected to walk one to two days after your operation. This is normal, and healthy. A physical therapist will assist you.

The goal is to get back to the pre-fracture level of function, but only about 50 percent of patients with hip fractures actually do this. The other 50 percent lose some function and independence. Therefore, it is important to attempt to become functional and self-sufficient as quickly as possible. Those who are able to walk within two weeks following surgery have a better chance of living at home one year after surgery. Again, hip fractures are a difficult problem, and should be viewed as such.

OSTEOARTHRITIS OF THE HIP

The hip is a ball-and-socket joint. The femoral head (the ball) fits into the pelvic acetabulum (the socket) with a high degree of exactness. Anything that distorts the round shape of the femoral head, or the smoothness of its socket, may lead to arthritis. Although "primary osteoarthritis" of the knee is common (arthritis from just wear and tear), arthritis of the hip in the absence of a preexisting deformity is very uncommon. The vast majority of osteoarthritis of the hip is caused by a preexisting deformity. The worse the hip deformity, the earlier arthritis strikes, and the more severe it is.

The most common ways the roundness of the hip gets distorted are from hip fractures, avascular necrosis (death of the femoral head's bone due to steroids, alcohol, trauma, sickle cell anemia, and other miscellaneous causes), and childhood disorders such as congenital hip dislocation, Perthes' disease, or slipped capital femoral epiphysis.

An extensive review of hip arthritis is beyond the scope of this chapter. However, there are a few things you may find helpful to know.

The less pressure you place on an arthritic hip, the less it may hurt. Using a cane in the *opposite* hand may decrease the forces across your hip by up to a third. Losing weight is also very helpful. Nonsteroidal anti-inflammatory drugs (Motrin®, Advil®, Naprosyn®) may be helpful in the early stages of hip arthritis, because the pain early on is often due, at least in part, to joint inflammation. No nonsteroidal medication has ever been found to be better than any other, and if one works for you, and doesn't produce any severe side effects (such as gastrointestinal difficulties), you should probably stay with it. If one or two don't work for you, the odds are that none of the others will either. And once the arthritis is advanced (bone on bone), it is highly unlikely that any of the nonsteroidal medications will help.

After trying the above, if your hip pain is still such that it interferes with your daily life and ability to function, you may want to consider getting a total hip replacement. This is actually one of the most successful operations in the entire history of surgery. It is one of the best, if not the best, operation we currently have for improving the quality of a patient's life. It is major surgery, but the rewards often justify it. Younger patients (below fifty or so years) are often not as good candidates for hip replacement, and occasionally hip fusions (fusing the joint so that it doesn't move) or osteotomies (cutting the bones around the hip to redirect the forces onto any good remaining cartilage) are done instead. Your orthopaedic surgeon can provide you with more information.

Conclusion

The foregoing is by no means an all-inclusive list of all the musculoskeletal ailments that can occur. In fact, it's a very select list of a few common ailments that you can actively do something about.

This chapter should not be construed as a text of self-diagnosis or home remedies. Any severe or long-standing musculoskeletal pain or problem should be evaluated by a musculoskeletal specialist, an orthopaedic surgeon who is trained and skilled in the diagnosis and treatment of these problems.

This chapter attempts only to explain the reasons behind some of the more common aches and pains that affect middle-aged and older people, of both sexes. It also tries to tell you that you *can* do something about them, and what that something is.

It is our sincere belief that the patient must take an active role in his or her own health and welfare. Too often, the message given by health care professionals is that the patient is a passive recipient of care that is administered to him or her: Take these pills and rest. Have someone massage you, or do something *to* you.

The patient must contribute. The patient must make the effort to understand his or her problem, and to learn what he or she can do about it. The patient must stay in, or get into, some kind of reasonable shape.

Even surgery is a team effort. The doctor's part is over in a few hours, at the most. The patient must do the postoperative rehabilitation, otherwise even the greatest surgeon in the world will not be able to produce an optimal result.

It used to be that patients would get upset when the doctor looked at them as just "an elbow," or "a knee," and didn't recognize that there was a person attached to that painful joint. Good physicians have learned that we don't treat "knee problems." We treat "a person who has a knee problem."

Well, the time has come for the patient to realize this too. Many patients come in severely overweight, smoking heavily, drinking too much, having not exercised in years, and they wonder why their leg hurts. Then they expect the physician to give them a pill, a shot, or an operation to cure them. They roll their eyes at even the suggestion that they exercise. They didn't come to the doctor to get exercise. They came to get "cured," without pain or effort.

Sorry. It doesn't work that way. The hipbone is connected to the thighbone, which is connected to the rest of you. You can't look at your sore arm as just a sore arm without taking your whole body into account. It's not realistic, and it doesn't work.

The good news, however, is that you *can* make a difference, you *can* take control of your own body. You've just got to make the effort.

You've only got one body. If you let it waste away you won't get another. Isn't it worth taking care of?

Chapter 6

OSTEOPOROSIS—PREVENTABLE AND TREATABLE

WITH STUART WEINERMAN, M.D.

Stuart Weinerman, M.D., an endocrinologist with a primary interest in osteoporosis, wrote this important chapter. He is always accompanied by a resident or medical student who sticks close to his side, hoping to learn more about this relatively new area of women's health. He is currently practicing at the North Shore University Hospital Women's Health Services in Bethpage, Long Island, New York. He is married and has two daughters.

Osteoporosis, a major health problem related to menopause, is a disease of decreased amount of bone, and loss of bone architecture, that increases the risk of fracture. I emphasize that *osteoporosis is a disease, currently preventable and treatable*. As you will see, there is *no reason for women to shrink with aging, or to experience a fracture, just because they get older.*

Why Worry?

Osteoporosis is one of the most frequent major health problems that the average fifty-year-old female will suffer in her lifetime. Approximately 40 percent of all white or Asian women will have an osteoporosis-related fracture unless some intervention is made. There are 1.3 million fractures occurring per year in this country due to this disease, and the number is expected to rise as the population gets older.

The fractures caused by osteoporosis include compression or wedge fractures of the vertebral bones in the spine, fractures of the hip, and fractures of the wrist. Wrist fractures generally heal well, and therefore are not the primary concern. Spine and hip fractures can be associated with much more significant problems. Spinal compression fractures, which occur at a rate of a half million per year in women, can occur even with minimal trauma—simply from coughing, sneezing, or picking up a grandchild. Unlike other fractures, the spinal vertebrae never fully heal and once fractured, their shape remains forever deformed. The cumulative effects of multiple vertebral fractures cause an increase in the normal curve of the spine. This results in loss of height and kyphosis (the dowager's hump) and serious changes in body mechanics—decreased space for the lungs, and loss of waistline—as the ribs fall into the pelvis. These problems are in addition to acute pain at the time of the fractures. Other women have progressive fractures that compress the vertebrae, but they never actually note any sudden, acute severe pain. These fractures also contribute to spinal postural difficulties and lead to chronic back pain over time.

Hip fractures in the elderly can have even more severe effects: 15 percent of elderly women with hip fractures die within the first six months of medical complications such as emboli (clots), which travel from the leg to the lungs, heart attacks, or pneumonias. Approximately 25 to 50 percent of elderly women with hip fractures lose their pre-fracture independence. Many are forced to enter nursing homes or rehabilitation facilities, or need assistance to continue living at home. For many women, this potential loss of independence is the most feared outcome. Hip fractures and their sequelae are the primary reason that osteoporosis is such a tremendous economic burden to our society. The combined costs of osteoporosis-related care—the costs of acute surgery and long-term nursing care—are currently estimated at $14 billion per year.

Hip fractures have been clearly proven to be caused by falling directly on the hip. It is a myth that most women first break the bone then fall. Therefore, anything that increases the risk of falls will also increase the risk of hip fractures. This includes poor vision, using sedative drugs, and lack of safety equipment in the house such as grab bars in the bathroom. Being in poor physical condition, with a reduced ability to break or cushion the fall if it occurs, also contributes. Thus our prevention strategies must include not only maintaining normal bone health, but encouraging normal muscular health and instituting fall prevention strategies. This includes regular exercises such as walking or running to help maintain strong muscles as well as good balance. Fall prevention strategies are discussed in detail later in this chapter.

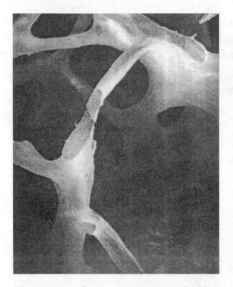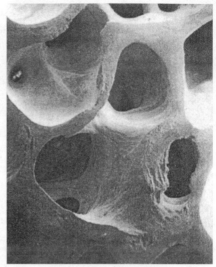

Figure 6.1. Osteoporotic bone (left) compared with normal bone (right).

Adapted from D.W. Dempster et al., "A Simple Method for Correlative Light and Scanning Electron Microscopy of Human Iliac Crest Bone Biopsies: Qualitative Observations in Normal and Osteoporotic Subjects," *Journal of Bone and Mineral Research* 1 (1986): 15–21.

WHY DO WE LOSE BONE?

Bone is a living tissue, constantly remodeling itself—old bone is removed, new bone is laid down. Osteoclasts, the bone-removing cells, are specialized cells that are programmed to dig out a certain, fixed amount of old bone and then stop. The osteoclasts then communicate with the bone-forming cell, the osteoblast, which goes to the site of remodeling. The osteoblast first deposits new bone matrix, which includes collagen and other protein. The osteoblast then helps calcium and other minerals stick to the matrix, filling in the defect left by the osteoclast. The two processes are normally tightly coupled; when resorption is increased, increased formation follows and if resorption is slowed, formation slows. Thus remodeling allows our bones to grow when we are young and to change shape as we add height. After the age of growth, remodeling allows for ongoing repair, i.e., repair of microscopic damage, so that the bone strength remains normal for decades.

YOUR BONE RETIREMENT BANK ACCOUNT

Although bone stops linear growth by age eighteen, it continues to get denser until the mid-twenties. At that point the bones are as strong as they will ever be, as if we put as much bone into our bone retirement bank account at age twenty-five as we ever will. This is an important fact, because women who do not maximize their bone health may never catch up later. Thus adequate calcium intake, normal exercise, avoidance of smoking, etc., are all critically important for children and teenagers. Women who do not have normal bone development, such as women who suffer from anorexia nervosa in this age group, may be at high risk for future fractures.

From the time of peak bone development until menopause, the bone density remains fairly steady, decreasing only slightly. However, estrogen deficiency at the time of menopause causes a fairly rapid rate of bone loss, up to 1 to 3 percent per year at some sites. One to 2 percent per year does not sound significant, but when added over many years results in this current epidemic.

The mechanisms by which estrogen deficiency causes bone loss remain somewhat unclear. Estrogen has a direct beneficial effect on bones. Lack of estrogen causes an increase in the rate of bone resorption. In attempt

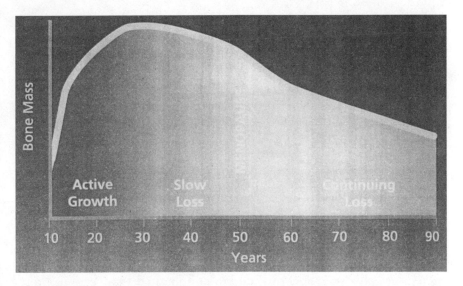

Figure 6.2. Bone mass in women.

Adapted from R.D. Wasnich et al., *Osteoporosis: Critique and Practicum* (Honolulu: Banyan Press, 1989), 179–213.

to keep up, osteoblasts try to increase bone formation but can't fully match the bone resorption. Thus bone loss occurs, due to mismatch in the rates of bone loss versus new bone formation, because the tiny defects left by the osteoclasts are never quite filled in. There may also be indirect effects of estrogen deficiency on calcium metabolism, so that the body does not handle calcium as efficiently. For example, without adequate estrogen, there may be impairment of calcium absorption from the intestines.

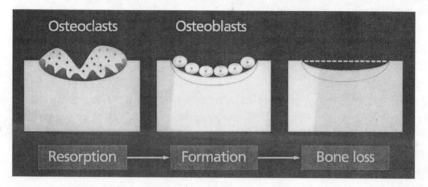

Figure 6.3. Bone remodeling in adults.

Adapted from A.M. Parfitt, "Bone Remodeling in the Pathogenesis of Osteoporosis," *Resident and Staff Physician*, December 1981, 60–72.

Different groups of people have different expected peak bone mass. Men have about 10 to 15 percent higher bone density at peak than women. Similarly, blacks have higher peak bone mass, on average, than whites or Asians. This explains why men and African Americans are relatively protected from this disease. However, osteoporosis can occur in men or blacks, especially if there is a specific cause, such as use of glucocorticoid medicines (see below). Women, especially white or Asian women, are generally at highest risk for developing osteoporosis.

OTHER CAUSES OF OSTEOPOROSIS

Menopause is the most common cause of osteoporosis, but not the only cause. Many other factors can contribute. For example, some patients have rare disorders, such as osteogenesis imperfecta, in which the bone protein or collagen is abnormal due to an inherited trait. Various problems of calcium balance—either too much or too little in the blood—can be associated with bone loss. Smoking and alcohol in excess both contribute to bone loss. Males, somewhat analogous to females, may develop osteoporosis if their hormone (testosterone) levels are too low. The most common secondary cause for bone loss is medications.

MEDICATIONS THAT AFFECT BONE HEALTH

Certain medications can cause or contribute to bone loss in some people. The most commonly encountered are glucocorticoids, excessive doses of thyroid hormone or vitamin A, and antiseizure medicines. The biggest problem, by far, is the effect of glucocorticoids, or steroids, such as hydrocortisone or prednisone. These are not to be confused with anabolic steroids, which are related to testosterone. Glucocorticoids are widely, and appropriately, used in many diseases, such as asthma, arthritis, inflammatory bowel disease, and after transplantation, because they remain the most powerful treatments for these disorders. Unfortunately, they can cause an early and rapid bone loss—up to 10 percent of the spine bone mass in the first six months! It is estimated that one-third to one-half of all patients on long-term steroid therapy will suffer fractures as a side effect. This can occur in anyone, white or black, male or female, young or old. It is therefore highly recommended that anyone being treated with these drugs discuss bone health with a physician, and consider specific evaluation and treatment as appropriate.

Thyroid hormone medications, when used in excess, can have small effects on bone density, but much less than previously published. Thyroid hormone has *no* harmful effect on bone when used in the right dose for the individual patient. It is easy to check that the correct dose is being given by doing a routine blood test called TSH (thyroid stimulating hormone). This test should be done at least annually. No patient should avoid treatment of hypothyroidism due to fear of osteoporosis. However, some patients, such as those with thyroid cancer, must take higher doses than normal in order to suppress the cancer and keep it from recurring. They should discuss bone health with their physician.

Phenytoin (Dilantin®) and other seizure medicines can sometimes interfere with vitamin D metabolism in the liver and contribute to bone loss. Vitamin A when taken in excess appears to have direct toxicity to bone. Vitamin A is present in many over-the-counter vitamin and antioxidant preparations; the dose should be reviewed with a primary care provider. In general, the dose should not exceed the RDA (recommended daily allowance) of 5,000 units. Many other drugs may cause osteoporosis, such as long-term heparin therapy, but are not commonly prescribed and will not be discussed here.

Risk Assessment: How Do You Know if You Are at Risk?

It is fairly easy to diagnose osteoporosis in the patient who has already lost significant amounts of bone or who has suffered spine or hip fractures due to the disease. *The challenge of medicine is to find the patients at risk for the problem and prevent the disease before it occurs.*

The first assessment is to review the risk factors for osteoporosis. This should ideally be done at the time of menopause, when the patient must make decisions concerning estrogen or other therapies.

Who then develops osteoporosis? Women who never achieve their normal peak bone density, who lose it too early, or lose it too quickly. The following are risk factors.

NOT ACHIEVING NORMAL PEAK MASS

- Genetics (family history)
- Inadequate calcium nutrition during childhood and adolescence
- Diseases or drugs that affect bone: anorexia nervosa, glucocorticoids

EARLY BONE LOSS

- Early estrogen deficiency, due to natural or surgical menopause
- Use of drugs that lower estrogen like GnRH agonists (Lupron®), used for endometriosis
- Loss of estrogen due to excessive exercise or anorexia nervosa

RAPID BONE LOSS

- Genetics
- Inadequate calcium intake and/or vitamin D deficiency
- Smoking, which causes estrogen levels to be low
- Alcohol excess, which is toxic to bones
- Inadequate exercise
- Medicines, such as glucocorticoids or excessive doses of thyroid supplements or vitamin A, which can affect bone directly
- Other diseases, such as rheumatoid arthritis or inflammatory

bowel disease, which are associated with a diffuse inflammatory
response in the body including the bones
- Diseases affecting calcium metabolism, such as primary hyper-
parathyroidism

TESTS FOR DETERMINING BONE LOSS

The risk factors are useful but not adequate to determine who is truly at
risk or not. Plain X rays are often not useful, as significant bone loss must
occur before it can be reliably seen on X ray.

The single best way to assess who is likely to suffer a fracture in the
future is a test called bone mineral densitometry (BMD). BMD can be
done by a variety of simple outpatient X-ray tests. The basic concept is
the same for all of them: A beam of energy is passed through the bone.
The denser the bone, the less X ray will pass, much like shining a light
through a curtain—the thicker the material, the less light that will cross.

The best technique uses two different levels of energy, to allow for differences in absorption across bone and soft tissues like fat and muscle.
Thus the test is called DEXA, for dual energy X-ray absorptiometry. This
is similar to an older technique that used an isotope of gadolinium, called
dual photon absorptiometry. It is now rarely used. DEXA allows the rapid
measurement of the bones that we are most interested in—the spine, hip,
and wrist—often is only twenty minutes or less. Ideally, several sites are
measured, because many people have significant differences in bone density between the various sites. The radiation exposure is very low, about
the amount received from natural radiation when flying to Europe and
back on a commercial airline, or about a third of a chest X ray. Current
machines are also very precise, to about 1 percent in the spine and 2 to 3
percent at other sites. Until recently the test was not widely available and
was often not covered by insurance. Fortunately, the number of DEXA
machines, and tests being performed, is rising rapidly as osteoporosis
awareness increases, and most insurers are now covering the procedure.

Several other similar tests are available. Quantitative computerized
tomography (QCT) can be used, but it uses a higher dose of radiation,
costs much more, and has a poorer precision. QCT was used more commonly in the past but less often today. Several new ways of measuring the
forearm or hand density have been developed to lower costs and make
testing more readily available in doctors' offices. These include peripheral DEXA, single X-ray absorptiometry, and radioabsorptiometry. These
tests are not as precise as DEXA and do not look at the sites that we are

most worried about—the spine and hip. Therefore, the tests are best used in communities where DEXA is not available.

BMD, by any of the techniques, gives three results for each site. These are an absolute value, expressed as grams of bone mineral per unit; a comparison to age- and sex-matched controls, or "normals"; and a comparison to young "peak" bone mass at age thirty. The results may be expressed as a percentage of normal, or as a standard deviation score, or distance from the mean value on the bell-shaped curve of normals. At first it does not make sense to compare a woman who may be fifty, sixty, or seventy years old with women aged thirty. The explanation is based on understanding that by age seventy to seventy-five, about 50 percent of all women already have thinned bones and are at risk for fractures. If we compare a seventy-five-year-old woman with other seventy-five-year-old women, she may

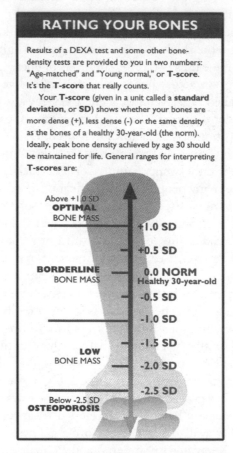

RATING YOUR BONES

Results of a DEXA test and some other bone-density tests are provided to you in two numbers: "Age-matched" and "Young normal," or **T-score**. It's the **T-score** that really counts.

Your **T-score** (given in a unit called a **standard deviation**, or **SD**) shows whether your bones are more dense (+), less dense (-) or the same density as the bones of a healthy 30-year-old (the norm). Ideally, peak bone density achieved by age 30 should be maintained for life. General ranges for interpreting **T-scores** are:

Above +1.0 SD
OPTIMAL
BONE MASS
                           +1.0 SD

                           +0.5 SD

BORDERLINE   **0.0 NORM**
BONE MASS   Healthy 30-year-old

                           -0.5 SD

                           -1.0 SD

                           -1.5 SD

LOW
BONE MASS   **-2.0 SD**

                           -2.5 SD
Below -2.5 SD
OSTEOPOROSIS

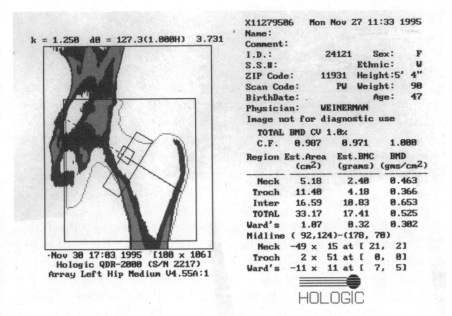

```
k = 1.250  d0 = 127.3(1.000H)  3.731
```

```
·Nov 30 17:03 1995  [100 x 106]
Hologic QDR-2000 (S/N 2217)
Array Left Hip Medium V4.55A:1
```

X11279506   Mon Nov 27 11:33 1995
Name:
Comment:
I.D.:   24121   Sex: F
S.S.#:   Ethnic: W
ZIP Code: 11931 Height:5' 4"
Scan Code: PW Weight: 90
BirthDate: .   Age: 47
Physician: WEINERMAN
Image not for diagnostic use
   TOTAL BMD CV 1.0%
   C.F.   0.987   0.971   1.000

Region	Est.Area (cm^2)	Est.BMC (grams)	BMD (gms/cm^2)
Neck	5.18	2.40	0.463
Troch	11.40	4.18	0.366
Inter	16.59	10.83	0.653
TOTAL	33.17	17.41	0.525
Ward's	1.07	0.32	0.302

Midline (92,124)-(178, 70)
   Neck   -49 x 15 at [21, 2]
   Troch   2 x 51 at [0, 0]
   Ward's -11 x 11 at [7, 5]

HOLOGIC

Figure 6.4a. Example of hipbone density by DEXA method.

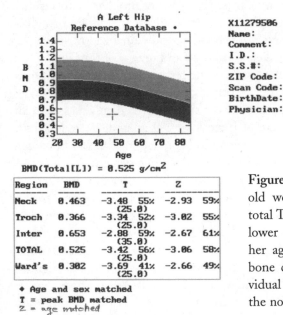

A Left Hip
Reference Database ·

BMD(Total[L]) = 0.525 g/cm²

Region	BMD	T		Z	
Neck	0.463	-3.48	55%	-2.93	59%
		(25.0)			
Troch	0.366	-3.34	52%	-3.02	55%
		(25.0)			
Inter	0.653	-2.88	59%	-2.67	61%
		(35.0)			
TOTAL	0.525	-3.42	56%	-3.06	58%
		(25.0)			
Ward's	0.302	-3.69	41%	-2.66	49%
		(25.0)			

♦ Age and sex matched
T = peak BMD matched
Z = age matched

X11279506   Mon Nov 27 11:33 1995
Name:
Comment:
I.D.:   24121   Sex: F
S.S.#:   Ethnic: W
ZIP Code: 11931 Height:5' 4"
Scan Code: PW Weight: 90
BirthDate: Age: 47
Physician: WEINERMAN

Figure 6.4b. This forty-seven-year-old woman has osteoporosis. Her total T-score is −3.42, a value much lower than would be expected for her age. The graph that plots her bone density shows that her individual bone density falls well below the norm (see +).

be "average" for her own age group—but average at seventy-five is already high risk for fractures! We therefore compare women with an ideal group, thirty-year-old women, who do not suffer from these fractures. This comparison, when expressed as a standard deviation, is called a T-score.

These concepts are quite difficult for many patients and health care providers to grasp. To simplify the interpretation, the World Health Organization (WHO) has published definitions of osteoporosis risk based on bone density results. The WHO uses the T-score to define osteoporosis risk, based on the concepts explained in the previous paragraph. A T-score of −1 or higher is normal, and the patient is considered at low risk. A T-score of −2.5 or lower is considered osteoporosis, or high risk. Between −1 and −2.5 is intermediate risk, called osteopenia (see pages 192 and 193).

Having a low bone mass and other risk factors puts the individual at higher risk. For example, simply having had a previous fracture, or having a mother who suffered a hip fracture, increases the future risk of fracture. Having a low bone density added to the equation results in a risk that is even higher. Many density testing centers will therefore have you complete a questionnaire to help the interpreting physician assess your own personal risk of fractures.

If a woman or a man is diagnosed with fractures or is found to have low bone density, additional testing may be indicated to exclude other diseases and to assess calcium status. Many other problems can result in bone loss, including thyroid disease, adrenal diseases, and abnormalities of calcium metabolism. The testing must be individualized for each person based on history, physical examination, and review of routine lab tests such as blood counts and chemistries. The testing can become complicated or expensive for some patients, but is fairly simple for most.

Many women ask if an initial bone density test, which only measures current bone density and not rate of bone loss, will accurately predict future bone status. In general, there is a very good correlation with low bone density at the time of menopause and having low bone density, and increased risk of fracture, later in life. Some patients may lose bone more slowly or more quickly than average women. For patients who are concerned, the test can be repeated after one, two, or several years to look for rapid bone loss.

A new technique which has received FDA approval is quantitative bone ultrasound. Ultrasound has been used for many years in medicine to obtain images of internal organs, and is completely safe to use. Structural engineers have been using ultrasound for many years for a different purpose—to test the strength of materials. Bone ultrasound is useful in determining bone quality, while BMD determines the amount of bone. Ultrasound has the potential advantages of being very quick, requiring no radiation, and being much less expensive than other BMD techniques. The portable device transmits sound waves through the patient's heel. The sonometer then calculates the speed and attenuation of sound through bone. This measurement then is used to assess the patient's risk for fracture.

Another new development in this field are blood and urine tests that can measure the rate of metabolic activity in the bone—biochemical markers of bone turnover. These tests indirectly measure the activity of the osteoclasts and osteoblasts discussed previously. The most promising of the tests, used frequently in our office, is called n-telopeptides collagen cross-links (Osteomark) assay. This test has the potential of estimating the current rate of bone loss. It measures levels of protein that are excreted in the urine as bone is removed by osteoclasts. The test is performed on a second morning urine sample. The higher the amount of bone protein in the urine specimen, the higher the risk of bone loss. Further, by using this test, doctors can monitor patients who are being treated to see if their bone loss is stopping. It is encouraging to see a normalization of this test very early in treatment, within one or two months, instead of having to wait the usual one to two years for repeat bone density results. The exact role for these tests remains somewhat controversial, but we are routinely using these tests to see if patients are responding to drug therapy.

Prevention of Osteoporosis

Calcium

Adequate calcium intake is absolutely critical for normal bone health. Without adequate calcium intake, your body will steal calcium from your bones to support day-to-day metabolic needs. After many years the slow loss of calcium can result in major bone loss. Unfortunately, most women in our society do not get enough calcium in their diet to meet their bodies' needs. The current recommended daily allowances, according to a NIH expert panel, is 1,000 mg per day, and 1,500 mg per day for postmenopausal women not on estrogen. The average intake for postmenopausal women, according to a large federal survey, is closer to 500 mg a day—or only one-third of basic nutrition. It is not surprising that fractures are so common if women are chronically not getting adequate amounts of this important mineral.

The average postmenopausal female needs to increase calcium intake by about 1,000 mg per day. This can be from dietary sources or supplements. Dietary sources that are rich in calcium include milk, yogurt, hard cheeses, fish with bones (like sardines), fortified products such as orange juice with added calcium, and some tofu products. Low-fat or skim milk products have all the usual calcium or more—there is no reason to increase fat to get calcium. Green vegetables like spinach and broccoli contain calcium but may contain other compounds, such as phytates and oxalates, that make it difficult for the body to absorb the calcium.

Many women can't increase dietary calcium enough to meet the requirements because of lactose intolerance, food allergies, or other reasons, or simply do not want to modify their diets so much. Calcium supplements can be reliably used to maintain adequate intake. Two types are recommended: calcium carbonate and calcium citrate. The type of calcium you take is less important than the fact that you take it. Remember too that, to date, the bulk of the literature or osteoporosis therapy is based on calcium carbonate. Calcium carbonate is cheaper and is effective for most people (see page 227). Calcium carbonate can cause bloating and constipation in some, and is not well absorbed in some very elderly or in those who lack stomach acid. Calcium citrate is a better choice in these cases as it will be somewhat better absorbed and cause less abdominal discomfort. Calcium carbonate is best taken with meals, and calcium citrate on an empty stomach. However, absorption is reasonable either way, so take them when you are most likely to remember on a daily basis.

Many other calcium preparations are available. Most are more expensive than carbonate or citrate and confer no health advantage. "Natural" preparations, such as dolomite, bone meal, or hydroxyapatite may be contaminated with lead and other heavy metals, and should always be avoided (see chapter 7).

Calcium is necessary but not sufficient to stop bone loss. Numerous studies have shown that calcium supplements can slow the rate of bone loss in menopause but do not stop it. Many women are surprised to learn of a low bone density despite faithfully taking adequate amounts of calcium since menopause. It should not be surprising. Remember: Calcium treats calcium deficiency, not estrogen deficiency!

Other minerals such as magnesium and boron have been studied and do not appear to have any significant benefit to normal women on well-balanced, healthy diets.

VITAMIN D

Vitamin D is necessary for adequate absorption of calcium from our diet. Most healthy people make enough vitamin D in the skin using energy from sunlight. Many elderly people, especially nursing home patients or shut-ins, may not make enough and will require additional vitamin D as a supplement. Similarly, people in northern locations may not get enough sunlight, especially in winter, and may require additional vitamin D. Some, especially those with bowel or liver disease, may require much higher doses. For most people, higher doses do not help prevent bone loss and may increase the risk of too much calcium in the blood. Actually, taking toxic doses of vitamin D can cause bone loss. Therefore, if you take more than one multivitamin, read your labels and avoid preparations that do not disclose vitamin D content. The new upper limit for vitamin D is 2,000 IU or 50 mcg. Vitamin D must first be processed in the liver and kidneys into an activated hormone—1,25 vitamin D—before it can function. It is not important to take vitamin D simultaneously with calcium, as long as the total daily vitamin D intake is adequate.

EXERCISE

Bone responds to stress. The pressure placed on the hipbone when you walk makes it stronger. If bone is not continuously stressed, rapid bone loss occurs. This can be seen in the extreme case of the astronauts in space: Without gravity, even these well-conditioned men and women suffer rapid bone loss. Regular exercise is necessary for normal bone health, preferably exercises that push the bone against gravity, like walking, dancing, or running. Swimming, which does not put gravitational strain on bones, has less benefit. Specific weight training may have some additional benefit for bones when added to routine aerobic exercises, but much less than many investigators had hoped. Like calcium, exercise is necessary but not sufficient. It may help slow bone loss, and has many other potential health benefits, but does not fully prevent bone loss due to estrogen deficiency. This is most clearly seen in situations where overzealous exercise and weight loss cause estrogen deficiency in premenopausal women and result in a syndrome called athletic amenorrhea. Exercise does not prevent the bone loss due to the lack of estrogen!

But exercise can reduce the risk of fractures by maintaining normal muscular health. Good strength and normal reflexes have been shown to reduce the risk of falls and of fractures related to falls. Exercise is helpful at any age;

it is never too late to begin, even for men and women in their nineties. It is recommended that anybody beginning a new exercise regimen consult with her physician to help design a safe and appropriate regimen.

FALL PREVENTION STRATEGIES

Falls are very common in the elderly, especially in patients who are frail, have other medical problems, use sedatives, have impaired vision, or live in nursing homes. Many of these falls and associated fractures can be prevented with simple strategies. The home environment needs to be reviewed. Adequate lighting is important, particularly on stairs and in bathrooms. Grab bars and nonskid mats should be installed in bathrooms. Kitchens should be organized so that no one is climbing on old chairs to reach for something on a high shelf. Impediments such as scatter rugs or worn carpeting should be removed. Proper visual care, with updated corrective eyeglasses, can prevent many falls. These simple commonsense approaches can prevent many tragedies.

Medical Therapy

There are three main classes of drugs that have been approved by the FDA for the prevention or treatment of osteoporosis: estrogen, bisphosphonates (Fosamax®), and calcitonin (Miacalcin®, Calcimar®, Cibacalcin®). The three classes have very different properties, but all affect bone by turning off the osteoclast and preventing further bone loss. There may be moderate initial gains in bone mass after starting therapy, especially with Fosamax®, but these agents do not directly increase bone formation.

ESTROGEN

Estrogen replacement therapy remains the "gold standard" for the prevention and treatment of postmenopausal osteoporosis. Numerous studies have shown that estrogen prevents bone loss and reduces the risk of fractures. The earlier the therapy is started, the more the benefit, as more normal bone mass is preserved before loss has occurred. Estrogen may result in a moderate initial increase in bone mass, but its major effect is on preserving existing bone and preventing further loss. This had led to a myth that estrogen can only be used in the first five to ten years after menopause, which is not true. Bones remain responsive to estrogen at any age, and can be used even in the elderly, to prevent further loss and even increase bone mass. This has been clearly demonstrated in several randomized, controlled trials in elderly women. However, the patients already have had major losses, and so therapy is not as effective as primary prevention.

Another myth is that estrogen protects every patient from bone loss. Unfortunately, at the low doses of estrogen that are commonly used, such as Premarin® 0.625 mg or Estrace® 1 mg, approximately 15 percent of patients continue to have some bone loss, especially at the hip. As with any drug, some patients may need a higher dose or different therapy to achieve the desired result.

The overall risks and benefits of estrogen, and different formulations and regimens, are discussed elsewhere in this book. In terms of osteoporotic effects, there is evidence that similar doses of oral or transdermal estrogens have similar effects on bone health. Progestins, which are used to protect the uterus, do not appear to add any bone benefit to estrogen in commonly used doses. Similarly, there are no major differences between cyclic or continuous regimens in terms of bone. High doses of progesterone alone may be beneficial to bone, but may cause other adverse effects and so need further research.

If estrogen replacement therapy is used for prevention of osteoporosis, a fairly long duration of treatment should be planned. Short-term use after menopause, e.g., for two to three years to help control symptoms, does not appear to confer persistent protection against fracture when women really need it—at age sixty-five to seventy. Women should consider staying on estrogen for at least five to ten years for long-term protection. That does not mean that a woman must make a ten-year decision at the time of menopause: Women are always counseled to reevaluate the use, or lack of use, of estrogen every year, based on their own lives and any new information about the safety and benefits of estrogen.

BISPHOSPHONATES

One of the most exciting classes of compounds is the bisphosphonates, which include etidronate (Didronel®) and alendronate (Fosamax®). Bisphosphonates are very effective at turning off osteoclasts (the bone cells that remove bone), and are effective in treating any bone disease characterized by high rates of metabolic activity in the bone. The oldest drug,

Didronel®, is the least potent of the class. Prior studies demonstrated that it is moderately effective in preventing bone loss and fractures when used in a cyclic regimen: Take 400 mg a day for two weeks, followed by eleven weeks of no drug, then repeat the cycle. The drug was not specifically approved by the FDA for osteoporosis, because of relatively small numbers of patients involved in the clinical trials, but remains a useful agent for many patients. Its major advantage is safety, as the drug has minimal side effects at this dose.

Fosamax® is the first of the truly potent oral bisphosphonates, and was approved in 1995 for the treatment of osteoporosis. It was approved in 1997 for the prevention of bone loss in early postmenopausal women who still have normal bone density. In several large clinical trials, involving thousands of patients, alendronate, 10 mg daily, has clearly been shown to not just prevent bone loss, but also increase bone mass by 8 percent in the spine, compared with placebo controls, and 5 percent in the hip. For the first time with any drug, alendronate has been proven to decrease the rate of hip and spinal fractures by 50 percent, and most other fractures by one third. A lower dose of alendronate, 5 mg daily, has been shown to be as effective as standard doses of estrogen in preventing bone loss in early menopausal women with normal bone density. This may be an alternative to estrogen for women who are at high risk for osteoporosis, due to a family history of the disease, or have previously suffered fractures from minor trauma, even if the bone density is currently normal.

There are no data yet available on whether alendronate adds to estrogen's effects on bone, or vice versa. Two large, randomized controlled studies are in progress and should fully answer the question. A small prior study showed that etidronate was additive to estrogen in the treatment of osteoporosis, demonstrating at least a theoretical basis for considering combination therapy.

Alendronate is fairly safe when used correctly. The major potential side effect is irritation to the esophagus or stomach causing heartburn or even ulcerations, if the pill stays in contact with the lining of the gut for too much time. To prevent this problem, Fosamax® must be taken with a full glass of plain water, on a completely empty stomach first thing in the morning. I often suggest that patients take a sip or two of water before putting the pill in their mouth. Wetting the entire passage before the pill is swallowed may help the pill slide down and avoid sticking along the way. Then follow the pill with an eight-ounce glass of water. In addition you must not remain in bed or go back to bed, but be upright. Therefore, take the pill even before you wash up, shower, or get dressed. Nothing can be taken by mouth for at least thirty minutes.

In the large clinical trials, when patients were carefully instructed and motivated to take the pill correctly, there were no differences in side effects in patients taking the active medicine or a dummy pill. The drug does accumulate in bone, and remains buried within the bone for many years, but appears to have no other significant side effects or risks. However, the longest experience with this drug is only five years of use, and questions remain concerning its long-term use. For example, we do not yet know the ideal duration of use.

The availability of alendronate has clearly been responsible for a great increase in interest in, and awareness of, osteoporosis. It represents the first nonhormonal therapy proven to be at least as effective as estrogen, if not better in some situations. Several additional bisphosphonates in research currently, including tiludronate, residronate, and ibandronate, appear quite promising for the future.

CALCITONIN

Calcitonin is a naturally occurring hormone, present in many animal species, that can turn off bone loss. Salmon and human calcitonin have both been used for the treatment of osteoporosis; the salmon form is more potent, molecule for molecule, and has been generally the drug of choice. Until recently, calcitonin had only been available by injection, like insulin, and was quite expensive. This limited the use of the drug. Salmon calcitonin by nasal spray (Miacalcin®) was approved for use in the treatment of osteoporosis in late 1995. The drug is much easier to administer, is well tolerated, and is lower in cost than the injectable form. However, nasal spray calcitonin is only moderately effective in treating osteoporosis. The percentage of patients who respond to this therapy is lower than with estrogen or alendronate. Miacalcin® does not work to prevent bone loss in the first five years after menopause when the rate of loss is highest. Also, its effect on hip bone loss is much less impressive than with Fosamax®. The effect on the reduction in the risk for fractures is still not certain; preliminary reports, as of 1997, of an ongoing trial suggest a small reduction in spinal fractures, again less than seen with the other agents. A potential advantage for Miacalcin® is analgesic, or pain-reduction, effect, seen in some patients when the drug is used after a recent fracture. Miacalcin® should be considered as an alternative therapy for patients who can't take estrogen or Fosamax®. It may be particularly useful in the patient who has recently suffered a spinal compression fracture.

RESEARCH: NEW THERAPIES

Many new therapies are currently in clinical research and appear promising; several of these may be available in the near future, others will require much more testing. The most important development will be drugs that can significantly *increase* bone mass, not just prevent further loss.

Sodium fluoride has been known for many years to increase bone density by up to 10 percent per year in the spine. However, the bone was not always normal, and the increased bone density did not reduce the risk of fractures. A slow-release preparation, using a lower dose of fluoride than previously studied, a modified cyclic regimen, and higher doses of calcium, appeared to increase spinal bone mass and decrease fracture risk. The compound received preliminary approval from an FDA committee in 1995, but final approval has been delayed pending the results of larger trials.

Testosterone is the prime example of the male hormones called androgens; others include the weak adrenal androgen DHEA and synthetic hormones such as nandrolone. Androgens are anabolic, in that they build up muscle and bone mass rather than just prevent further loss. Unfortunately, doses of androgens that are effective in bone also cause unwanted side effects in women: worsening of cholesterol levels and heart disease risk, masculinization of voice, and excessive male pattern hair growth. Many researchers are investigating potential agents that may help bone without causing the unwanted effects. Dehydroepiandrosterone (DHEA) is a steroid hormone secreted by the adrenal gland. DHEA has received enormous publicity as an "anti-aging" compound and can be bought without prescription in health food stores. Studies have shown that the level of this hormone decreases with aging, and lower levels appear to be associated with changes in body composition, immune function, etc. However, as there are no long-term studies of safety or benefit, it is prudent not to use this hormone until the studies are completed (see page 120).

Selective estrogen-receptor modulators (SERMs) are drugs that work like estrogen in some organs but are anti-estrogens in other tissues. The best recognized is tamoxifen, which is an anti-estrogen used in patients with breast cancer. It has partial pro-estrogen effects on bone, and is moderately effective in preventing spinal bone loss. Evista® (raloxifene) was approved in December 1997 for the prevention of osteoporosis. In early postmenopausal women who had normal bone density, raloxifene was very effective in preventing bone loss. The use of this drug in patients who have already lost bone is still being studied. Raloxifene lowers cholesterol levels, like estrogen, but does not improve the good HDL levels. The research studies have not yet proven a reduction in the risk of heart attack. The major benefit is that raloxifene does not stimulate the breast or uterus. Women had no increase in breast tenderness, and preliminary data show a possible decrease in the risk of breast cancer. Long-term studies are planned to study the potential role of this drug in reducing the risk of breast cancer. Because there is no stimulation of the uterus, there is no menstrual bleeding associated with the use of raloxifene, and there is no need for a progestin. There is a slight increase in the frequency and severity of hot flashes with this drug. This anti-estrogen effect on the brain raises potential concerns about the long-term effect on mental function; studies are looking at effect on memory and mood. Raloxifene appears to be well tolerated, with few side effects. There is a small increase in the risk of deep vein thrombosis, or clots in the legs, but this is a relatively rare problem.

Raloxifene is a reasonable alternative to estrogen for select postmenopausal women. The exact role of this drug will certainly be better understood as clinical experience grows with time (see page 112).

Phytoestrogens are plant hormones that mimic some of the effects of estrogen. Epidemiological studies suggest that women in countries (such as Japan) that consume large amounts of phytoestrogens (found in soy products) may be healthier than women in countries with lower intakes. However, there are many other dietary, lifestyle, and genetic variables that need to be considered. There are no large, controlled, prospective studies on the use of phytoestrogens at this time. (See chapter 3 on alternative therapies).

Parathyroid hormone (PTH) causes bone loss if given continuously or at high doses. However, when given in intermittent boluses, PTH causes increases in bone density and strength. Several trials are now using intermittent injections of fragments of the PTH protein and appear to be successful in reversing bone loss. Other therapies may offer the potential to cause intermittent secretion of PTH from the normal parathyroid glands, and thereby stimulate bone growth. Growth hormone and related hormones, such as insulin-like growth factors, also may be able to significantly increase bone mass.

Various analogs, or modifications, of vitamin D are also being investigated. The active form of vitamin D, 1,25 dihydroxycholecalciferol, can increase bone mass but also raises blood calcium, which can be dangerous. Analogs that increase bone mass without increasing blood calcium are being developed.

Other researchers are investigating the molecular biology of the communication between the osteoclast, the bone-removing cell, and the osteoblast, the bone-forming cell. Researchers are designing novel therapies to change the cellular communication to decrease bone loss and simultaneously increase bone formation. This approach is still quite early in research, and may not be applicable to clinical medicine for many years.

The purpose of reviewing future therapies is not simply to list new developments, but to remind readers of the very optimistic future for the treatment of this syndrome. The current drug options are very good, and will be expected to continually improve as new therapies are identified, studied, and become clinically available.

Additional Resources

Many resources are available to help women learn more about osteoporosis. The premier source is the National Osteoporosis Foundation, 1150 17th Street NW, Suite 500, Washington, D.C., 20036, telephone (202) 223-2226. The NOF has three major missions: patient education, physician education, and lobbying to support research. Many educational materials are available from them, including a newsletter with information on the disease. Many local hospitals and community groups have support groups for women with osteoporosis; you should ask your primary physician or contact area hospitals for more information. Many other women's organizations, such as the Older Women's League or Hadassah, have local educational programs.

Summary

Osteoporosis is a common and serious disease that has been mostly ignored in our society in the past. It is a preventable and treatable problem, not an inevitable consequence of aging. All women should meet RDAs for calcium and vitamin D intake and should exercise regularly. Many women should consider bone densitometry to assess the risk of future fractures at the time of menopause, especially if they are undecided about hormone replacement therapy. There are reasonable nonhormonal alternatives now available for patients who do not want estrogen, or who should not take estrogen. The choice of agents should be discussed in detail with the physician and should be based on each individual's specific needs and concerns. With increased awareness of osteoporosis and improved early diagnosis and treatment, women should no longer ever suffer from loss of height or fractures.

Table 6.1. Comparison of Prescription Drugs Available for Osteoporosis

	Hormone replacement	Alendronate	Nasal calcitonin	Raloxifene	Etidronate
Spine BMD	↑	↑↑	minimal effect	↑	↑
Spine fractures	50% ↓	50% ↓	36% ↓	no data	↓ preliminary data
Hip BMD	↑	↑	no effect	↑	↑
Hip fractures	50% ↓ no randomized data	50% ↓	no data	no data	no data
Analgesia (relief of fracture pain)	no	no	+	no	no
Adverse effects	breast tenderness, cancer risks, menses	upper GI irritation	rhinitis	hot flashes, clotting	minor GI irritation
Other benefits	cholesterol and heart, symptoms, etc.	no	no	improved cholesterol, ↓ breast cancer	no
Approved for prevention or treatment	prevention and treatment	prevention and treatment	treatment only	prevention only	no
Cost relative to ERT	+	++	++	++	++

Chapter 7

VITAMINS AND CALCIUM—SPECIFICALLY FOR WOMEN

This chapter will focus on the role of vitamins and minerals and their function and importance to women. In truth, we will hardly scratch the surface of what is known about this rapidly evolving topic. Because of its potential benefits, it would be wrong to leave this subject out of a woman's health book. In spite of this, vitamin and mineral supplements remain one of the most controversial areas in nutrition today.

Never think, even once, that a poor diet can be overcome by taking a vitamin pill. Foods contain vitamins and minerals and complex mixtures of hundreds of substances that just can't be put into a tablet. We generally take nutrition for granted—few of us consume five servings of fruits and vegetables daily. Scientists are only now beginning to understand how very much our very lives, health, and longevity depend on proper nutrition.

Nutritional needs vary for all of us with our stage of life: childhood growing years, adulthood, and old age. Women's needs are even more complex than men's, with our unique nutritional needs during menstruation, pregnancy, lactation, and menopause. It is therefore not possible to make one blanket recommendation for women of all ages.

Although vitamins and minerals are grouped together, they are very diverse in their structure and function. In general, both facilitate various body processes, acting as coenzymes and cofactors, i.e., as catalysts. They also have specialized functions essential to the body. An overview is given in the following table.

TABLE 7.1. VITAMINS AND MINERALS: FUNCTION AND ROLE IN HUMAN HEALTH

Vitamin/mineral	Function	Role in health
Vitamin A	Growth, reproduction, cell differentiation	Vision, healthy skin and hair
Beta-carotene	Provitamin A, antioxidant converts as needed into vitamin A	Immune function, possible reduced risk for cancer
Vitamin D	Regulation of calcium metabolism	Healthy bones
Vitamin E	Antioxidant/free radical scavenger	Reduced risk for heart disease, cataracts
Vitamin K	Blood clotting proteins necessary for bone protein	Regulation of clotting, bone protein
Vitamin C	Reductive reactions, free radical quenching	Immune function, wound healing, iron absorption, reduced risk for cancer/heart disease, cataracts
Vitamin B_1	Energy-releasing reactions	Normal functioning of nervous system/muscles
Vitamin B_2	Oxidation-reduction reactions	Physical performance, cataracts
Niacin	Oxidation-reduction reactions	Normal functioning of nervous system
Vitamin B_6	Metabolism of amino acids, lipids, and certain hormones	Normal functioning of nervous system
Folic acid	DNA synthesis, cell division	Blood cell formation, reduced risk for birth defects, cancer, and heart disease
Vitamin B_{12}	One-carbon metabolism	Blood cell formation, normal functioning of central nervous system
Biotin	Carboxy group transfer, lipid synthesis	Healthy skin and hair
Pantothenic acid	Carbohydrate, fat and amino acid metabolism	Growth and development
Calcium	Cell membrane function, signal transduction	Healthy bones and teeth, muscle function, nerve transmission
Phosphorus	Energy transfer and storage, phospholipids, acid-base balance	Healthy bones and teeth
Magnesium	Energy metabolism	Normal neurological, neuromuscular, and myocardial function
Chromium	Potentiation of insulin action	Regulation of blood sugar
Copper	Activation of enzyme systems in several pathways	Connective tissue, iron metabolism, melanin formation, neurological function, protection against oxidative stress
Iron	Heme-containing proteins and enzymes	Hemoglobin production, immune function, work performance, mental function
Iodine	Component of thyroxine	Thyroid function
Manganese	Activation of several enzyme systems	Normal growth, bones, reproduction, protection against oxidative stress
Zinc	Activation of enzyme systems in various pathways	Growth, reproduction, immune function, skin, hair, and nervous system
Selenium	Component of antioxidant enzyme system	Reduced cancer risk
Molybdenum	Activation of enzymes	Normal growth

Recommended Dietary Allowances

Many of us are familiar with the term RDA, which stands for recommended dietary allowances. These *minimum standards* were set by the Food and Nutrition Board of the U.S. National Academy of Sciences in 1968 and were designed to reflect the amounts of essential nutrients required by most healthy Americans *to prevent nutritional deficiency diseases* and maintain normal health. These recommendations are revised every few years, and in recent years this process has become rather controversial. The latest recommendations[1] are shown in table 7.2 as they pertain to women. As you look over the table, you should be aware that not all scientific agencies or physicians agree with this table.

One major problem is that many Americans, especially young women and most older men and women, don't even eat to RDA amounts of many micronutrients. When we pass up specific food groups, it's kind of like running a car on low oil pressure. The car will be fine at first, but over time, a car that should have lasted and not caused trouble will need to be taken for repairs frequently and soon will not run at all. Well, you can trade in your car and buy a new one, but you're stuck with only one little body. Better take care of it by starting with a good diet!

In the case of some nutrients where there is not enough data to set an RDA, the board set a range called estimated safe and adequate daily dietary intake (ESADDI). There is now accumulating evidence that taking certain nutrients in higher than RDA/ESADDI amounts (often several times the RDA) can decrease the risk for certain diseases. There are numerous examples: antioxidant vitamins, especially vitamin E, offer some protection against heart disease; B vitamins, in particular folate, vitamin B_6, and vitamin B_{12}, can also decrease the risk of heart disease; folate and multivitamins can help prevent some birth defects; and antioxidant vitamins may lower the risk of some precancerous conditions. Remember, the RDAs, which I believe are outdated, were not and are not meant to reflect the higher intakes that provide these health benefits. As we go into the next millennium, let us hope that the concept and definition of RDA will change to amounts needed for "optimum" health. Several leading scientists have realized that chronic diseases cause many deaths and much disability in this country.[2] They have proposed higher intakes of the antioxidant vitamins to help prevent chronic diseases such as heart disease, cancer, and osteoporosis, and to improve the quality of life as well as decrease health care costs.

TABLE 7.2. 1989 RECOMMENDED DIETARY ALLOWANCES

Females   *Vitamins*

(age group)	A mcg RE*	D mcg†	E mg TE‡	K mcg	C mg	B₁ mg	B₂ mg	Niacin mg NE§	B₆ mg	Folate‖ mcg	B₁₂ mcg
11–14	800	10	8	45	50	1.1	1.3	15	1.4	150	2.0
15–18	800	10	8	55	60	1.1	1.3	15	1.5	180	2.0
19–24	800	10	8	60	60	1.1	1.3	15	1.6	180	2.0
25–50	800	5	8	65	60	1.1	1.3	15	1.6	180	2.0
51+	800	5	8	65	60	1.0	1.2	13	1.6	180	2.0
Pregnant	800	10	10	65	70	1.5	1.6	17	2.2	400	2.2
Lactating to 6 mo	1,300	10	12	65	95	1.6	1.8	20	2.1	280	2.6
7–12 mo	1,200	10	11	65	90	1.6	1.7	20	2.1	260	2.6

Minerals

	Calcium mg	Phosphorus mg	Magnesium mg	Iron mg	Zinc mg	Iodine g	Selenium mcg
11–14	1,200	1,200	280	15	12	150	45
15–18	1,200	1,200	300	15	12	150	50
19–24	1,200	1,200	280	15	12	150	55
25–50	800	800	280	15	12	150	55
51+	800	800	280	10	12	175	65
Pregnant	1,200	1,200	300	30	15	175	65
Lactating to 6 mo	1,200	1,200	355	15	19	200	75
7–12 mo	1,200	1,200	340	15	16	200	75

*Retinol equivalents. 1 retinol equivalent = 1 mcg retinol or 6 mcg ß-carotene. 800 RE = 2,667 IU.

†As cholecalciferol. 10 mcg cholecalciferol = 400 IU of vitamin D.

‡α-Tocopherol equivalents. 1 mg d-α-tocopherol = 1 α-TE = 1.5 IU of vitamin E.

§1 NE (niacin equivalent) is equal to 1 mg of niacin or 60 mg of tryptophan. (Tryptophan is a dietary precursor for niacin.)

‖The Institute of Medicine now recommends 600 mcg folic acid for pregnant women, 500 mcg for women who are breast-feeding, and 400 mcg for adults over fourteen years of age.

RDIs or Reference Daily Intakes

U.S. RDIs are set by the U.S. Food and Drug Administration (FDA). They represent a modified version of the RDAs set by the Food and Nutrition Board of the National Academy of Sciences. They were created for purposes of nutrient labeling of food and vitamin and mineral formulations. Many of you may remember seeing percent USRDA values on the labels of food products. Those values were easy to understand. But just when we were all getting comfortable with their use, the FDA switched to the use of RDIs (reference daily intakes), DRVs (daily reference values), and percent DV (percent daily value) for nutrition labeling purposes. It may take some time before we are comfortable again with nutrition labels. The RDIs for vitamins and minerals are shown in table 7.3. Even experts get confused by the discrepancy between the many different numbers quoted by various governmental agencies.

TABLE 7.3. REFERENCE DAILY INTAKES (RDIs) OF VITAMINS AND MINERALS (ADULTS)

Vitamins		*Minerals*	
Vitamin A	5000 IU	Calcium	1000 mg
Vitamin C	60 mg	Iron	18 mg
Vitamin D	400 IU	Phosphorus	1000 mg
Vitamin E	30 IU	Iodine	150 mcg
Thiamine	1.5 mg	Magnesium	400 mg
Riboflavin	1.7 mg	Zinc	15 mg
Niacin	20 mg	Copper	2 mg
Vitamin B_6	2 mg	Selenium	70 mcg
Folate	400 mcg	Chromium	130 mcg
Vitamin B_{12}	6 mcg	Manganese	3.5 mg

The role of vitamins and minerals in several conditions of importance to women follows.

PREGNANCY AND LACTATION

Vitamin A

Pregnant and lactating women have increased requirements for many nutrients, as shown in the RDAs (see table 7.2). Vitamin A requirements remain at 800 RE (retinol equivalents) (2,667 IU) during pregnancy; however, other vitamins and minerals are increased. During lactation, requirement for vitamin A is also increased. It is interesting to note that while the allowance for calcium increases to 1,200 mg daily, the National Institutes of Health recommends 1,500 mg daily.

Folic Acid

During the last few years, research has focused on folic acid for its role in the prevention of two of the most common and severe birth defects, spina bifida (open spine) and anencephaly (absence of brain tissue).

The average intake of folate in the U.S. is about 0.2 mg a day, half the amount that is needed to help prevent birth defects. The significance of the problem is great, for there are about 60 million American women who are of childbearing potential and who are at risk for having a child with birth defects.

It is estimated that 40 to 50 percent of women are not sure when or if they are going to become pregnant; i.e., as many as half of all pregnancies are unplanned. It is further estimated that about four thousand pregnancies a year involve neural tube defects, and approximately 50 percent of these defects might be prevented by simply consuming 0.4 mg (400 mcg) of folic acid starting a month *before* conception.[3] Because neural tube defects occur very early in pregnancy, taking this dose of folic acid before conception and continuing for three months after conception may help prevent some of these devastating birth defects.[4] Other research in the *American Journal of Clinical Nutrition* (1996) showed that taking folic acid during pregnancy in a daily vitamin and mineral supplement reduced the risk of preterm labor and low-birth-weight infants. In addition, antioxidants are now thought to decrease the incidence of preeclampsia. *Interestingly, the synthetic folic acid in vitamin formulas is highly bioavailable as contrasted with the naturally occurring forms in food, which are tightly bound and therefore less efficiently absorbed.* Here is one example of when a vitamin is more efficient than food.

WOMEN AND WEIGHT-LOSS DIETS

Dieting is a way of life for millions of American women. While caloric restriction is sometimes a must, exercise and behavior modification are equally important. Weight-loss diets for women usually suggest 1,000 to 1,600 calories per day. Several years ago the U.S. Department of Agriculture issued a report that stated that *diets providing less than 1,600 calories a day fall short of the RDAs for several vitamins and minerals.* For this reason alone, it is prudent for dieters to take a daily multivitamin supplement to help make up for any shortcomings in their diet. One additional point: Those who do aerobic exercise should be aware that free radical damage may occur because of increased oxidative stress. However, there is evidence that this damage can be minimized or possibly prevented by increased ingestion of antioxidant vitamins. In addition, prescription drugs will be available soon that block fat uptake in the intestine. They will probably also decrease the absorption of the fat-soluble vitamins. Therefore, it will be necessary to take extra fat-soluble vitamins to make up for those that may be lost due to the action of these drugs.

SOME REASONS WHY AGING WOMEN HAVE POOR NUTRITION

Many factors contribute to poor nutrition, especially in older women. You may recognize some of the following in your everyday life, or in an older relative's life.

Living alone is a common cause of poor nutrition. Many women feel that it's not worth the time or effort to shop and cook just for themselves. This can be a special problem after the loss of a spouse.

Physical disability due to chronic disease such as rheumatoid or osteoarthritis makes it difficult to cope with bundles of groceries and shopping carts, to say nothing of bending and lifting pots full of water, slicing, opening bottles and cans, or removing a heavy turkey or chicken from the oven.

Poverty is all too present among seniors. On fixed incomes, many women are forced to decide between food and medications. If this is the case for yourself or anyone you know, please refer to page 101, as free medication is available from many pharmaceutical companies for those who can demonstrate limited resources and insufficient or no insurance coverage.

Dental problems, loss of teeth, and denture pain and problems often make it difficult to eat raw, healthy, firm fruits and vegetables. Because of dental problems, or even no teeth at all, many elderly are forced to switch to soft, less varied, and less nutritious diets.

Educational level may cause lack of understanding of the importance of good nutrition. Actually, this should read "food education level," because often wealthy women with college degrees have worse diets than women of lesser means.

Medications may interfere with vitamin and mineral absorption and metabolism, may decrease your appetite, or may make you less alert, even to your everyday nutritional needs.

Depression, more common in women than in men, may contribute to lack of appetite or increased appetite. Also, medications to control depression may alter desire for food.

In addition to the above difficulties, according to most experts, the elderly have increased requirements for many vitamins and minerals. The current RDAs do not address their needs,[5,6] because for the most part, everyone over the age of fifty-one has usually been lumped together. Recently, the issue of RDAs specifically for the elderly or people who are ill, smokers, etc., has been raised.

Antioxidants

Research shows that increasing the intake of antioxidant vitamins and minerals above RDAs may help reduce the risk of chronic diseases associated with aging. Aging is presumed to be the result of cumulative oxidative stress from exposure to free radicals* from our diets, from the environment, as well as from our own cellular metabolism. If we do not maintain adequate antioxidant protection throughout our lives, free radicals can begin to take their toll. These very active substances cause damage to DNA, proteins, and lipids. There are many types of free radicals and our antioxidant defense system of enzymes and antioxidant nutrients tries to balance them and keep them under control. Vitamins E and C, carotenoids, and selenium are among the potent antioxidant nutrients that help neutralize the free radicals, allowing normal cell function to continue.

---

*Free radicals—highly reactive compounds that can cause injury to genes and cell membranes or transform innocuous chemicals into destructive ones.

CHRONIC DISEASES

Many debilitating diseases that occur as we age may stem in part from our nutritional past as well as present nutrition. Examples are heart disease, various types of cancer, osteoporosis, diabetes, arthritis, and obesity. Nutrition has a definite effect on the health of our brain and state of mind, i.e., our ability to learn, think, concentrate, and remember. So it is sad that so many people with depression, arthritis, heart disease, and diabetes eat so poorly that their illness actually may worsen. It is startling to note that only about *half* of all Americans eat a piece of fresh fruit on any given day.

Menopause: Osteoporosis

Osteoporosis is a common health problem in 25 million older women and older men (see chapter 6). Several factors, both nutritional and nonnutritional, play a part in the development of osteoporosis. Among the nonnutritional factors are genetics, age, sex (females are at higher risk), exercise, illness, smoking, alcohol, estrogen levels during the reproductive years, and whether or not a woman takes hormone replacement or other bone-preserving medications. Among nutritional factors, the most important are calcium and vitamin D, along with vitamins C, B_6, and K. A postmenopausal woman has to make doubly sure that she is ingesting adequate amounts of these important nutrients in particular.

Calcium is the principal mineral in our bones. Not only is it important for our bones, but also muscle and nerve activity depend upon it. For example, if our calcium levels get low, several body systems assure that speedy contributions are made from our bones to keep critical blood levels within normal range.

In general, women have lower than recommended intakes of calcium throughout their entire teens and adult lives. Because prevention is best, we must make sure that our daughters and granddaughters get enough calcium. Calcium is the stuff that builds a bone bank that is full to capacity. Our ability to create this bone bank exists primarily in our early years. We build bone only until age twenty-five to thirty! From then on, we borrow against it for the rest of our lives. If we fully supply our daily metabolic calcium needs through diet and/or supplements, only then does stealing calcium from our bone calcium bank *not* have to occur.

We are beginning to study young women who put themselves on strict diets or have anorexia. Bone densities show that they already have lost bone and have abnormally low bone density levels. Unfortunately, it is probable that their bone bank will remain shortchanged and increase their early risk of fracture. High sodium intake and consumption of fast foods, processed foods, and excess salt added from salt shakers are another set of problems that occur in teenagers and result in an increased urinary loss of calcium. It may make the difference between those who fracture later in life and those who don't. Actually, most of us continue to have excess salt in our diets. Therefore, it would be a good idea for most of us to decrease our salt intake, especially if our calcium intake is less than optimum to begin with.

Although American women generally have low intakes of calcium, there has been a recently established upper limit of 2,500 mg per day. Above this level, there may be excess calcium in the bloodstream, which may increase the risk of forming kidney stones. Excess calcium can also interfere with the absorption of magnesium, zinc, and iron. It is always a good idea to take a full eight ounces of fluid, preferably water, with your vitamins and minerals.

Vitamin D (produced in the skin by sunlight) is necessary for the absorption and metabolism of calcium.[7] Most of us who live in the more northern latitudes do not get sufficient sunlight during winter to produce sufficient amounts of vitamin D. Therefore, we experience increased bone loss over the winter months. In addition, older skin has a decreased capacity to synthesize vitamin D.[8-11] Therefore, average men and women aged fifty-one to seventy are advised to take 400 IUs or 10 mcg of vitamin D. After age seventy, the recommended dose of vitamin D is 600 IU or 15 mcg, while some physicians are recommending 800 IUs or 20 mcg. In addition, as with calcium, there has been an upper limit added for vitamin D, which is 2,000 IU or 50 mcg. Over that upper limit, excess amounts of vitamin D can actually be detrimental to bone.

Phosphorus and magnesium have been recognized as playing an important part in specific aspects of bone growth. Phosphorus tends to be in excess in our diets. It is found in high amounts in proteins, such as meat, chicken, fish, and in soft drinks, which we tend to overconsume. It should *not* need to be supplemented. Therefore, the new recommendations for phosphorus are much lower than in the past. The RDA for magnesium has recently increased to 420 mg/day for the average man and 320 mg/day for the average woman over thirty. It may interest you to know that *magnesium has not been shown to have an effect on calcium absorption,* although it is usually found added with calcium to mineral supplements. Magnesium is easily absorbed while calcium absorption is under the control of vitamin D and its hormones. Vitamins C, B$_6$, and K also have a role in bone formation and maintenance.

Vitamin B$_6$ and vitamin C are essential for the proper synthesis of a bone protein called collagen. Actually, vitamin C may play a significant role in improving bone density. Using food frequency questionnaires and bone density data on 775 postmenopausal women in the PEPI Trial (Postmenopausal Estrogen/Progestin Interventions), which was sponsored by the National Institutes of Health, women who consumed large amounts of vitamin C–rich foods such as broccoli and oranges had better hipbone densities. They found that for every additional daily 100 mg of vitamin C, there was an overall increase in total bone mineral density of 2 to 2.5 percent. Since a 3 percent increase is associated with a 50 percent reduction in hip fractures, this is important news. Women in the study who had the high intakes of vitamin C and calcium had the best bone mineral density of the women studied. The authors of this study from Loma Linda University School of Medicine explained that vitamin C is quickly excreted from the body, pointing to the importance of replenishing adequate amounts of vitamin C from foods. Supplements of vitamin C taken several times over the course of the day might also fill this need.

Vitamin B_6 is also required for the synthesis of osteocalcin, another important bone protein. Vitamin K is also directly involved in the production of this protein. This is another example of interplay between the various micronutrients in maintaining proper functioning of our body.

Heart Disease: Antioxidants

Cardiovascular disease is the leading cause of morbidity and mortality in the industrialized world, and many developing countries are catching up with us in this regard. Although men, at a younger age, are at higher risk than women, heart disease has now become the number one health problem for women. Lifestyle factors such as stress, smoking, and poor diet often increase the risk. While total cholesterol is still considered a risk factor, the emphasis on cholesterol has now shifted to the ratio of HDL cholesterol to LDL cholesterol. Actually, the consensus among experts is that LDL is not detrimental until it becomes oxidized due to inadequate intake of antioxidant nutrients.[12] Once oxidized, LDL starts a sinister sequence of events that eventually injures the cells lining our blood vessels. This results in plaque formation and clogging of our arteries.

There have been a number of studies in recent years, both epidemiological and intervention trials, that show an inverse relationship between antioxidant intake and risk for heart disease. Increased intake of antioxidants protects us from early blood vessel damage and may also decrease the progression of coronary artery disease after it has already occurred.[13–16] However, the benefits of vitamin E in nearly all of the studies were primarily limited to study subjects who took large amounts of d-alpha-tocopherol (vitamin E) supplements.[17] Because vitamin E is expensive, many daily multivitamin formulations contain less vitamin E than many experts would consider desirable.

Perhaps the best known study on vitamin E was the Harvard Medical School Study, which involved 39,910 male physicians who enrolled in the study in 1986. Those who took higher levels of vitamin E, 60 to 100 IU per day, had a 40 percent decreased risk of coronary artery disease at long-term follow-up.

The Nurses' Health Study, which studied 87,245 female nurses, found that the risk of heart disease was about 40 percent lower among women who took vitamin E supplements (at least 100 IU per day) compared with the risk in women who took none.

A study published in the *Lancet* (1996) showed that 100 IU of vitamin E reduced the risk of heart attack by one-third. Vitamin E has also been shown to decrease the risk of stroke and peripheral vascular disease. Other studies show that people who already have atherosclerotic disease and who took high doses of vitamin E had a decrease in repeat heart attack and other cardiac complications. They were also shown to have less coronary artery lesion progression on angiogram and a 50 percent reduced risk of cardiovascular death. Dr. Nigel Stephens from England concluded that for most patients who already have angina, he would encourage the use of high doses of d-alpha-tocopherol to reduce their risk of death.

Because the average American diet provides only about 8 to 12 IU of vitamin E a day, the additional vitamin E needed can only be obtained by taking a supplement. It is interesting to note that many doctors take antioxidant supplements, and many researchers feel that there is already sufficient evidence to recommend routine vitamin E supplementation for everyone, especially the older population. Of interest too is the finding that countries with high incidence of coronary artery disease, such as Scotland and Finland, have been shown to have low levels of vitamin E in blood sampling studies. France and southern Italy, where risk is low, showed higher levels of vitamin E.

Diabetics are another group of patients who often suffer vascular complications from their disease. Impaired vascular function in diabetics may be caused by dysfunction of the cells that line the blood vessels due to excess free radical production and subsequent oxidative damage. Most diabetics are at high risk of oxidative damage because high blood sugars cause excess free radicals, especially when blood sugar control is poor. Researchers from the Joslin Clinic in Boston suggested the use of antioxidants in diabetics to improve insulin action, decrease painful symptoms, help with diabetic eye problems, and help decrease kidney damage and renal protein loss as well as to minimize blood vessel damage. Vitamin C has also been shown to improve circulation in diabetics. Lipoic acid may be another important antioxidant for some diabetics.

Smoking, of course, is a major risk factor for coronary artery disease. Basically, smoking is thought to result in oxidant damage to blood vessels. Vitamin C has been shown in several studies to help counter this effect in some people.

Our lungs are normally protected against free radical damage by their own production of antioxidants as well as by dietary vitamins C, E, and carotenoids. Oxidative injury from smoking and pollution can cause the development of lung disease. Cigarette smoking actually lowers levels of vitamin C. Asthma, chronic obstructive lung disease, and many other pulmonary problems may relate to oxidant stress and therefore may be able to be improved through good diet and antioxidant supplements. Much of this research is just in its infancy.

Heart Disease: Folic Acid

Another vitamin that is emerging as a key player in reducing the risk for cardiovascular disease is folic acid.[18] Increased blood levels of an amino acid called homocysteine have been shown to be a powerful risk factor for vascular disease, coronary artery disease, peripheral vascular disease, and cerebral vascular disease.[19] Postmenopausal women have significantly higher levels of homocysteine than premenopausal women. In the June 11, 1997, issue of the *Journal of the American Medical Association (JAMA)*, a large study from Europe showed that *increased homocysteine levels are a risk factor for vascular disease that is as important as smoking or high blood cholesterol!* The researchers found that increased levels of homocysteine caused even greater risk in men and women who smoked and was associated with the worst prognosis in women with hypertension. The hypothesis is that these elevated levels increase clotting or exert an adverse effect directly on the lining of the blood vessel walls, both of which lead to vascular disease.

A fourteen-year follow-up of 80,082 women in the Nurses' Health Study done by the Harvard School of Public Health showed that "the risk of coronary heart disease was reduced among women who regularly used multiple vitamins as the major source of folate and vitamin B_6 . . . and among those with higher dietary intake of folate and B_6." They found that the women at "lowest risk had intakes of folate above 400 mcg and vitamin B_6 above 3 mg per day." Commentary in the same *JAMA* (February 4, 1998) stated, "These findings show that large segments of this population of 80,000 women have insufficient intake of these nutrients to prevent cardiovascular disease. . . . Women with the lowest intakes of folate and vitamin B$_6$ have the greatest risk of mortality and myocardial infarction. . . . These results support the view that the current recommended dietary allowances for these nutrients are too low to provide optimal protection against cardiovascular disease and need to be revised."

Blood homocysteine levels are determined by genetics as well as folate intake. Many elderly people who have normal folate, B$_6$, and B$_{12}$ levels in their blood actually have decreased levels in their cells. We ascertain this from the fact that their metabolism was only normalized by giving supplements of these vitamins.

In about 30 percent of coronary artery disease cases studied the patients have increased blood levels of homocysteine. Average blood levels for homocysteine are between 5 and 15 micromoles per liter. According to Dr. Graham, a cardiologist from Dublin, the risk of cardiovascular disease appears to increase when homocysteine levels reach 8, double at 12, and are fourfold higher at the highest levels. With suboptimal intake of folic acid, homocysteine levels rise, as it cannot be cleared or properly metabolized by the body. It therefore seems logical that an increased daily intake of folic acid, along with adequate amounts of vitamin B$_{12}$ and vitamin B$_6$, which are needed for the enzymatic reactions, would help reduce homocysteine levels in our blood and decrease the risk for cardiovascular disease.[20] As we can now measure homocysteine levels in the blood, this may become as routine as measuring blood cholesterol. By the way, while safety of folic acid per se is not an issue when higher amounts are ingested over time, some worry about the possible masking of vitamin B$_{12}$ deficiency. This concern can be addressed by simply increasing the intake of vitamin B$_{12}$ somewhat.

A strong relationship between coffee drinking and blood homocysteine levels was made in the January 1997 issue of the *American Journal of Nutrition*. A large study from Norway of 16,175 men and women showed that coffee raises homocysteine levels and therefore risk of heart disease. The more cups of coffee consumed, the higher the homocysteine level. Coffee drinkers who also smoked heavily had the highest homocysteine levels. This study may help provide some answers as to why coffee drinkers are at higher risk than what their cholesterol levels seem to predict, but additional studies are needed to confirm this phenomenon.

SELENIUM

Researchers from the University of Arizona did a four-year study of 1,312 men and women, all of whom had basal cell or squamous cell types of skin cancer. They were given 200 mcg of selenium or placebo to see its effect

on the future development of a second skin cancer. People who participated lived in the eastern plains area of the United States, an area where
there is low selenium in the ground and in the crops. Half the study subjects given selenium supplements were found to have a 63 percent reduction in their risk for colon cancer, a 70 percent reduction in the risk for
prostate cancers, as well as a 52 percent overall reduction in cancer mortality. Because women composed only 25 percent of the group, data on
breast and gynecological cancers were not significant. Oddly, the only
cancers that seemed not to benefit from selenium supplementation were
the skin cancers. While selenium supplements are generally safe at this
dose (200 mcg), much higher doses (above 910 mcg) can be toxic.

CHROMIUM

Chromium is another essential element in human health. Chromium is
necessary for insulin function and thus plays an important role in glucose
metabolism. Adequate amounts of chromium help maintain and normalize proper glucose levels. There is growing evidence that chromium supplementation may be beneficial in some middle-aged subjects with glucose
intolerance and in patients with type II diabetes. Therefore, it is important
that we ingest adequate amounts of chromium especially as we get older.
The estimated adequate and generally safe daily dose for chromium is
from 50 to 200 mcg—with variability according to the individual.

OTHER SUBSTANCES

There are other trace elements, such as molybdenum, which are essential
to human health. For other elements, such as boron, nickel, and silicon,
while there is some evidence that laboratory animals have a requirement,
deficiency or health benefits in humans has not been established.

Coenzyme Q_{10} facilitates enzyme activity in our bodies. It is important for energy production, especially in the heart muscle. There is current research on supplementing coenzyme Q_{10} in congestive heart failure
and other conditions such as cardiomyopathy and hypertension.

Iron

In elderly men and women, the presence of low levels of iron is a risk factor for heart disease and for all causes of mortality. A study that appeared

in the *American Journal of Cardiology* on January 15, 1997, showed that in 3,936 people seventy-one years of age and older, those who had the lowest levels of iron in their bloodstream had the highest risk of death from all causes and the highest risk of death from heart disease. Iron is a major component of hemoglobin, the molecule responsible for carrying oxygen throughout our bodies and our hearts. This does *not* mean that you should arbitrarily begin to take iron supplements. However, it does mean that a good well-balanced diet is important to the maintenance of normal iron and hemoglobin levels, which can easily be checked by your doctor.

Actually, iron deficiency anemia is the most common nutritional deficiency in the United States and in the world. Lack of iron most commonly occurs in young menstruating women who often lose more iron each month than they replenish in their diets. On the other hand, for the postmenopausal women who take hormone replacement, some will menstruate again, and although flow is normally light, the possibility of iron deficiency could increase for them.

The average American diet contains only 5 to 6 mg of iron per 1,000 k/cal. Therefore, many women do not consume enough calories, or enough red meat or dark chicken meat, to meet their iron requirements. If you are a strict vegetarian, you may be at risk for iron deficiency because only 2 to 5 percent of the iron in vegetables and grains can be absorbed, while lean red meat and dark chicken contain 10 to 35 percent bioavailable iron.

When we develop anemia, we feel fatigued, our heart rate increases, and it is exhausting to work. Actually, by the time anemia shows up on our lab tests, we have already depleted our iron stores. Anemia occurs late, after hemoglobin production fails. If your doctor finds that you are anemic, it is usually necessary to take iron supplements for several months in order to restock your iron reserves even *after* your hemoglobin has returned to normal. Simple blood tests will guide your doctor's recommendations. Ferrous sulfate or gentler ferrous gluconate are most often prescribed for this purpose.

Iron and Athletes

Both male and female athletes who run may lose iron through their gastrointestinal tract and may test positive for fecal blood after long runs. Iron can also be lost in tiny amounts in sweat and urine. The continual impact of feet hitting the pavement also causes red cells to break down and this also adds to iron loss. In addition, if you are a real athlete, you may have something that is called sports anemia. This condition can be hard to diagnose, because athletes often have lower hemoglobin levels, not because they are anemic, but because their bodies dilute their total blood volume by conserving salt and water. This "pseudo-anemia" creates increased protection against dehydration and aids sweating.

MISCELLANEOUS: MENTAL FUNCTION/IMMUNE FUNCTION

Some studies have shown that high doses of vitamin E may slow the progress of Alzheimer's disease. Mental function, in particular cognitive studies, have shown the importance of vitamin B_{12} and folic acid. Two recent reports document the prevalence of vitamin B_{12} deficiency in the elderly in the U.S.[21, 22]

Increased amounts of antioxidant nutrients—vitamin E and beta-carotene—and zinc have been shown in some recent studies to improve immune function in the elderly. The *Journal of the American Medical Association* (1997) stated that those who took 200 mg per day of vitamin E produced six times more antibodies after being given a vaccine for hepatitis B or for tetanus infection. (Remember, our immune system is also the key to resisting cancerous growths.) It is important to understand that this benefit can only be achieved by increasing ingestion *above* the current RDAs. Whether you should increase ingestion and by how much is an individual decision to be reached in consultation with your personal physician. This is important, as vitamin E may interact with other medications you are currently taking.

Drug-Nutrient Interactions

Interactions between various drugs we take (both prescription and over-the-counter) and vitamins and minerals occur daily. We must pay attention to even commonly used nonprescription medications such as antacids, laxatives, and painkillers because each can alter nutrient levels. In the prescription drug category, diuretics are among the most commonly prescribed, especially in the elderly. While they enhance the excretion of sodium from the body, in that process some of the water-soluble vitamins are also lost! We have learned a great deal during the last three decades about drug-nutrient interactions, primarily due to the pioneering

TABLE 7.4. INTERACTION BETWEEN DRUGS AND NUTRIENTS

Class	Generic name	Nutrient affected
Antibiotics	Tetracyclines	Vitamin B_2 Vitamin C Calcium Iron
Laxatives	Mineral oil	Vitamin A Vitamin D Vitamin E Vitamin K
Anti-inflammatory drugs	Aspirin	Vitamin C Folic acid Iron
	Indomethacin	Iron
	Sulfasalazine	Folic acid
Cholesterol-lowering drugs	Cholestyramine	Vitamin A Folic acid Vitamin B_{12}
	Colestipol	Vitamin D Vitamin K Folic acid
Anticonvulsants	Phenytoin	Vitamin D Vitamin K Folic acid
Tranquilizers	Chlorpromazine	Vitamin B_2
Antihypertensives	Hydralazine	Vitamin B_6

work of scientists such as Dr. Daphne Roe[23] and Dr. John Hathcock.[24] An example of a few such interactions is shown in table 7.4.

INTERRELATIONSHIP AND SYNERGY AMONG MICRONUTRIENTS

In a metabolic sense, none of the micronutrients works alone. In the body, all metabolic pathways consist of a sequence of events requiring several vitamins and minerals working together. There are other interactions too, such as one nutrient facilitating the absorption of another, or the metabolism of one requiring the action of another. This is why one more time, "balance" is important, i.e., one should ingest appropriate balanced amounts of all the essential nutrients.

Vitamin-Mineral Supplements

In theory, we are all supposed to get all the necessary vitamins and minerals in adequate amounts from a "balanced" diet. But how many of us really know what that is or even think about it while we are eating? "Balanced diet" is a mystery to most of us. Only 15 percent of Americans eat five fruits and vegetables daily. This is why many nutritionists and medical professionals believe that it is a good idea to take a multivitamin-mineral supplement just to be sure.

It is ironic that some of the agencies setting nutritional guidelines advise against taking vitamin-mineral supplements above the RDAs. They have generally ignored the titillating research supporting the potential health benefits of several vitamins and minerals in higher than RDA amounts. If we depend entirely on our diet for the daily needs of micronutrients, most of us will be getting only sustenance amounts of most of them, just enough to prevent developing deficiency states!

Unless you are "educated," shopping for vitamin-mineral supplements can indeed be a frustrating experience, with so many products and combinations to choose from. Here are a few tips: Divided doses are generally better (such as A.M./P.M. formulas). This will enable more efficient absorption and metabolism of the micronutrients. As a general rule, take your vitamins with food; absorption of the nutrients works better this way.

In 1982, there were no specifically formulated vitamin products for women. Patients came to my office with shopping bags full of vitamin bottles, overdosing on some separate vitamins, neglecting others completely. The majority of my patients, however, took none.

Because I believed that almost all women need to supplement their diets, I resolved to create a complete and balanced formula for my patients to simplify their lives. I have always felt that a balanced formula was important because taking too much of any single nutrient may create artificial deficiencies of others or create other adverse effects. It soon became apparent that a once-a-day multivitamin tablet containing twenty-five ingredients in full amounts would be too big to swallow. The required dose of calcium alone was too bulky! Furthermore, taking all of the recommended calcium and vitamins at one time is not advisable. The amount of calcium absorbed in the intestine is usually limited to approximately 300 mg at any one time. Tablets containing more than that simply leave the remaining calcium unabsorbed sitting in your gut, where leftover calcium carbonate may be broken down into gas and produce bloating in some people, according to J. Chris Gallagher, M.D., Professor of Medicine at Creighton University in Omaha, Nebraska, one of the foremost experts on osteoporosis in the country. Therefore, by taking vitamins and calcium in smaller doses with meals over the course of the day, you absorb and metabolize them best and your body can utilize the nutrients more efficiently.

Furthermore, B-complex vitamins, which are good for morning energy, belong in a daytime formula, while calcium, magnesium, and vitamin B_6 and E create a more calming night formulation and help get rid of pesky night leg cramps. It was also apparent that younger women needed more iron to compensate for menstrual blood loss and lower levels of vitamin A (to help avoid birth defects that can come from excess levels of vitamin A). Mature women needed more micronutrients, calcium, and less iron. In addition, I recommend to patients that the B-complex vitamins not be made from yeast, as many people have allergies to yeast; that zinc, copper, and manganese be derived from amino acid chelates so that they are readily absorbable; and that iron be in the gentle form of ferrous gluconate.

Table 7.5 shows my formula for women over forty, and can serve as a guide as to what I hope you would look for in a formulation for yourself.

Two day and two night caplets are taken daily; one day caplet is taken after breakfast and one after lunch, then one night caplet is taken after supper and the last night caplet at bedtime with a small glass of water or with milk and a cookie or a snack of your choice. This night caplet provides sufficient calcium for critical body functions during sleep, when you would not be eating. This nighttime dose therefore protects your bones, which otherwise would be the source for this necessary mineral.

To ensure that I don't forget a dose, I leave one set of vitamins in the bathroom and one in the kitchen. In addition, I keep my vitamins in a beautiful pillbox in my purse. For women who cannot tolerate B-complex vitamins in the morning because of acid breakfasts, e.g., ones that consist primarily of coffee and juice, I recommend taking a night caplet after breakfast. The calcium it contains will buffer the acid, calm your stomach, and protect your bones. The day caplets then are taken after lunch and supper, and the remaining night caplet at bedtime.

TABLE 7.5. VITAMIN AND MINERAL FORMULA FOR WOMEN OVER AGE FORTY

Ingredients	2 day vitamins provide	2 night vitamins provide	DAILY TOTAL
Vitamin A	4,000 I.U.		4,000 I.U.
Beta-Carotene*	2,500 I.U.	2,500 I.U.	5,000 I.U.
Vitamin D$_3$	200 I.U.	200 I.U.	400 I.U.
Vitamin E	100 I.U.	100 I.U.	200 I.U.
Vitamin K$_1$	50 mcg		50 mcg
Vitamin C	250 mg	250 mg	500 mg
Vitamin B$_1$	10 mg		10 mg
Vitamin B$_2$	10 mg		10 mg
Vitamin B$_6$	20 mg	30 mg	50 mg
Niacinamide	25 mg	25 mg	50 mg
Folic Acid	400 mcg		400 mcg
Vitamin B$_{12}$	50 mcg		50 mcg
Biotin	100 mcg		100 mcg
Pantothenic Acid	20 mg		20 mg
Calcium†	450 mg	550 mg	1,000 mg
Magnesium	150 mg	150 mg	300 mg
Potassium	25 mg	25 mg	50 mg
Iron	9 mg		9 mg
Zinc	7.5 mg	7.5 mg	15 mg
Copper	2 mg		2 mg
Manganese	2 mg		2 mg
Iodine	25 mcg	25 mcg	50 mcg
Chromium	50 mcg	50 mcg	100 mcg
Selenium	25 mcg	25 mcg	50 mcg
Molybdenum	25 mcg	25 mcg	50 mcg

*Vitamin A activity.
†USP precipitated calcium.

Reading Calcium Labels and Understanding Purity and Amounts

It is interesting to note that while the RDA for calcium for elderly women is 800 mg, the National Institutes of Health recommends 1,500 mg for postmenopausal women who do not use estrogen, and 1,000 mg for those who do. Actually, 1,500 mg is hard to get just in your diet, so most women not on hormone replacement need to supplement. Because the average intake of calcium among U.S. women is only 500 mg, all of us need to try harder to increase our dietary calcium intake. In reality, many women on hormone replacement need to supplement also, often because they are unable to tolerate milk and milk products, the major dietary source of calcium. Furthermore, whether you take hormones, calcitonin, or Fosamax®, calcium potentiates their effect on bone.

Dolomite and bone meal have been known to be contaminated with lead, arsenic, and other unwanted substances for many years and consumer groups have demanded their removal from store shelves. They should never be used for long-term therapy and never given to children. More than a decade ago, I became aware that there was also a slightly increased amount of contaminants in oyster shell calcium, which comes from the ocean floor. Limestone (calcium carbonate rock) mined in the United States provides some of the inherently purest raw product available. Processing and cleaning the mined limestone further improves its purity.

First, mined limestone is crushed, and impurities removed. This is all that is required for the grade of FCC calcium carbonate. FCC-grade calcium is used in many current calcium products and also in animal feed and paint products. If the label reads FCC calcium, or if there is no USP noted before the word *calcium* on the label, this is what you are getting. *USP calcium is what you should request* for yourself and for your children or grandchildren. USP calcium is a precipitated calcium that has been further purified by boiling and slaking the limestone to remove impurities three separate times.

The process also creates tiny molecules that have large surface areas, making them easy to absorb. As of 1997, only 30 percent of calcium products contain this improved product. It is upsetting to know that cheap FCC-grade calcium is still used by major chains. Because of public pressure, these companies will soon be forced to change this practice.

In 1997, Californians proposed California Proposition 65, which will try to limit the amount of exposure to lead in supplements to 0.5 micrograms a day. This has upset some scientists. They fear that women will stop taking calcium supplements altogether because of their fear of lead. I just think that it is time women were told which supplements are the best. It is important to realize too that sufficient calcium intake protects against lead accumulating in body tissues.

Different calcium sources contain different percentages of elemental calcium. The table below will help you read your labels.

Source	Percentage calcium
Calcium carbonate USP	40.0
Calcium carbonate FCC	40.0
Oyster shell powder	34.5
Dibasic calcium phosphate AN	29.5
Calcium sulfate, USP AN	29.4
Dolomite, white	19.1
Calcium citrate	19.0
Calcium lactate, USP	14.7
Calcium gluconate	9.0

The smaller the percentage of calcium, the more tablets you must take to get the dose you need. For example, while it is possible to put 1,000 mg of calcium from calcium carbonate in two tablets because it contains 40 percent calcium, it would take ten to eleven tablets of calcium gluconate to provide the same 1,000 mg of elemental calcium, because calcium gluconate contains only 9 percent calcium. Learn to read labels. The label should read: USP calcium 1,000 milligrams (mg) or USP elemental or USP precipitated calcium 1,000 mg. If it reads 1,000 mg calcium gluconate, for example, you are only getting 90 mg of calcium.

Closing Thoughts

We all recognize the importance of healthy diet and healthy lifestyle in maintaining good health and minimizing the risk for chronic degenerative diseases. Our ailing health care system can reduce health care costs by putting greater emphasis on disease prevention. Nutrition is a key player in any disease prevention strategy. There is growing evidence for the potential benefits of balanced intakes of essential nutrients in adequate amounts. With respect to vitamins and minerals this may often reflect intakes above the RDAs or what most of us get from our typical diet. Therefore it seems wise to consider an appropriate supplement. In this regard, we may not want to wait for our national policy-making bodies to develop new guidelines for optimum intakes of nutrients in terms of disease prevention and perhaps treatment. We should make our own judgment now based on good science and common sense and include our doctors in this decision.

Notes

1. *Recommended Dietary Allowances*, tenth edition, Food and Nutrition Board, National Research Council, National Academy of Sciences, Washington, D.C., 1989.

2. P. A. Lachance, "Future Vitamin and Antioxidant RDAs for Health Promotion," *Preventive Medicine* 25 (1996): 46–47.

3. L. E. Daly, P. N. Kirke, A. Molloy, D. G. Weir, and J. M. Scott, "Folate Levels and Neural Tube Defects," *Journal of the American Medical Association* 274 (1995): 1698–1702.

4. W. C. Willett, "Folic Acid and Neural Tube Defect: Can't We Come to a Closure?" *American Journal of Public Health* 82 (1992): 666–68.

5. I. Jialal and S. M. Grundy, "Effect of Combined Supplementation with Alpha-Tocopherol, Ascorbate and Beta Carotene on Low-Density Lipoprotein Oxidation," *Circulation* 88 (1993): 2780–2786.

6. P. Knekt, A. Reunanen, R. Jarvinen, R. Seppanen, M. Heliovaara, and A. Aromaa, "Antioxidant Vitamin Intake and Coronary Mortality in a Longitudinal Population Study," *American Journal of Epidemiology* 139 (1994): 1180–89.

7. D. R. Fraser, "Vitamin D," *Lancet* 345 (1995): 104–7.

8. M. F. Holick, "Vitamin D—New Horizons for the 21st Century," *American Journal of Clinical Nutrition* 60 (1994): 619–30.

9. R. P. Heaney, "Bone Mass, Nutrition and Other Lifestyle Factors," *American Journal of Medicine* 95, suppl. 5A (1993): 29s–33s.

10. B. Dawson-Hughes, S. S. Harris, E. A. Krall, G. E. Dallal, G. Falconer, and C. L. Green, "Rates of Bone Loss in Postmenopausal Women Randomly Assigned to One of Two Dosages of Vitamin D," *American Journal of Clinical Nutrition* 61 (1995): 1140–45.

11. F. M. Gloth, III, C. M. Gunberg, B. W. Hollis, J. G. Haddad, Jr., and J. D. Tobin, "Vitamin D Deficiency in Homebound Elderly Persons," *Journal of the American Medical Association* 274 (1995): 1683–86.

12. R. A. Riemersma, D. A. Wood, C. C. Macintyre, R. A. Elton, K. F. Gey, and M. F. Oliver, "Risk of Angina Pectoris and Plasma Concentrations of Vitamins A, C and E and Carotene," *Lancet* 337 (1991): 1–5.

13. H. N. Hodis, W. J. Mack, L. La Bree, L. Cashin-Hemphill, A. Sevanian, R. Johnson, and H. P. Azen, "Serial Coronary Angiographic Evidence That Antioxidant Vitamin Intake Reduces Progression of Coronary Artery Atherosclerosis," *Journal of the American Medical Association* 273 (1995): 1849–54.

14. L. H. Kushi, A. R. Folsom, R. J. Prineas, P. J. Mink, Y. Wu, and R. M. Bostick, "Dietary Antioxidant Vitamins and Death from Coronary Heart Disease in Post Menopausal Women," *New England Journal of Medicine* 334 (1996): 1156–62.

15. M. J. Stampfer, C. H. Hennekens, J. E. Manson, G. A. Colditz, B. Rosner, and W. C. Willett, "Vitamin E Consumption and the Risk of Coronary Disease in Women," *New England Journal of Medicine* 328 (1993): 1444–49.

16. C. J. Boushey, S.A.A. Beresford, G. S. Omenn, and A. G. Motulsky, "A Quantitative Assessment of Plasma Homocysteine as a Risk Factor for Vascular Disease: Probable Benefits of Increasing Folic Acid Intakes," *Journal of the American Medical Association* 274 (1995): 1049–57.

17. M. J. Stampfer and M. R. Malinow, "Can Lowering Homocysteine Levels Reduce Cardiovascular Risk?" *New England Journal of Medicine* 332 (1995): 328–29.

18. J. B. Ubbink, W.J.H. Vermaak, A. Van der Merwe, P. J. Becker, R. Delport, and H. C. Potgieter, "Vitamin Requirements for the Treatment of Hyperhomocysteinemia in Humans," *Journal of Nutrition* 124 (1994): 1927–33.

19. R. M. Russell and P. M. Suter, "Vitamin Requirements of Elderly People: An Update," *American Journal of Clinical Nutrition* 58 (1993): 4–14.

20. J. Blumberg, "Nutrient Requirements of the Elderly—Should There Be Specific RDAs?" *Nutritional Review* 52 (1994): s15–s18.

21. J. Lindenbaum, I. H. Rosenberg, P.W.F. Wilson, S. P. Stabler, and R. H. Allen, "Prevalence of Cobalamin Deficiency in the Framingham Elderly Population," *American Journal of Clinical Nutrition* 60 (1994): 2–11.

22. L. H. Allen and J. Casterline, "Vitamin B_{12} Deficiency in Elderly Individuals: Diagnosis and Requirements," *American Journal of Clinical Nutrition* 60 (1994): 12–14.

23. D. A. Roe, *Drug-Induced Nutritional Deficiencies,* second edition (Westport, CT: Avi Publishing, 1986).

24. J. N. Hathcock, "Metabolic Mechanisms of Drug-Nutrient Interactions," *Federation Proceedings* 44 (1985): 124–29.

PART II

Specific Health Problems of Women

Chapter 8

URINARY TRACT INFECTIONS—PREVENTION AND THERAPY

WITH JOHN MIKLOS, M.D., AND LAWRENCE R. LIND, M.D.

John R. Miklos, M.D., is a fellowship-trained physician in the important new medical specialization known as urogynecology. While in the past, the urologist would look at the bladder, the gynecologist at the vagina and pelvic organs, and the general surgeon at the rectum, urogynecologists are trained to provide comprehensive evaluation of all of these organs. Since problems are often interrelated, it makes sense to have physicians who are experts in all of these organs. Dr. Miklos is a widely published author and lecturer and is well known for his expertise in minimally invasive (laparoscopic) reconstructive pelvic surgery.

Urinary Tract Infections

Each year in the United States, lower urinary tract infections (UTIs) account for approximately five million physician visits and carry a health care cost of about $1 billion. It is estimated that between 10 percent and 20 percent of women will experience a UTI at some time in their lives and approximately 80 percent of women who have one infection will experience another one within a year. If you have an infection, you may experience pain, burning during urination, or frequency of urination. Don't be alarmed. Fortunately, there is much to be optimistic about. Recent medical advances have resulted in more simple tests to diagnose UTIs, improved treatments, and have made it easier to prevent these infections. Sometimes the treatment of UTIs is based upon unproven opinions that health care providers have taken for granted and passed on from generation to generation. It is important to know what the facts are regarding this common problem.

An understanding of generally accepted definitions is essential, as the commonly used terminology can, at times, be confusing. The upper urinary tract consists of the kidneys, which produce urine, and two tubes (ureters) that carry urine from the kidneys to the bladder (the organ that holds urine). The lower urinary tract consists of the bladder and the urethra (the tube through which urine passes from the bladder and the urethra (the tube through which urine passes from the bladder to the outside). Urethritis refers to inflammation of the urethra. Cystitis indicates inflammation of the bladder, and pyelonephritis refers to infection of the kidneys.

UTIs are eight times more common among women than among men. The most common times for UTIs to surface in women are either in the first year of life or with the introduction of sexual activity and pregnancy. UTIs are more common as women age. Alarming discomfort accompanies many infections and, generally, the infecting bacteria are confined to the bladder. Most bacteria are easily treated with antibiotics and the risk of serious complications to an otherwise healthy woman is small.

I THINK I HAVE AN INFECTION

Symptoms of UTIs can vary quite a bit. Most commonly, you will experience a sudden onset of pain or burning with urination. The pain, known as dysuria, is pronounced when urine passes through the urethra and often worse during the final moments of bladder emptying. You may also notice "frequency" and "urgency," and experience the urge to void often despite only a small amount of urine in the bladder. Other signs or symptoms encountered include bloody urine (hematuria), cloudy urine, nighttime urination (nocturia), lower belly discomfort, foul-smelling urine, and, occasionally, urine leakage (incontinence). Take these symptoms seriously! UTIs have the potential to harm your kidneys, which are essential life organs. Under proper care, UTIs can remain uncomplicated and isolated to the lower urinary tract, but if neglected, very serious consequences may develop. A health care professional will often distinguish lower urinary tract infection (cystitis and urethritis) from upper tract infection (pyelonephritis) before recommending therapy because upper infections can be more threatening to the kidneys and require different treatments.

An untreated lower UTI may progress to an upper urinary tract infection. A woman with pyelonephritis will usually have fever, chills, malaise, and occasionally experience nausea and vomiting. Lower back and flank pain (pain in the side of the torso) that is exacerbated with movement is also common.

Why Do Women Get UTIs?

The bacteria usually responsible for UTIs are often the same as those normally found in feces. They all have complicated long names including *Escherichia coli (E. coli), Staphylococcus, Klebsiella, Proteus, Enterobacter, Enterococcus, and Pseudomonas.* The problem is that while they normally are found in the intestines, they don't belong in the bladder. While many bacteria can cause UTIs, *E. coli* accounts for about 80 percent of uncomplicated UTIs, and *Staphylococcus* is the culprit in another 5 to 15 percent. UTIs often get started when bacteria normally found in the stool, or around the anus or the vagina, find their way into the bladder and stick to the bladder lining. The opening to the urethra, unfortunately, is only a few inches away from the rectum and contamination is common from bacterial stool remnants around the anus. At times, these same bacteria can be found contaminating the vagina, which lies immediately below the urethra and is another source of contamination.

The primary pathway in which bacteria enter the urinary tract is through the urethra. A closer look at the female urinary tract provides a second possible reason why women are more prone to UTIs than men. The female urethra is much shorter, providing less resistance to bacterial ascension into the bladder. We don't know if urethral length is the key factor. Also, trauma and, at times, nerve damage to the urethra during childbirth may be important factors in decreasing the long-term defenses against infection. Certainly, no male urethra has ever experienced a vaginal childbirth, which is another explanation for why women experience UTIs more often than men do.

SEXUAL INTERCOURSE

Perhaps the most common way the bacteria move into the urethral area is through sexual intercourse. The risk of UTI in young women rises dramatically with the start of sexual activity. Several studies show that women with UTIs are more likely to have had intercourse within the previous twenty-four to forty-eight hours than are women without UTIs. It is presumed that intercourse spreads bacteria around the genital area; this is especially true if the woman is engaging in both vaginal and anal intercourse. As we discussed earlier, the vulvar areas are commonly contaminated with bacteria. Even the most conventional sexual activities bring skin of the vulva in close contact with the urethra. Furthermore, any bacteria present on the partner's penis or genital area is certain to be in contact with the urethra. UTI risks in some ways are similar to sexually transmitted disease risks. Multiple partners or infected partners will increase the risk of urinary, vaginal, and cervical infection. This is definitely a situation where more is not better!

Fingers can also spread bacteria from the rectal and vaginal area to the urethra. In cases of anal sex, your partner should use a condom, then throw it away and wash his penis and hands before engaging in other sexual activity. If bacteria enter the lower urinary tract during sexual activity, urinating promptly will usually wash them out. You should drink enough fluids before sex so you can urinate within ten to fifteen minutes afterward. Voiding after intercourse will help wash out bacteria that may have entered the urethra and is a useful preventive measure. You can also take a warm bath or use a bidet or a movable shower head to cleanse the vulvar and perianal areas. These are all good cleansing methods to prevent the contamination of the urethra by bacteria from the vulvar and anal areas. More forceful streams, such as a Jacuzzi jet, theoretically can force bacteria from the vagina into the urethra and are therefore not recommended.

Douching has been shown in several studies to *increase* the risk of vaginal and cervical infections. Presumably, the normal and protective bacteria (lactobacilli) are washed out in the douching process, leaving the vagina more vulnerable to contamination. The studies do not look specifically at UTIs but if the vaginal area is more susceptible to infection, then the urethra and bladder are also more susceptible. In general, douching is not recommended.

BIRTH CONTROL METHODS

Certain types of birth control (i.e., diaphragms and spermicide) make women more prone to UTIs. Using a diaphragm may increase the risk of UTIs by as much as four times. Research has suggested that this may be due to trauma to the urethra, decreased sensation to void, and poor bladder emptying, all of which can happen with diaphragms because they must remain in place for at least six to eight hours after sex. Bacteria may also enter the urethra during insertion and removal of the diaphragm, or if it is left in place too long.

Just as douching may wash out the protective bacteria in the vagina, spermicide can also kill the protective lactobacilli in the vagina, encouraging infection and causing bacteria to multiply and possibly to contaminate the urethra. Use of a diaphragm, which traps spermicide in the vagina for long periods, in addition to having its own harmful effects, presumably intensifies this effect.

It is important to receive a balanced message: Spermicide and diaphragms may increase UTIs but unprotected sexual relations carry major risks. There are many contraceptive methods available. If UTIs are a frequent problem, you should seek counseling about other methods.

How Can I Prevent Recurrent UTIs?

Approximately 25 percent of women who have had cystitis will have a recurrent infection. Health care providers commonly counsel patients on various voiding, hygiene, and dietary habits in hope of preventing UTIs. Behaviors that may cause recurrent UTIs include: long intervals between emptying the bladder, inadequate fluid intake, direction of wiping after defecation, tight undergarments, bathing habits, and topical irritants. Also, certain dietary substances erode the bladder lining, making it more vulnerable to bacteria. Despite widespread practicing of these common hygienic and dietary habits, however, research has not proven that UTIs can be prevented with these techniques.

Prevention strategies include the following: urinating within one hour of the urge to void (rather than postponing voiding); drinking eight glasses of water a day (preferably spring water rather than chlorinated, acidic tap water); wiping from front to back after a bowel movement to avoid spreading bacteria from the rectal area to the urethra; changing underwear every day; using cotton underwear; changing sanitary napkins frequently and tampons at appropriate intervals; avoiding hot tubs and highly chlorinated pools; avoiding perfumed toilet paper, powders, and bubble baths; and avoiding feminine hygiene products such as deodorants, sprays, and douches, which can contribute to UTIs by irritating the urethra. When considering studies of many women, these factors were not individually shown to change the risk of a UTI. However, it is possible that in the individual patient, one or more of these behaviors may play an important role. Since there is little risk or cost involved in implementing these changes, it is therefore reasonable for a woman with recurrent UTIs to practice drinking lots of water, regular bladder emptying, and front-to-back wiping in order to decrease her risk of subsequent infections.

Regarding dietary substances thought to be bladder irritants (caffeine, all artificial sweeteners, citrus fruits and juices, chocolate, tomatoes, spicy foods, alcohol, carbonated beverages, and heavy sugar loads), the digestion of these substances makes the urine more acidic and irritating. Acidic urine may damage the bladder lining and cause irritation of nerve endings, resulting in pain or the urge to urinate. Patients who drink large quantities of acidic fruit juices should consider diluting them with an equal amount of water. Water is an excellent substitute for acid-containing fluids and women should be encouraged to drink six to eight glasses a day. The easiest way to estimate if you are getting enough fluid is to look at the voided urine. If it is nonodorous and pale yellow, then generally fluid intake is adequate.

Another dietary supplement recently receiving a great deal of attention is cranberry juice. A six-month study performed at Harvard Medical School showed that the risk of having bacteria in the urine was 42 percent lower in women who drank cranberry juice when compared with women who drank a red-colored drink that was not cranberry juice (placebo). The results of this study and others appear to support drinking cranberry juice.

You may be confused because cranberry juice is acidic (and in general acidic juices are to be avoided), yet it is being recommended to prevent UTIs. By the time cranberry juice reaches the bladder, it does not change the acidity of the urine much at all. Certain substances in cranberry juice help prevent adherence of bacteria to the bladder wall; however, once the bacteria adhere, cranberry juice will not kill or eradicate the infection. Most cranberry juice contains only 25 percent real cranberries, and some cranberry cocktails contain just 2 percent. Based on the studies, cranberry juice drinks containing 20 to 30 percent cranberry juice offer as much protection against UTI as pure cranberry juice, but keep in mind that they are more fattening (each 8-ounce glass contains 145 calories). Another sensible remedy is to take nonacidic cranberry pills, which are available without vitamin C, with esterified vitamin C, or in buffered form. Cranberry pills are most commonly sold over the counter at most health food stores.

A common misconception about prevention of UTIs is that eating or drinking specific dairy products, especially yogurt, can prevent infection of the urinary tract. Certain brands of yogurt and milk that contain live cultures of *Lactobacillus acidophilus* may have a role in fighting yeast in the vagina, but do not prevent UTIs.

SEEING THE DOCTOR

Most women who experience a UTI will see their doctor for diagnosis and treatment. Most physicians will obtain a urine sample to specify the exact type of infection. If you are without symptoms, or symptoms are mild, a brief office test is a reliable screening tool for UTIs. However, if you have strong symptoms and a history of recurrent infections, then it is necessary to know exactly which bacteria are causing the infection. The laboratory doing the urine culture will usually also test for "sensitivity." Bacteria grown from the infected urine are matched against different antibiotics until the most effective antibiotics are found. Because the results of urine cultures often take twenty-four to forty-eight hours to return, doctors will often initially treat the symptomatic patient with a broad-acting antibiotic while waiting for lab results. If the test shows the presence of types of bacteria that may respond better to a different antibiotic, your doctor may change the prescription.

In many patients, no causative bacteria are detected. This does not mean that you do not have an infection, or that a virus explains the infection. One possible reason is that symptomatic women drink a copious amount of water in hope of decreasing symptoms or eliminating the infection. This process makes the urine specimen and its concentration of bacteria extremely dilute, making it difficult for the bacteria to grow in the lab. Though present methods of urinary tract infection investigation are good, they remain less than perfect. One solution is to give a urine specimen first thing in the morning, when the urine is most concentrated. If a patient continues to be symptomatic despite negative cultures and antibiotic therapy, the physician should consider other possible causes.

Contrast dye X-ray studies or cystoscopy (looking inside the bladder) are not routinely performed in the diagnosis and management of uncomplicated UTIs. However, if you experience any of the following, contrast dye X-ray studies and cystoscopy may be important in finding the cause for the infection: (1) more than three or four UTIs in a twelve-month period, (2) an infection with specific organisms; e.g., *P. mirabilia, Pseudomonas sp.*, (3) symptoms suggesting pyelonephritis, e.g., fever, flank pain, (4) poor response to antibiotic therapy, (5) kidney stones, or (6) persistent blood in the urine. An intravenous pyelogram (IVP) is a contrast dye X-ray study. This study may be needed to determine abnormalities of the genitourinary tract, such as a kidney stone, kidney and ureter defects, or obstruction that prevents complete clearing of the infection.

Some patients have an abnormality in the urinary tract that causes improper emptying of the bladder. Cystoscopy can help confirm whether this is a result of stenosis (narrowing) or from a diverticulum (outpouching) of the urethra or bladder. Cystoscopy can also determine whether foreign bodies (stones, or sutures from previous operations, for example) are present. Foreign bodies can be a constant source of infection and should be removed to decrease the incidence of infection.

It is important to provide urine specimens when having repeated bouts of UTIs. Persistence of an infection means that the offending bacteria was never fully eliminated. Recurrence of infection usually means that the first infection was cleared and a new infection (usually with a different bacteria) has started. The doctor handles these situations differently as far as what tests are needed and length of treatment. The only way to distinguish these is to have the specimen analyzed by a professional laboratory.

Treatment for Simple UTIs

Usually, UTIs can be treated successfully with a variety of antibiotics. The antibiotics most commonly prescribed for patients with UTIs fall into four categories: sulfonamide and trimethoprim, penicillin and cephalosporin, nitrofurantoin, and quinolones. Many treatment plans have been studied for initial treatment of simple cystitis, ranging from a single dose to two or more weeks of medication. One of the most common misconceptions regarding UTIs is that all patients must be kept on antibiotic therapy for ten to fourteen days—despite research showing that 80 percent of the time an uncomplicated UTI can be treated with a single large dose of certain antibiotics.

The duration of antibiotic therapy has been a source of debate for decades. While most infections can be treated with a single dose, a slightly longer course (three days) can be 5 to 20 percent more effective. There is a growing consensus between urogynecologists and urologists that for most women with uncomplicated cystitis, a three-day antibiotic course is the regimen of choice. The three-day course has about half the relapse risk of single-dose therapy. Compared with a seven- to fourteen-day regimen, it has fewer side effects, better compliance, decreased risk of the emergence of resistant bacteria, and of course less cost.

Three-day antibiotic courses eradicate 90 to 95 percent of urinary tract infections in young women. However, short regimens are appropriate only for women who are not pregnant, do not have diabetes, and have had symptoms for less than a week. Postmenopausal women are more prone to relapse for undetermined reasons, and should be treated with a minimum three-day course for initial infection and seven to fourteen days for recurrences. It is important that you complete the entire prescription as provided by the physician. All too often patients stop taking their medication early because they feel better and are no longer experiencing symptoms. By stopping medication early the woman puts herself at risk for recurrence of a hardier and stronger infection. Stopping the medication early kills the weakest bacteria and leaves the most resistant bacteria behind to begin the reinfection process all over again. Recently, a single-dose packet of orange-flavored granules has been developed for urinary tract infections. Made into a drink, the medication remains in the body for three days. This new antibiotic is known as Monurol™ (fosfomycin). One dose certainly makes therapy easy.

Recurrent UTIs

The first recurrent infection can be handled in essentially the same manner as initial infections. If a patient does not respond to treatment or has a recurring infection within a few days or weeks after the initial therapy, a longer course of treatment is justified. If a patient develops three to four UTIs in twelve months, a comprehensive investigation is warranted. Several strategies are available to help women prevent recurrences.

Long-term, preventative treatment with low doses of an antibiotic is often recommended when infections occur frequently. This method consists of taking an appropriate antibiotic daily or every other day for approximately six months. Then the antibiotic should be stopped to see whether the woman can go without continuous therapy. If the patient develops a UTI, therapy should resume.

A second method is prophylaxis after sexual relations. This option is for women whose infections may be associated with sexual activity. The patient takes a dose of antibiotic after each sexually active session. In comparison to conventional (daily) therapy this method often requires less antibiotics, unless you are sexually active more than once daily!

Self-start or self-treatment therapy is a third option. For the most part, patients can correctly diagnose UTIs based on recurring symptoms. In some situations patients are instructed to begin treatment immediately after symptoms of the UTI occur. In a study conducted several years ago, patients correctly self-diagnosed bacterial UTIs 90 percent of the time. The patients who reported symptoms indeed had documented bacteria in the urine. The bacteria cleared with self-start medication. Although this method of therapy is not suitable for all women, it is safe, effective, and inexpensive. It is important that a physician instruct you to use the self-start method and that you not implement it on your own. Behavioral changes, like those mentioned earlier, should also be considered.

Postmenopausal UTIs

Postmenopausal women should consider estrogen replacement for prevention of UTIs. Estrogen is essential in making genital and urinary tract tissue thicker and allowing for better lubrication—two factors that inhibit the progression of bacteria into the lower urinary tract. Estrogen may also improve resistance to UTIs because it increases vaginal acidity, making it a poor habitat for infection-causing bacteria. To clarify, acid is irritating to the bladder but is favorable for infection prevention in the vagina.

As women age, the lack of estrogen may be one of the causes of vaginal relaxation and the bladder may drop (cystocele), creating a reservoir of urine that encourages the growth of bacteria. Estrogen can be taken by mouth or vaginally using a cream. Daily application of a topical vaginal estrogen cream has better effects on the urinary and genital tract than oral estrogen. However, the well-established benefits to bone and heart are not proven when estrogen is given only by the vaginal route.

Conclusion

Urinary tract infections continue to be a major health problem for women in the United States. Recent advances focusing on simpler diagnosis, treatment, and prevention have resulted in shorter length of required treatment, higher patient compliance, and less cost. Short-term therapy consisting of a single dose or a three-day course of antibiotics is very effective for simple UTIs. However, for patients who have complicated infections (e.g., pyelonephritis), known structural abnormalities of the urinary tract, recurrent UTIs, or have had previous urinary tract surgery, longer-term antibiotic treatment and/or prophylactic antibiotic therapy has been shown to be most beneficial. Physicians and patients should also consider altering behavior that may be causing recurrent UTIs. Despite a lack of conclusive research, it still makes sense to try to decrease chances of recurring infection by practicing good hydration, regular bladder emptying, good hygiene habits, and avoidance of irritants. With knowledge of prevention and treatment techniques you can employ on your own and regular communication with your physician, you should be able to minimize urinary tract infections.

Chapter 9

URINARY INCONTINENCE—PREVENTION AND NEW THERAPY

WITH LAWRENCE R. LIND, M.D.

Lawrence R. Lind, M.D., is fellowship trained in a new, much-needed specialty called urogynecology. This specialty will make life much better for women with urinary incontinence. It focuses on the often-related problems of dropped pelvic organs, pelvic pain, pain with urination, and reconstructive surgery for abnormalities of the female genital organs. It makes sense to have urogynecologic physicians who can offer surgical and nonsurgical options for treating incontinence. Problems with control of urine and with dropping of the pelvic organs have been taboo subjects until very recently. In years past, women thought that daily soiling of themselves was a part of the normal "aging" process. Physicians often did not ask about these problems because few knew how to treat the problems effectively. But finally these concerns are coming out of the closet.

Am I the Only One?

Incontinence is not a normal part of aging! More than two-thirds of women over the age of sixty-five have control of their urine and their dignity. You should be satisfied with nothing less! Television and magazine advertisements would have you believe that wearing diapers is the best way to deal with incontinence. Don't let the money-hungry marketers of absorbent products keep you from reality: Incontinence is not a normal part of aging. Almost every type of incontinence can be treated and often cured.

Incontinence is a major cause of disability, dependency, and social embarrassment. Athletes give up their healthy and rejuvenating activities because of incontinence. Other women become social hermits for fear of soiling themselves in public. Still others sleep with towels and rubber sheets. In severe cases, the soiled skin becomes irritated and ulcerated. Embarrassment and depression are common. This is not the dignity you deserve. At last, there is hope. Thanks to the growing field of urogynecology, there are experts available to provide caring and modern evaluation and treatment.

There are over thirteen million incontinent Americans of all ages. What does this cost the American health care system? Conservative estimates place the cost of caring for incontinent women to be over $25 billion annually!

The likelihood of incontinence becoming a problem increases as women age but there are many additional factors that affect the chances of becoming incontinent. Numerous studies show that 10 to 30 percent of women between fifteen and sixty-four years of age experience embarrassing accidents as a result of incontinence. For noninstitutionalized women over the age of sixty, the frequency of incontinence ranges from 15 to 35 percent, and within nursing homes, about 50 percent of the 1.5 million occupants are incontinent.

The problem is twice as common in women as in men. There are some differences in anatomy between the sexes, but the most significant difference, as far as incontinence goes, is that only one of the two sexes experiences vaginal childbirth with the associated trauma to the pelvic organs.

Despite these remarkable statistics, research has shown that less than half of women with incontinence seek professional help. It is time the public understands that although there are aspects related to aging and childbirth that increase the chances of becoming incontinent, it is not a normal part of aging. While the figures presented above make it clear that many women will become incontinent, the other side of the coin is that more than two-thirds of women over sixty-five have control of their urine. As with other medical problems, there are known causes, established methods of evaluation, and many surgical and nonsurgical treatments.

Women nowadays live longer and maintain excellent activity levels through their sixties, seventies, eighties, and even nineties. This is quite a change from twenty-five years ago. The increasing population of older women and their better health in the senior years essentially dictate that education and care of incontinent women must be recognized as an important health care issue. We can look forward to increased numbers of urogynecologists educating the public and caring for this devastating but correctable problem.

If $25 billion in costs impressed you, the latest information about the aging population certainly will also. Based on 1995 data from the U.S. Census Bureau, the "over sixty-five" population will increase from 8 percent in 1950 to almost 13 percent in the year 2000, representing more than a 50 percent increase. More significant is the projection that between the years 2000 and 2050, the senior population is projected to increase from 13 percent to 20.5 percent. In addition to the sheer increase in numbers, these more active seniors are appropriately demanding complete health into their eighties and nineties. Incontinence evaluation must be an integral part of caregiving. Women have the right to say, "I feel healthy, I want to be active, I want my bladder problem fixed."

There are several definitions related to incontinence and pelvic organ prolapse that readers must understand if they want to be informed about incontinence. With the proper vocabulary laid out, we can discuss the causes of incontinence and the most up-to-date methods for evaluating and treating incontinent women. There are many new nonsurgical treatments available. On the surgical side, there have been exciting advances in minimally invasive surgery, which requires little or no recovery period. By the conclusion of this chapter, you should have a comfortable understanding of the problems of pelvic prolapse and incontinence and understand what methods are available for prevention, evaluation, and treatment. This topic has therefore "come out of the closet."

Causes of Dropped Pelvic Organs and Incontinence

Prolapse and incontinence are generally problems related to weakness of the floor of the pelvis. Some anatomy and several terms must be clarified. The pelvic organs and tissues that are essential to this discussion include the uterus, cervix, vagina, bladder, urethra, rectum, and intestines. In addition, there are ligaments, muscles, and bones that support the pelvic organs. Figure 9.1 shows a view of these structures from the side as they appear in a normal woman in the standing position. In the center of these structures is the vagina.

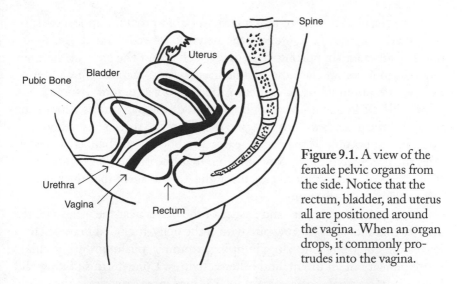

Figure 9.1. A view of the female pelvic organs from the side. Notice that the rectum, bladder, and uterus all are positioned around the vagina. When an organ drops, it commonly protrudes into the vagina.

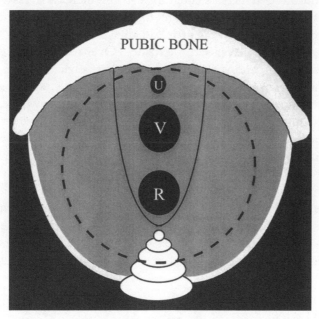

Figure 9.2. A view of the female pelvis looking down from above. The white areas are the bony structures of the pelvis. The shaded area is the muscular "floor" of the pelvis, which is important for supporting the pelvic organs. Note that the muscular layer has openings to allow the urethra, vagina, and rectum to pass through. These openings, especially after the vaginal opening has been stretched from childbirth, are potential weak points. The dotted line indicates the average size of a newborn's head, to emphasize the necessary stretching of the vagina in childbirth.

The pelvis has a sheet of muscular tissue that provides important support for the organs. In figure 9.2, the pelvis is viewed from above, showing the muscular supporting layer of the pelvis and the gaps in the floor required to accommodate the vagina, urethra, and rectum. These "perforations" are potential weak points in the support structure. Imagine carrying a plastic bag of groceries. The bottom of the bag carries a lot of the weight of the groceries. Now imagine that there are three reasonably sized holes in the bottom of the bag. Clearly, the bottom of the bag is weaker after the holes are present. Now imagine that one of the holes is stretched to allow a newborn infant to pass through. All will agree that the bag now has a major weakness in its floor!

The supporting muscles and tissues of the pelvis bear the weight of any activity that increases the pressure within the belly. Included in these challenges are coughing, sneezing, jumping, running, pushing during childbirth, delivery of an infant, and other activities. Long-term smoking and lung conditions that increase coughing can also increase stress to the pelvis.

An often-overlooked challenge to these structures is the straining associated with constipation. It is sad that in our "hurry up" society all activities, including defecation, are rushed. Over time, pushing with every bowel movement can increase the chance that pelvic organs may drop. It may surprise many readers to learn that pushing and straining are not part of a normal bowel movement. Intestinal gas, involuntary pulsation of the wall of the intestine, and relaxation of the pelvic muscles are involved with normal evacuation. Significant straining should not be involved.

Obesity increases the weight of the belly contents and theoretically causes an increased challenge to the supporting tissues. In some women there are inborn weaknesses in the connective tissues, and therefore, an increased risk of failure of pelvic supports. Data has shown that women with laxity of the joints have a higher risk of incontinence, suggesting that there is a generalized weakness of connective and support tissues in some women. Tobacco use may also decrease the actual strength of supporting structures.

DEFINITIONS

1. *Urethra*
The urethra is the short tube through which urine passes to exit the body. It begins at the base of the bladder and opens just beneath the clitoris. Normally, when you see urine exiting the body it is coming from the urethra. Sometimes, as the result of trauma or surgical injury, urine may exit directly from the bladder with the patient having no control.

2. *Urethral Hypermobility*

Urethral hypermobility occurs when, under conditions of straining, lifting, or coughing, the bladder and urethra drop. When the bladder drops, women may experience a sensation of tissue moving, a bulge sensation, or loss of urine. Normally these structures are prevented from dropping during strenuous activities.

3. *Prolapse (General)*

Failure of pelvic supports (the muscles and ligaments attached to the uterus, bladder, vagina, and other organs) allows the pelvic organs to drop. The movement of any organ or tissue down toward the outside is termed prolapse. It is similar to hernias of the belly wall, with which many women are more familiar. Hernias of the belly wall usually represent movement of the intestines into the front of the belly wall through a weak spot. A common place for hernias is at the belly button. You may notice a common theme here as the belly button was the exit point of the umbilical cord early in life. This is a "perforation" of the front of the belly just as the vagina and rectum are "perforations" of the floor of the belly. Most of the hernias discussed in this chapter represent movement of something into or through the floor (bottom) of the belly. Remember the paper bag whose contents are too heavy and which overcome the strength of the bottom of the perforated bag. Fortunately, the pelvic organs will not tear through and fall out. They may, however, push out so far that they appear outside of the body. The first sight of this can be alarming but it is rarely an emergency situation.

Most women are familiar with prolapse of the uterus. You should know that the rectum, urethra, bladder, and vagina may prolapse as well. There are some terms related to each of these problems.

3a. *Prolapse of the Uterus*

Uterine prolapse is the dropping of the uterus and cervix. There can be minimal prolapse, which you would not be aware of, or it can be advanced such that you may be able to feel the cervix at the opening of the vagina. Some say this feels like the tip of a nose. In severe cases the entire uterus may be outside of the inverted vagina.

3b. *Prolapse of the Bladder (Cystocele)*

Cystocele is the dropping of the bladder, which then bulges into the vagina. The patient often feels a sensation as if a ball were in the vagina, or, if it is advanced, may notice soft tissue outside the vagina, which is most noticeable when standing, walking, or straining. It is usually more noticeable when the bladder is full. Cystocele is often present when incontinence is a problem.

3c. *Prolapse of the Rectum (Rectocele)*

Rectocele is the protrusion of the rectum into the vagina. The bulging sensation may be indistinguishable from a cystocele, but may also cause difficulties with bowel movements including either constipation or lack of control of flatus or stool. Some women have to push on their rectocele in order to empty their rectum when defecating.

3d. *Prolapse of the Urethra (Urethrocele)*

Urethrocele is the dropping of the urethra, which is the short tube that connects the bladder to the outside.

3e. *Prolapse of the Vagina*

Vaginal vault prolapse is the dropping of the innermost part of the vagina (the part that usually is farthest inside, near the cervix).

Incontinence

Incontinence is the inability to control either urine or feces until a socially appropriate time at which urination or defecation is voluntarily performed. There are several types of incontinence. It will take several repetitions of the following details to truly understand the subtle differences between types of incontinence.

The muscle in the bladder wall is called the detrusor muscle. Detrusor instability is a form of urinary incontinence in which the bladder muscle squeezes involuntarily, resulting in partial or complete bladder emptying. The bladder normally receives a continuous message from the brain to stay relaxed and not to squeeze. When seated on the toilet, and the time is appropriate, normal people are able to interrupt the continuous relaxation signal and let the bladder do what it wants to do, which is to squeeze. Detrusor instability happens when the voluntary control of bladder activity, as described, is lost.

The uncontrolled squeezing of the bladder muscle may be provoked by coughing, sneezing, walking, running water, or other stress maneuvers, or without provocation. This type of incontinence is important because it is common, causes large amounts of urinary loss, and often *does not* respond to standard surgical treatments. A typical patient gets a strong urge to urinate and as she approaches the toilet the urgency becomes so severe that urine escapes before she reaches the toilet. When the bladder contracts in this situation, it will often contract until the bladder is completely empty, thus causing large amounts of urine loss. If voiding is postponed because of a busy schedule, or lack of proximity to a bathroom, the larger amount of urine that collects makes an involuntary bladder contraction much more likely. Another common scenario is urine loss that begins a few seconds after a cough and continues for anywhere from one to several seconds. Other women experience the sensation that when they put their keys in the lock to enter the house the urgency to urinate becomes so strong that control is impossible. Some women have urinary loss at the time of orgasm, which has been mistaken in the past as female ejaculation. This may represent an abnormal detrusor activity but the mechanism is not clearly understood.

Stress incontinence refers to urinary loss from the bladder under conditions of increased belly pressure. It also implies that the increased belly pressure did not trigger the bladder muscle to contract (which would be detrusor instability). In other words, if the increased pressure has triggered detrusor instability and the bladder is squeezing to cause leakage, it is not stress incontinence. Although there is some overlap, it is helpful to think of detrusor instability as a problem with the bladder muscle and the nerves that tell it to squeeze, and to think of stress incontinence as a problem of the support of either the bladder and/or urethra.

The problem with lack of support can be difficult to understand. Consider a garden hose with water running through it. If you step on the hose it is like a cough. If the hose is on a firm surface, the water will stop flowing when you step on it. Now consider the hose on a soft surface, like mud or clay (which is like not having support). When you step on the hose, the hose simply sinks into the mud without getting compressed. The water continues to leak through the hose if the foundation below is not strong. That is the problem in stress incontinence.

A typical patient with stress incontinence notices short, nonsustained leakage that starts exactly when the cough starts, and stops immediately when the cough is over. Lifting heavy objects is another common situation in which stress incontinence is likely. So-called giggle incontinence is urinary loss associated with laughing, and can be due to stress incontinence, detrusor instability, or both.

Can I Tell if I Have One Type of Incontinence as Opposed to Another?

It is important to know that the symptom of urine loss after coughing or sneezing is not an accurate way to distinguish stress incontinence from detrusor instability. The scenarios described above are the classic, most pure descriptions of patients with each type of incontinence. The overlap in symptoms is great, which is why detailed evaluation is necessary to distinguish between them. This point cannot be overemphasized as it is common for many types of urinary loss to be incorrectly labeled as stress incontinence. Incorrect diagnosis is a major reason for improper treatment, suffering, and treatment failure. Remember, urine loss after a cough does not necessarily mean the problem is stress incontinence.

Subdivisions of "Stress Incontinence"

Sorry, but to be true to the promise of demystifying incontinence, some of the details have to get technical. If you do not have severe incontinence you may want to skip this section.

Stress incontinence has already been described as a problem of loss of support of the bladder and/or urethra. The pelvic muscles may be weak and/or the other supports of the bladder and urethra may have weakened. In the past ten to fifteen years we have come to realize that loss of support is not the only factor involved with stress incontinence. The urethra itself may contribute to or explain the problem. The urethra is normally closed except when voluntarily urinating. In some women the walls of the urethra are not closed tightly enough and incontinence may occur. Your physician must evaluate the urethra as well as the supports in order to provide the proper treatment.

Stress urinary loss may occur if either the urethral tube has lost its ability to close, termed intrinsic (urethral) sphincter deficiency, or when the muscular support of the bladder base is insufficient, termed genuine stress incontinence. Thus the popular term "stress" incontinence really has subdivisions into genuine stress incontinence and intrinsic (urethral) deficiency. With genuine stress incontinence, the problem is that the bladder and urethra are not well supported. With intrinsic sphincter deficiency, the problem is not support but rather that the tube through which urine passes is open rather than closed. In reality, many women with stress incontinence probably have a combination of these problems. It is also possible to have both stress incontinence and detrusor instability.

If you have more than one type of incontinence, treatment is more sophisticated and the chances surgery will fail are greater. This is especially true if one of the types of incontinence has not been found prior to surgery. Again, one of the most common reasons for surgical failure is error in diagnosis or incomplete diagnosis. Too often, all incontinence is incorrectly labeled stress incontinence.

Overflow incontinence is a less common type of incontinence. It refers to a condition where the bladder does not empty adequately and therefore is often overfilled. When the bladder is full, straining, coughing, or lifting are likely to result in loss of urine. This is analogous to walking with a full pot of water. Even a healthy person is likely to spill small amounts of water if the pot is filled completely to the brim. The symptoms may be similar to classic stress incontinence, but here the problem is not the support of the bladder but rather that it does not empty completely and is on the verge of spilling all the time. The symptoms of stress incontinence and overflow incontinence are quite similar. A detailed incontinence evaluation is necessary to distinguish the two problems. A surgical treatment intended for classic stress incontinence when the patient actually has overflow incontinence would make the problem worse.

Urinary fistulas are a rare type of incontinence. This is an abnormal pathway of urine that can be created as a complication of gynecologic surgery or radiation. In addition to exiting at the urethra, urine may also exit at the top of the vagina. An analogy would be when water drains down a sink. All the water should go into the drainpipe, and then to the drainage system outside the house. A fistula is similar to a leak under the sink that occurs when there is a defect in the pipe.

Looking again at figure 9.1, it is clear that the vagina is central to all of the structures involved in problems of prolapse and incontinence. Prolapse of any of these organs can cause discomfort, a sensation that there is a bulge or ball in the vagina or outside the vagina, or low back pain. Depending on the degree of prolapse of the bladder and urethra there may be urinary frequency, difficulty voiding, or conversely, incontinence.

Incontinence and Prolapse

HOW IS INCONTINENCE RELATED TO PELVIC ORGAN PROLAPSE?

An important concept is that stress incontinence in many cases is a symptom of the more general problem of prolapse. As a result of lack of support of the bladder, the bladder drops under conditions of stress or simply from gravity. Genuine stress incontinence is urinary loss resulting in part from the bladder dropping at times of stress (hypermobility of the bladder and urethra).

IS IT DANGEROUS IF THE PELVIC ORGANS ARE DROPPING?

Women who are aware of a bulge are often fearful that one of the organs is falling out. It is extremely rare for this situation to represent an emergency; however, medical evaluation is advised any time there is a protrusion. In almost all cases, the bulge is either the cervix, or the vaginal wall with one of the other organs (bladder, rectum, or intestines) behind it, pushing it outward. A frequent question is whether it is safe to continue sexual relations when a prolapse is present. In most cases, women with prolapse are able to continue enjoying normal sexual activity. Sexual activity is not likely to harm the protruding organ. Usually, when the woman lies on her back, the bulge recedes into the vagina. If it does not, it can be pushed in safely prior to sexual relations. If there is discomfort, irritation, or urinary loss with the sexual activity, then evaluation is recommended.

With regard to long-term effects, a bulge is likely to bulge farther with progression occurring slowly over several years. In rare cases, severe dropping of some of the pelvic organs can kink the normal urine pathway from the kidneys to the bladder. This situation is urgent, and although patients may experience back pain that brings them to medical evaluation, some women may not have any symptoms. Once again, help is available and a woman should not hesitate to seek proper evaluation.

WHAT CAUSES PELVIC ORGAN PROLAPSE AND INCONTINENCE?

You can now understand why certain factors cause incontinence or prolapse. A large number of correctable causes can be remembered with the mnemonic "DIAPPERS," as coined by Resnick; however, there are these other causes as well.

Some Causes of Incontinence

Vaginal Childbirth
Pelvic Trauma (e.g., automobile accident)
Back Trauma or Spinal Disease
Chronic Lung Conditions
Connective Tissue Weakness
Head Injury or Neurological Problem

More Causes of Incontinence: "DIAPPERS" Mnemonic

Delirium
Infections
Atrophic Vaginitis
Pharmacology (drugs)
Psychological Disorders
Endocrine Disorders
Restricted Mobility
Stool Impaction

Delirium

Delirium is a confusional state. It may result from drugs or medical illness and is commonly associated with incontinence. If the cause of the delirium is identified and treated, often the incontinence will cease. For example, some medications cause confusion and subsequent incontinence. Infections can cause delirium and when treated for the infection, the delirium and incontinence improve.

Infections

Women with urinary tract infections often are incontinent. *E. coli* is the most common bacteria causing urinary tract infections. There is a toxin produced by the bacteria which relaxes the urethra, making it easier for urine to escape. In many cases treatment of an active urinary tract infection will resolve the incontinence problem. There are a number of theories for this but the essential message is that extensive evaluation of incontinence should not be performed until the reversible problem of a urinary tract infection is either treated or proved not to be present. (Treatment of urinary infections is discussed in chapter 8.)

Atrophic Vaginitis

Menopause occurs when the ovaries cease to produce the usual levels of hormones. The urethra and vagina are sensitive to estrogen; their linings thicken in response to the hormone, estrogen. Studies, however, are divided as to whether giving a menopausal woman estrogen has any effect on incontinence. In general women with incontinence and signs of atrophic vaginitis (thinning of the walls of the urethra and vagina) should be treated with estrogen replacement but only after full counseling about all the risks and benefits. It may improve the incontinence and will usually decrease irritation, dryness, and discomfort if present.

Pharmacology

Drugs are a common cause of incontinence. For example, diuretics (water pills) result in an increased volume of urine and therefore an increased challenge to the urinary control mechanism. The comprehensive list of medications that affect the urinary tract is many pages long. The most common categories include medicines for blood pressure control, diuretics (water pills), antidepressants, and sleep medications. Some of the commonly used offenders include Minipress®, Parlodel®, Propulsid®, Humorsol®, Lasix®, hydrochlorothiazide, Prozac®, and Zoloft®. This is certainly not a comprehensive list and your physician should evaluate your medication list. Always have your full list of medications and vitamins when seeing a physician for any reason. A pharmacist can also inform you if certain medications may have an effect on the urinary system.

Psychological Disorders

Patients with psychological disorders may use incontinence as a mechanism for gaining attention. Women may have urinary symptoms related to the psychological effects of sexual abuse. Some patients with depression simply do not care whether or not they soil themselves. Treatment of the psychiatric disorder often results in improvement of the incontinence problem.

Endocrine Disorders

Endocrine disorders that affect the urinary system include diabetes mellitus, diabetes insipidus, and hypercalcemia. These conditions cause production of a large amount of urine, thereby challenging the continence mechanism. Many women have control of their urine but only by a small margin. Medical problems that increase the amount of urine produced will push these women "over the edge." In addition, some diabetics lose the ability to sense that the bladder is full and therefore may not use a toilet frequently enough to avoid overflow incontinence.

Restricted Mobility

Restricted mobility is a common, reversible cause of incontinence. Some patients simply need assistance to reach a toilet safely and in a timely manner. Patients with arthritis, gait problems, and other ambulation problems need to have nearby facilities available so they may use their normally functioning bladders. This cause of incontinence is common among the elderly and debilitated, but with effort can be easily resolved.

Stool Impaction

The long-term straining associated with chronic constipation can place excessive stress on the bladder and its supports. Proper defecation involves relaxation of the pelvic floor and not straining. If constipation is an ongoing problem and has not responded to dietary changes, medical evaluation is recommended. Many women can be cured of their incontinence with simple dietary changes.

There are studies that document a higher incidence of incontinence in obese patients but it is not certain whether weight as an independent factor causes incontinence.

OTHER CAUSES OF INCONTINENCE

Increasing age is most definitely associated with incontinence. There are probably many contributing factors including gravity, which over time causes the organs to drop, hormone changes associated with menopause, and neurological changes. Furthermore, injuries originally sustained to nerves and muscles decades before may only become obvious later in life.

Chronic lung conditions associated with smoking, asthma, pneumonia, and bronchitis are risk factors for incontinence. The increased abdominal pressure associated with coughing over many years places an increased stress to the pelvis. In addition, tobacco may have a direct detrimental effect on the lining of the urinary tract.

Head injury and neurological problems may also be a factor. Following a stroke, it is very common for the victim to have poor urinary control. Most commonly, the patient develops detrusor instability and therefore experiences large amounts of leakage because of involuntary squeezing of the bladder muscle. The incontinence improves in the majority of patients in the first year, so encouragement and treatment should be offered. It is common for women with neurological disorders such as multiple sclerosis to have incontinence. In some women, incontinence may be the first sign that there is a neurological problem. A physician should be seen in these cases as soon as possible.

Physical injury to the head, or any part of the spinal cord, can cause urinary problems. In some situations the result is an inability to urinate while at other times the result is incontinence. Head and spinal cord injuries require expert evaluation as the urinary problems can be complex.

Childbirth and the Pelvis

WHAT IS THE EFFECT OF VAGINAL CHILDBIRTH ON THE PELVIS?

Vaginal birth is the most significant risk factor associated with incontinence and pelvic organ prolapse. What has not been clarified is the relative role of each component of the delivery process in causing damage to the pelvic floor. In other words, the delivery process involves carrying a growing fetus for nine months, early labor, active labor, a pushing period, delivery, and recovery.

We know that women who do not enter labor at all have significantly less chance of developing prolapse or incontinence (although the risk is not eliminated). Women who have had cesarean deliveries have been shown to have greater pelvic muscle strength after delivery compared with women who have had vaginal births. The first vaginal delivery appears to carry the greatest increased risk of incontinence. The incontinence rates in women with one, two, or three vaginal births do not increase in a step-wise manner; this suggests that the major injury to muscles, ligaments, and nerves occurs with the first delivery. This statistic should not be misunderstood to mean that if a woman is continent after a first vaginal birth that she will always be continent.

Some women may be incontinent immediately after delivery and in many cases this resolves. Other women may have no incontinence associated with the pregnancy or immediate postpartum period but suffer incontinence years later. Physical trauma of vaginal delivery and resultant pelvic nerve damage have been documented in studies and in clinical experience. Some or all of the pelvic muscle strength can be recovered with appropriate pelvic floor strengthening programs after vaginal delivery, a subject discussed later in this chapter.

It is not known what fraction of the damage occurs at each stage of the labor and delivery process. What is clear is that discussion of prolapse and incontinence issues with respect to the labor process is alarmingly missing from the prenatal counseling process. Pregnancy lasts nine months and hundreds of issues are discussed; surprisingly, however, in childbirth preparation books there are only brief sections regarding the pelvic floor and incontinence.

As women are becoming more educated on this subject, they may question whether to spare the pelvis the trauma of vaginal delivery and undergo cesarean delivery. It is known that serious complications, although still rare, are more likely to occur with cesarean delivery than with vaginal delivery. These include bleeding, infection, and surgical damage to pelvic organs. In addition, the recovery period is longer following a cesarean delivery. At this stage, it is not recommended that women undergo cesarean delivery to prevent incontinence. However, in the future, obstetricians may change the way that labor and delivery is managed if the strength of the pelvic supports can be preserved. For example, many doctors encourage their patients to push as hard as they can from the moment they reach full cervical dilation to the point of delivery. Instead, perhaps women should be taught to "push" with their abdominal muscles while at the same time relaxing the pelvic muscles. Coordination of muscles may turn out to be more important than maximal straining, which is currently encouraged. Many obstetricians have already acted on these ideas by encouraging patients to push only when they feel the natural urge, rather than at an exact amount of dilation at the cervix.

Those who have gone through labor remember the exhausting pushing that was required. It is unlikely that any of you were coached regarding the subtle details of pelvic relaxation. The normal response of the pelvic muscle when you maximally strain is for the muscle to tighten. If you are straining, the body responds by tightening the muscular opening through the pelvis. This is the opposite of what is desired. We may soon see prenatal classes that focus on pushing with the belly muscles but relaxing the pelvic floor muscles. Someday, pelvic strengthening classes may be started before delivery and resumed afterward to prevent incontinence. Unfortunately, exercises are usually recommended when incontinence has already become a problem. Prevention is always the best strategy. Some of these ideas are already in practice; however, research in this area is still in its infancy (no pun intended).

In the future, we hope to be able to develop criteria prior to delivery that will help to predict who will or will not suffer significant damage to the muscles, nerves, and ligaments of the pelvis, bladder, vagina, and rectum. (Editor's note: Dr. Lind is currently involved with research to identify ways to predict which women will experience prolonged labor, or future incontinence.)

Vaginal Birth after a Cesarean Delivery: What Are the Issues?

Another controversial issue is the delivery method if a cesarean delivery was required in the first pregnancy. For medical and financial reasons there is extreme pressure on doctors to decrease cesarean delivery rates. Studies have indicated that attempting vaginal delivery after previous cesarean birth is relatively safe, provided the physician has checked for certain qualifying factors. The medical rationale is that a successful vaginal birth avoids the inherent surgical risks of cesarean delivery. Current thinking is that medically, the vaginal route is favored but remember, sometimes another cesarean section is the better choice. In fact there are certain complication risks that are higher when having a vaginal birth after a previous cesarean delivery. Put simply, each type of delivery carries unique benefits and risks. You should be fully informed of all the pros and cons of each choice.

With regard to pelvic support issues, there is little scientific data to guide deliveries after cesarean section. In some situations, a little common sense is perhaps an adequate substitute for lack of scientific data. If the first pregnancy resulted in a cesarean delivery because the infant would not fit through the birth canal, and the present pregnancy has an infant of equal or greater size, it may be appropriate to consider a cesarean delivery. In some situations, a cesarean was required during the first pregnancy before labor proceeded far enough to tell if the fit was tight. If the adequacy of the space has essentially not been tested, then pelvic floor issues are identical to the situation of a first pregnancy. It is the first infant passing into the vaginal canal that brings with it the most significant increased risks of urinary, gas, and stool incontinence.

FORCEPS: FRIEND OR FOE?

With regard to forceps-assisted vaginal deliveries, what is known is that vaginal tears, including lacerations that extend to the rectum, and pelvic nerve damage are increased with forceps-assisted deliveries. The extent of damage is a risk for both urinary and fecal incontinence. There are, however, factors that contribute to the need for forceps delivery. Most commonly, they are used when the infant's head is too large for the birth canal. Unfortunately, the addition of forceps requires the head and forceps to pass through the canal together, and often this means even more space is needed.

It is important to receive a balanced message. Forceps may increase pelvic floor damage but they may also at times be the best option for delivery. The issue again is proper informed consent. Again, the way that labor and delivery are managed may change over the next several years with regard to issues of preserving the pelvic floor.

Seeking Evaluation and Testing for Prolapse or Incontinence

If a bulge, pain, or incontinence is making you concerned, you should seek evaluation. It is never too early and it is never too late. Unfortunately, not all physicians inquire about incontinence and other related problems. It is therefore up to each woman to be educated regarding available treatments, to seek proper evaluation, and to have no fears regarding discussion of these problems. Traditionally incontinence has been evaluated by urologists or gynecologists. Urogynecologists are a new group of specially trained physicians available to women with such problems. An excellent source for physician referrals in the specialty of urogynecology is the American Urogynecologic Society (401 N. Michigan Ave., Chicago, IL 60611, tel. (312) 644-6610), which lists doctors by geographic locations.

PHYSICAL EXAMINATION

The evaluation of incontinence is more involved than the standard yearly gynecologic evaluation. At your office examination, you should expect an evaluation of prolapse and incontinence. It is a detailed process that may take two to four physician visits. One of the problems with brief evaluations is that they fail to diagnose all of the problems. Remember, a problem with loss of urine may be silently accompanied by problems with the vagina, uterus, or rectum as well. It is quite common for women who have incontinence to also have prolapse of one or more of the other pelvic organs. It is essential to understand that if there are two components to the problem and only one is corrected, there may be no improvement whatsoever. Surgery for one problem may also unmask a second problem that could be worse than the one that was corrected. A common scenario is the woman who has a vaginal hysterectomy for prolapse of the uterus and finds that after the surgery the prolapse of the uterus is gone but she is incontinent. The concept is complete pelvic evaluation and it rarely can be accomplished in a single ten-minute evaluation.

EVALUATION

1. The evaluation usually begins with completion of a detailed urinary diary, which is usually sent to your home by mail. You will be asked to record all fluid intake for twenty-four to forty-eight hours. In addition, the amount and frequency of voids as well as any accidents should be recorded.

2. At the first visit a thorough history and physical examination will be performed. The examination includes a detailed pelvic examination, neurological examination, and several special tests.

3. The patient is asked to void into a container while a scale beneath

the container measures the speed of the urinary stream. A very slow urinary stream suggests either that the path of urine is blocked or that the bladder muscle does not squeeze adequately.

4. When voiding is completed, a sterile urine specimen is obtained by passing a small catheter (tube) into the bladder via the urethra. The urine is evaluated for possible urinary tract infection. If there is discomfort, it is mild, and most women have no pain at all during this evaluation. The amount of urine left in the bladder is an important measurement. The residual amount of urine indicates adequacy of the bladder muscle for emptying, or can suggest blockage of the urethra.

Many women are confused with the extensive evaluation of the bladder in situations where there is prolapse but they have no urinary complaints. The bladder may work well for you while it is prolapsed, but after repair, an incontinence problem may be uncovered. It is important to recognize that in most situations of prolapse, the bladder is not in the normal position and therefore the evaluation includes manually putting the bladder in the normal position to see if it still holds urine effectively. In fact, the bladder sits on the uterus and if the uterus changes position, so does the bladder. In most situations, the evaluation of a bulge and the evaluation of incontinence will be similar.

5. The bladder will often be filled by a small sterile tube in order to see how much water is tolerated. If the bladder contracts involuntarily during the filling process, it is suggestive of detrusor instability, as described earlier.

6. After the bladder is full and the catheter removed, the patient is asked to cough in order to visualize the force necessary to cause urinary loss and to see the character of the leakage. Short, nonsustained urine loss with each cough is suggestive of stress incontinence.

7. An assessment of the mobility of the urethra and bladder (how much they drop with straining) is generally performed by placing a narrow Q-Tip swab or sterile tube in the urethra and asking the patient to strain. Normally, in the lying position the Q-Tip swab is horizontal. If it moves too much when the patient is bearing down, then urethral hypermobility is present. In order to choose the appropriate treatment for incontinence, it is essential to know if the urethra is hypermobile.

8. If the prolapse or incontinence problem is not demonstrated in the lying position, the examinations or tests may be repeated in the standing position. It is important for the patient to realize that it is the doctor's job to re-create the problem in the office. Therefore, if incontinence is the problem, then you will be provoked to leak urine. This is a point of understandable anxiety. No one wants to leak urine while someone is watching.

Be aware that the only way to have the problem intelligently evaluated is to demonstrate it in the presence of a trained observer.

Usually a diagnosis is derived from the above evaluation and a preliminary treatment plan initiated. If the doctor is at all uncertain of the cause of the problems, subsequent tests may include cystoscopy, urodynamics, or X-ray testing. This sequence varies among many well-trained physicians; the sequence at your first visit may be different.

SPECIAL TESTING

1. In cystoscopy, the doctor views the urethra and bladder through a sterile narrow telescope. The procedure is performed in the doctor's office and usually causes no pain.

2. During urodynamics, two small catheters (flexible tubes) are used, one placed in the vagina or rectum, and one in the bladder. The tubes are about the diameter of spaghetti and have pressure sensors at the tips. With the catheters in place, accurate measurements can be recorded during bladder filling, during cough and stress maneuvers, and during voiding. In addition, two sticky pads may be placed near the rectum to record muscle activity. In some situations X rays of the bladder during rest and with straining are useful in the evaluation. The sequence of tests allows the physician to distinguish between the various types of incontinence. This procedure, like cystoscopy, is performed in the doctor's office. Urodynamics is the gold standard for assessing complex voiding and incontinence disorders.

As can be seen from the details above, the evaluation of prolapse or incontinence is detailed, and uses several special maneuvers and tests. It requires patience and cooperation to allow the proper evaluation. Despite all the details and all the tubes, the evaluation usually causes no discomfort and women generally are glad to have a thorough evaluation of their problem. While the extent of evaluation may vary, if surgery is recommended for prolapse or incontinence, then urodynamics must be performed.

Treatment of Incontinence: Good News!

IS TREATMENT NECESSARY?

The severity of incontinence is for each patient to judge. If recurrent urinary tract infections or an annoying rash secondary to urinary soiling are present, then certainly treatment is recommended. In general, there are no life-threatening dangers associated with incontinence. When the problem is unacceptable to the patient then it should be evaluated and tested.

When prolapse is severe, the entire uterus and cervix along with the attached vaginal walls may appear outside the vagina. This may cause pain, infection, incontinence, or the inability to empty the bladder. This apparent contradiction is caused when the prolapse is so great that the urethra becomes kinked like a garden hose that is bent too sharply. In rare situations, severe prolapse may block the passage of urine, which is a serious problem. In these situations, prolapse should be treated immediately.

A brief word on what *not* to do: There is a procedure called urethral dilations, which is painful and may worsen incontinence. There are extremely specific situations when this treatment is appropriate and you should obtain two or three expert opinions that are in agreement prior to undergoing urethral dilations.

NONSURGICAL OPTIONS FOR INCONTINENCE AND PROLAPSE

There are many nonsurgical treatments for incontinence and the availability of products and methods is encouraging. Treatment should begin only after the appropriate urogynecologic evaluation as described previously. If after this sequence, a clear diagnosis of genuine stress incontinence or detrusor instability is established, then a preliminary, nonsurgical treatment plan may be started. Treatments include pelvic floor training (Kegel exercises) with or without biofeedback assistance, medications, dietary changes, and social changes. There are other noninvasive treatment options; however, only qualified specialists have significant experience with incontinence pessaries, external and internal devices to occlude the urethra, electrical stimulation, and collagen urethral injection therapy. Each of these modalities is detailed below.

If your physician cannot obtain a clear explanation for incontinence after the basic workup, or if there is no improvement after the initial treatment, then referral to a qualified specialist is recommended. There are medical conditions and certain patient characteristics that should be evaluated only by a qualified specialist without a preliminary attempt at treatment by a generalist. While most causes of incontinence do not represent significant medical urgency, there are some conditions that are either complex or are associated with medical urgency and dictate evaluation by a qualified specialist. These include diabetes, neurological problems, inability to urinate, previous surgery for incontinence, previous radical pelvic surgery, previous radiation to the pelvis, and incontinence associated with recurrent urinary tract infections.

Biofeedback/Pelvic Strengthening

Kegel pelvic muscle exercises were originally described by an obstetrician, Dr. Arnold Kegel, for the purpose of helping pregnant women decrease the involuntary loss of urine. The exercises strengthen the pelvic floor muscles so that during times of stress (coughing and sneezing), the muscle layer will maintain the position of the bladder and prevent leakage. This muscle group is always used when stopping urination, preventing a bowel movement, or when tightening the vagina voluntarily during intercourse.

Studies document that incontinence significantly improves as a result of a properly executed Kegel exercise regimen. Unfortunately, the exercises have a poor reputation in the general public because they are often not taught and supervised correctly. Like the biceps, the pelvic floor muscles are voluntary muscles. The important difference is that everyone knows how to use their biceps but few know how to use their pelvic floor muscles efficiently.

How many women gain their desired physique when attempting to train their muscles at health clubs? It is difficult to be disciplined, to exercise properly, and to do it regularly. It is absurd to expect that a brief explanation of Kegel exercises and an instruction sheet are going to result in a satisfactory exercise program. Studies demonstrate that even in an educated population, after an office session in which Kegel exercises were taught, half of women returned after one month doing them wrong. These women were straining rather than, or in addition to, doing Kegel exercises. Straining, as mentioned earlier, increases the risks of pelvic prolapse and incontinence. One-quarter of women, then, are not only doing the exercises improperly but are doing maneuvers that make the problem worse!

The solution is simple. There are qualified specialists in some urogynecologists' offices and in some physical therapy practices who are experts in pelvic floor strengthening. It is like having a personal trainer for the pelvic floor muscles and, fortunately, such training is at least partially covered by insurance. These specialists regularly monitor exercise techniques and provide technical and emotional support.

There are several methods that can help women perform these exercises correctly. Small sensors may be placed near the rectum or in the vagina which monitor muscle activity as the exercises are performed. In some situations, the muscle activity will be visually recorded on a meter or computer screen so that women can observe the effectiveness of their pelvic squeezing.

Vaginal cones are small cylindrical weights that can be placed in the vagina to assist in muscle training. Some women have difficulty understanding how to squeeze but understand the idea of holding a cone so it will not fall out. As success with one cone is achieved, a cone of heavier weight is used (just as you would lift heavier weights to build up your biceps).

The technique of providing visualization of muscle activity to assist in working toward a better performance level is referred to as "biofeedback." For some women a portable small biofeedback unit may be recommended so the visualization of performance can be done at home. Some of the more sophisticated equipment will actually record your home exercise sessions, allowing the trainer to review your performance. This technique is helpful for many women who find the visual documentation of the exercise to be a confirmation that they are achieving the proper method.

Women who have difficulty even under direct supervision may benefit from electrical stimulation. This technique is safe and not painful. A small probe is placed in the vagina and gives an electrical signal that automatically contracts the correct muscles. As the muscle contracts, you become familiar with the sensation of the correct muscle doing a correct contraction. Eventually, you perform the contraction without the assistance of the electrical stimulation.

When pelvic floor exercises are performed properly, they can be extremely effective. The important factors are to have the proper trainer and to be committed to doing the exercises regularly.

Behavior and Dietary Modifications

Urinary control can be improved with simple changes in behavior. These changes cost nothing and require only knowledge, dedication, and commitment. Many diets intended for weight loss recommend large amounts of fluid intake, often in excess of fifteen or twenty glasses of fluid daily. It is important to remember that all liquids are fluids and that includes ice cream, yogurt, Jell-O, milk shakes, and soups. The "correct" amount of fluids depends on several factors. If you honestly feel you are thirsty all the time, an evaluation by an internist is in order. Fluid requirement is affected by weight, physical activity, salt intake, and other factors. In general, your natural thirst should dictate fluid intake. If the urine is pale yellow and nonodorous, then generally fluid balance is normal. Do not be persuaded to think that gallons of water washes away medical problems.

The frequency of voiding varies considerably. Excluding nighttime, normal frequency for adults is seven to eight times daily. For people under the age of sixty-five during sleep hours, waking once to void is normal. As people age, bladder capacity generally decreases and both day and night voiding frequencies increase.

The bladder has a most unfortunate position in pregnancy, sandwiched between the pubic bone and the growing uterus. It is quite common for pregnant women to void frequently and to have incontinence. Less commonly, they experience urine blockage. If this happens, the woman will have severe pain and be unable to void as the bladder fills with an increasing amount of urine. Pregnant women who feel they are unable to urinate should seek immediate evaluation and not wait for severe pain.

In nonpregnant women, daytime voiding is usually every two to four hours. Waiting extended periods of time to urinate may result in overstretching of the bladder muscle, which eventually results in decreased ability of the bladder muscle to contract properly. The urine that is not excreted lies in the bladder, becomes stagnant, and is at risk for urinary tract infections. The other extreme, voiding very frequently, is also detrimental. Frequent voiding in order to avoid leakage episodes can result in a "small" bladder, which gives the sensation of being full at progressively lower volumes, therefore exacerbating the problem.

There are a number of foods that act as dietary irritants, resulting in a severe urge to urinate, urinary frequency, incontinence, or pain. A brief list includes alcoholic beverages, caffeine, spicy foods, milk products, sugar, carbonated drinks, cheese, chocolate, citrus fruits or juices, NutraSweet, saccharine, soy sauce, tomatoes, and onions. As many of these foods have nutritional value, the goal is not to eliminate all of them, but to eliminate one category at a time to see if there is a particular category that is particularly irritating to your bladder. More complete lists are available from your physician.

Bowel habits: Failure to empty the bowel can cause varying degrees of constipation that can have differing effects on the urinary process. If constipation is severe, the enlarged rectum can actually compress the urethra, making it difficult to empty the bladder. A diet rich in fiber and with the right amount of fluid intake should produce a soft, well-lubricated stool that is easy to pass. If you feel your fiber and fluid intake are adequate but are still constipated, consult your physician. There are some stool softeners that if used too frequently can exacerbate the problem.

There are a number of medications and foods that cause constipation. Often, permanent relief of constipation can be obtained by avoiding these foods and discontinuing or changing medications. Any medication change should be done with a doctor's supervision. Note that caffeine and alcohol act as diuretics (increasing water output). Therefore, while you may feel your fluid intake is adequate, if a significant amount of the intake is diuretics, they will aggravate constipation by causing you to lose excessive amounts of fluid. Oatmeal and rice are examples of foods that may cause constipation. Most painkillers, when used often, increase constipation (acetaminophen does not).

Behavioral changes and environment: Waiting extended periods of time to urinate can also contribute to incontinence. There are many reasons why some women delay voiding. Professionals may not feel they have the time to seek a rest room. Women who have dementia may simply not be aware of their bodily functions or the timely need to use a toilet. The bladder is normal in many of these women but the mental capacity or social arrangements are deficient. These women may need to have reminders to use bathroom facilities on a regular basis or require facilitated access to facilities.

Incontinent women should plan to have a bathroom within reasonable distance of the living or work area if their disorder cannot be corrected. In most cases, the longer the delay in voiding, the more likely it is that an accident will happen. Some bladder problems can be corrected with simple attention to accessibility to a toilet. Another problem is women who do not have the normal sensory awareness of a full bladder which would let them know that they should seek rest room facilities in the near future. For these women, a regular, timed schedule of voiding may resolve the problem. There are time clocks with discreet beepers or vibrations to remind patients to void at regular intervals. A bedside commode will help those women who are aware that they need to void but can't quite get to the bathroom in time.

Clothing: Clothing actually plays a significant role in good toileting habits. Clothes should be easy to manage when attempting to get to a toilet in a hurry. There are many women who are able to get to the bathroom only to wet themselves as they attempt to remove layers of clothes and open difficult buttons. If there are problems with dexterity, there are many clothes available with Velcro closures or elastic waists. A good source of information for these products is the National Association for Continence (tel. (864) 579-7902, or toll-free 1-800-BLADDER).

Medications: There are a vast number of medications that affect the lower urinary tract. A complete list of all medications and doses should be available from your doctor, but the most common offenders are diuretics, some antidepressants, and some hypertension medications (as mentioned previously). Certainly control of hypertension, body fluid balance, and heart function are more important than controlling incontinence. Nevertheless, with the large number of medications available, often physicians can alter doses or choose alternative medications that will maintain the essential systems and be less likely to exacerbate incontinence.

Numerous medications are used to control incontinence. Some over-the-counter cold medicines can be helpful with some types of incontinence but none should be taken without the advice of a physician. Both the over-the-counter and prescription medications can be very effective but close supervision is necessary to minimize side effects and drug interactions. Nonprescription drugs that may help incontinent women by tightening the urethra include Comhist LA®, Entex LA®, and Ornade®. These and other cold medications may also cause difficulty in emptying the bladder if the urethra becomes too tight to allow urine to pass. There is abundant research in progress concerning improved drugs for urinary control. Women can expect some excellent options over the next few years.

Estrogen Replacement and Vaginal Estrogen Cream

Estrogen has several beneficial effects on the lower urinary tract and vagina. As a result of estrogen deficiency in menopause, women may have symptoms including dryness, frequent urination, itching, and pain. Women with these symptoms may benefit from either oral or vaginal estrogen. Women who have "atrophic" changes associated with menopause may benefit from estrogen replacement. Symptoms include dryness, frequency of urination, itching, and pain. It is important to note, however, that the life-protecting benefits to the bone and heart are all documented with oral dosing and not with vaginal cream.

Some women will benefit from using estrogen cream vaginally. Vaginal or oral estrogen increases the thickness of the walls of the urethra, resulting in a tighter closure of the urethra. Theoretically, this improves the ability of the urethra to keep urine from escaping from the bladder. The literature is varied as far as how much success to expect from vaginal estrogen cream. Given that the risks are minimal, a trial of vaginal estrogen cream is reasonable for any woman with incontinence or vaginal irritation. The absorption of the vaginal estrogen cream into the blood varies. In some women the level can be as high as with oral estrogen and therefore, all the issues regarding risks and benefits of estrogen replacement apply to vaginal estrogen cream. A typical regimen uses one gram of cream nightly for two weeks and then one gram twice a week for lifetime maintenance. Many women will continue to have relief using even smaller maintenance doses. A new option for vaginal estrogen replacement is a small ring that stays in the vagina and releases small amounts of estrogen for three months. This eliminates the need to apply any creams and is therefore quite convenient.

Pessaries and Other Barrier Devices

Pessaries are devices worn in the vagina that elevate dropped organs and treat incontinence. Pessaries are usually made of silicone and come in varying sizes. They are somewhat similar to contraceptive diaphragms in consistency, insertion, and removal. The variety of shapes allows for comfortable elevation of dropped pelvic organs and for individualized fitting. Pessaries are generally inserted and removed by the patient after instruction from a physician or nurse, but some women prefer to have the physician remove and insert their pessaries every two months or so. The length of time they may remain in place between changing and cleaning varies from patient to patient. Some women can go for up to three months between changes while other women either require or prefer daily changes. The latest pessaries, specifically designed for women with incontinence, provide support to the area of the vagina that is immediately under the bladder. Here they can help prevent urinary leakage associated with coughing, straining, and other maneuvers. Pessaries have the advantage of having minimal risks but the disadvantage of requiring frequent changing and physician visits. Some women can have sexual relations with the pessary in place but most remove it prior to sexual activity. Nevertheless, if the symptoms are cured by a pessary many women are thrilled to avoid surgery.

Urethral insertion devices: There is one FDA-approved urethral occlusion device, the Reliance Insert® (Uromed), and one device in the investigative stage. The Reliance® device is a silicone plug with a small balloon at the end. After professional sizing and instruction, the patient places the device in the urethra and inflates the balloon, which will be on the inside of the bladder holding the device in place. This device has the advantage of providing immediate continence but must be removed each time to urinate and can cause an increased frequency of urinary tract infections. It is necessary to change and dispose of the small device each time you have to void. Some women choose to use this device at special social events or athletic activities while other women prefer to have the device in place more often. There certainly is a learning period with this device and many women find the insertion and removal too difficult to perform regularly. On the upside, it provides immediate nonsurgical control of involuntary urine loss. The devices that are still in research evaluation will not require removal to permit voiding.

Urethral "caps" or barriers: Two barrier devices are available that are placed over the opening of the urethra rather than into the urethra. The Fem Assist® device (Applied Medical) is a simple cap that is placed over the urethra. A gentle suction keeps the device in place and keeps the walls of the urethra closed. The Impress® device (Uromed) has a soft, cushioned, triangular flat surface covered with a special gel. The flat surface covers the urethra and acts as a simple barrier. Initial studies with each of these devices have demonstrated increased urinary control and little to no infection risk. It is too early to recommend one of these devices over the other as general use of these devices is just starting. Some patients find it difficult to apply or use these devices effectively, but since there is essentially no risk, you may want to try either or both.

Surgical Treatment

There are a large number of surgical procedures performed for incontinence. Before undergoing surgery, you should know a few essential pieces of information. First, there are different causes for incontinence and the same procedure is not effective for every type of incontinence. A qualified specialist must perform urodynamic studies prior to surgery in order to choose the proper procedure and to determine if you have characteristics that decrease the chances for a successful procedure. If urodynamic studies (history and physical examination alone cannot yield this information) prove that the problem is the classic genuine stress incontinence, the procedure on which there is the most data, and which has the most favorable and long-lasting results, is the Burch colposuspension. There are other procedures available, but when evaluated over time, they do not demonstrate as consistent or long-lasting results when compared with the Burch. One procedure, called the "sling" procedure, usually compares with the Burch with regard to curing incontinence but in most studies carries a higher complication rate. Based on the urodynamic evaluation, however, for some women, the sling may be advised over the Burch.

The Burch procedure historically required a five- to seven-inch horizontal incision in the pubic hairline (a "bikini" incision). This procedure can now be performed via the laparoscope (small telescope requiring two to four small skin punctures, each less than one-half inch) or by a reduced single two-inch incision in the hairline. Both approaches allow the patient to go home the day of surgery or the following day. These modifications of the Burch procedure are promising, noninvasive, and attempt to duplicate the standard Burch procedure. Data are not yet available concerning the long-term success of these less invasive approaches.

Alternative vaginal procedures are promoted by many physicians because they are less invasive and require a shorter recovery time than the standard Burch, and there may be situations when speed is essential and the vaginal approach may be favorable. The less invasive methods available for the Burch procedure may decrease the differences in recovery time that previously existed between the Burch and the vaginal procedures. Overall, the abdominal Burch approach is advised.

While the argument for the Burch procedure has been presented strongly, the procedure still has about a 5 to 10 percent initial failure rate, and about a 15 percent failure rate after five years. It is thus important to recognize when opting for surgery that cure is not guaranteed. In addition, a small fraction of women undergoing surgery for incontinence will have difficulty emptying the bladder following surgery. The amount of time to establish normal voiding varies. About half of women are able to urinate after a few days but it is not uncommon for women to be unable to void for seven to fourteen days. In extremely rare circumstances, the overcorrection is significant enough that a reoperation may be necessary to take out sutures that are too tight. The theme cannot be repeated often enough: Complete evaluation and completely informed decision making is necessary.

Collagen injections: While the problem in genuine stress incontinence is mainly a lack of support of the bladder, less frequently the problem is that the walls of the urethra simply are not closed tightly enough to hold urine (poor coaptation of the walls). When intrinsic sphincter deficiency is the problem, a collagen injection may be performed. The same substance that is injected by plastic surgeons to bulk up a small chin or cheekbones can be used to provide bulking to the urethra and stop involuntary urine loss. The procedure is performed either in the office or in an ambulatory surgery setting and the patient goes home the same day. There are no incisions, just injections. This is an excellent noninvasive treatment method, but patients must fall into a small, special category of incontinence in order to expect good results. In addition, women should know that it is not uncommon to require more than one session to achieve the desired results. Even physicians with excellent experience with the procedure require more than one session for success with some patients. Again, one hundred percent success cannot be guaranteed.

Conclusions

Urinary incontinence and other problems of pelvic organ prolapse are common. They are not part of the normal aging process and should be treated whenever the problem becomes unacceptable to the individual woman. Many aspects of everyday life, stress activities, medical problems, and childbirth affect the likelihood of developing incontinence. There is a need for increased education so that women can be informed about this problem that has been "taboo" for so many years. There may be some simple dietary or social habits that can be changed that will cure incontinence in some women. For others, a medication or pelvic exercises may be all that is needed. New ideas about managing labor and delivery may provide insight into decreasing the damage caused by vaginal childbirth. A vast array of incontinence pessaries, urethral occlusion devices, exercises, and injections are available that can cure incontinence. Established surgical procedures and a wide array of nonsurgical alternatives are available to incontinent women. Educated decision making is the rule for incontinence evaluation and treatment.

Chapter 10

BREAST CANCER—DIAGNOSIS AND NEW SURGICAL OPTIONS

WITH ERNA BUSCH, M.D.
ILLUSTRATIONS BY ERNA BUSCH, M.D.

Erna Busch, M.D., a cancer surgeon at North Shore University Hospital in Manhasset, New York, grew up in a family of five girls. She was expecting her first child when she agreed to write this chapter. Since then, she has given birth to a baby girl, whom she and her husband describe as a pretty little miracle.

We have come a long way with regard to breast cancer diagnosis and treatment. Too often women are overwhelmed, not only by the diagnosis, but by the specter of what will follow. Therefore, women should be presented with diagnostic steps that are easy and relatively noninvasive. New, minimally invasive surgical and radiological techniques make the diagnostic process easier, both mentally and physically. What is important is to get diagnosed and know whether or not more needs to be done. Should you be in the small percentile that actually turns out to have cancer, there is still more good news. It is now possible to have your breast surgery and avoid extensive axillary dissection for lymph nodes. Sentinel node biopsy makes the surgical process less painful and shortens recovery. Because damage to lymph drainage causes most postoperative problems, such as swelling of the arm and increased potential for infection, I am very excited about this new technique, although it must still be proven to be safe and as accurate as complete axillary dissection.

Nothing creates more anxiety and fear for a woman than finding a lump in her breast or learning her mammogram is abnormal. Breast problems are extremely common. But, unfortunately, so too is breast cancer. Over 180,000 women will develop breast cancer in 1997, one in every eight women, and nearly 40,000 women will die from it.[1] Yet it is a disease that can be cured in the vast majority of women when it is detected early.

Early Detection

The American Cancer Society recommendations for early detection include a combination of three screening methods: (1) routine monthly breast self-examination beginning at twenty, (2) breast examination by a health care provider every three years between ages twenty and forty, and yearly after age 40, and (3) yearly mammography beginning at age forty. All three of these are complementary and should be used together since each by itself can still miss a cancer.

Evidence suggests that cancers found by women who perform routine monthly breast self-examination are smaller than those cancers found by physicians. Smaller cancers mean higher rates of cure. Yet many women still do not perform the self-exam. Women who don't examine themselves say they aren't sure they're doing it right, they're too lumpy to know what's abnormal, they see their doctor regularly (and the doctor is better at it), or they're just too scared they'll find something. Some of these worries disappear after having instruction in breast self-examination by a trained health professional. (For the basics, see figure 10.1.) Doing self-examination is also one way of taking responsibility for your own health. The exam itself costs no money but is potentially lifesaving.

There are several signs of cancer to look for on examination of the breasts. Many of these signs can arise from other, noncancerous changes but any of these should be promptly evaluated by a physician. Finding a lump is the most common sign of breast cancer. Many women have lumpy breasts and no one can know a woman's breasts better than the woman herself. Breasts vary during the monthly menstrual cycle and a woman who becomes familiar with her normal monthly changes can spare herself a great deal of anxiety when she feels differences. Even a doctor who sees a woman once or twice a year can have a difficult time knowing what's normal for her. The truth, although not very reassuring, is that a physician may not always be able to distinguish a cancer from normal breast tissue, which is why a woman who knows her own breasts can help. A woman can be less concerned about something a physician feels if the woman knows her breasts have felt that way for a long time. On the other hand, a subtle change in what a woman herself feels, so slight that it might not seem significant to an examiner, can sometimes be an important sign of a problem that should not be ignored.

Other less common signs of breast cancer include new inward retraction or puckering of the nipple (inverted nipple), dimpling in the skin of the breast, discharge from the nipple (particularly if bloody or clear), ulceration of the skin, redness or swelling, pain, or a lump under the armpit. Nipple scaling and crusting may be a sign of a special condition called Paget's disease, which can be an indication of an underlying cancer. Remember, these signs do not always mean breast cancer and can indicate benign (noncancerous) conditions as well, but it is extremely important that a physician evaluate any of these.

Figure 10.1. Breast self-examination.

WHY DO THE BREAST SELF-EXAM?

There are many good reasons for doing a breast self-exam each month. One reason is that it is easy to do and the more you do it, the better you will get at it. When you get to know how your breasts normally feel, you will quickly be able to feel any change, and early detection is the key to the successful treatment and cure. Remember, a breast self-exam could save your breast—and save your life. Most breast lumps are found by women themselves, but in fact, most lumps in the breast are not cancer. Be safe, be sure.

WHEN TO DO BREAST SELF-EXAM

The best time to do breast self-exam is right after your period, when breasts are not tender or swollen. If you do not have regular periods or sometimes skip a month, do it on the same day every month.

NOW, HOW TO DO BREAST SELF-EXAM

1. Lie down and put a pillow under your right shoulder. Place your right arm behind your head.
2. Use the finger pads of your three middle fingers on your left land to feel for lumps or thickening. Your finger pads are the top third of each finger.

Finger Pads

3. Press firmly enough to know how your breast feels. If you're not sure how hard to press, ask your health care provider. Or try to copy the way your health care provider uses the finger pads during a breast exam. Learn what your breast feels like most of the time. A firm ridge in the lower curve of each breast is normal.

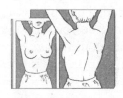

4. Move around the breast in a set way. You can choose either the circle (A), the up and down line (B), or the wedge (C). Do it the same way every time. It will help you to make sure that you've gone over the entire breast area, and to remember how your breast feels.

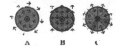

A   B   C

5. Now examine your left breast using right hand finger pads.
6. If you find any changes, see your doctor right away.

For added safety, you should also check your breasts while standing in front of a mirror right after you do your breast self-exam each month. See if there are any changes in the way your breasts look: dimpling of the skin, changes in the nipple, or redness or swelling.

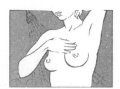

You might also want to do a breast self-exam while you're in the shower. Your soapy hands will glide over the wet skin making it easy to check how your breasts feel.

MAMMOGRAPHY

Routine mammography is a critical component of early detection. Mammography is widely available and screening programs are common. The Food and Drug Administration now certifies mammogram facilities. Accreditation is also offered by the American College of Radiology. This helps to ensure that the mammogram meets the standards for quality, including the radiation dose and the interpretation of the result.

Screening mammograms are those mammograms performed as a routine evaluation of otherwise normal breasts. A mammogram consists of compressing the breast tissue between two flat plates and taking an X ray. It is important to have adequate compression so the X rays can penetrate through the breast well and give an optimal image. Two images of each breast are routinely taken. By current estimates, a cancer can be seen on a mammogram more than two years before it would be able to be felt. Screening mammograms have clearly been shown to lower the mortality rate (risk of dying) from breast cancer in women over the age of fifty by 20 to 30 percent. It's somewhat more controversial whether regular mammograms benefit women between the ages of forty and fifty. However, one fact is clear: Incidence rates for breast cancer sharply rise after age forty, and women in this age group can and do die from breast cancer. Early detection is still the best hope to find cancer in order to treat it at a curable stage.

Mammography should also be performed at other times as recommended by a physician. Diagnostic mammogram refers to a mammogram performed because there is an abnormality present on physical examination; it also refers to additional mammographic X rays performed when an abnormality is detected on a routine screening mammogram. Additional images are often taken to better define specific areas of concern. Spot compression views are used to better delineate questionable masses, and magnification views help characterize hard-to-see microcalcifications. These extra images can help the doctor to decide if an abnormality is likely to be benign or is potentially malignant.

As with breast self-examination, many women have reasons why they don't have mammograms: They are afraid of getting exposed to radiation, afraid of the discomfort during the examination, or afraid of having something found. Sometimes a woman's doctor simply hasn't told her she should have a mammogram. And even today, many women remain unaware of the benefits. The dose of radiation from a routine mammogram has decreased with improvements in mammography equipment and is very small. The discomfort of having the breast compressed is quite real in many women, but in general having a mammogram should not be a painful experience. Remember the importance and benefits of the test in comparison to the very brief time of discomfort. If you are still having menstrual cycles, it's a good idea to try to plan your mammogram for a time during the monthly cycle when the breasts aren't so tender—usually right after the menses has finished—to minimize the chances of discomfort. Avoiding caffeine the week prior to the exam may help to reduce discomfort in some women.

Some of the abnormalities looked for on mammograms are masses, nodules, microcalcifications, densities, and asymmetries. Characteristic masses that are suspicious for cancers can have a stellate or sunburst appearance on the mammogram. Sometimes cancers can also form smoother nodules. Microcalcifications, which are tiny deposits of calcium, can also be a sign of an early cancer. The majority of findings and microcalcifications occurring in women's breasts are not due to cancer. However, it is not always possible to tell just by their appearance which abnormalities are cancerous and which are benign.

In cases where the suspicion for cancer is very low but there is concern because the area cannot be definitely classified as benign, a repeat mammogram in four to six months may be advised. In cases where the suspicion is greater, a biopsy may be advised. Be reassured, however, that of the abnormalities found on mammograms for which biopsy is recommended, only about 20 percent turn out to be cancers. If a cancer is found, remember most tend to be small and in an early stage.

Despite well-performed mammograms, some cancers are missed by mammography. This fact underscores the vital importance of manual breast examination in addition to routine mammography. It cannot be emphasized enough that if a lump is felt or other abnormality is present despite a negative mammogram, evaluation by a physician is critical.

OTHER IMAGING TESTS

Ultrasound is also being used more frequently to evaluate the breast. However, it does not and should not replace mammography for routine breast screening. It is used to help further define specific abnormal masses seen on mammograms or lumps felt on examination. It can help to differentiate a lump being caused by a cyst (fluid-filled lump) from one that is solid, something that cannot be done by mammography alone. It can also define the character of a cyst, if it is anything other than a simple cyst. For example, if a cyst is complex, either with debris floating in it or with multiple septations (separate pockets of fluid), then aspiration or drainage of the cyst by placing a small needle in the cyst is generally advised (see section on cysts page 285).

Computerized tomography (CT) has been disappointing as a breast-imaging test and is not generally used. Magnetic resonance imaging (MRI) is still an investigational test as far as breast imaging is concerned. Its main value is in detecting leakage from silicone implants, but studies are still in progress to further define its role in imaging other breast problems. Positron emission tomography (PET) scans are also investigational, but encouraging preliminary results are being obtained. Digital mammography is a promising type of mammogram being evaluated. It uses computer-enhanced images but many technical aspects need to be improved upon before it can replace standard mammogram imaging. A new test was recently approved for breast imaging, called the technetium-99m sestamibi scintimammography. It does not replace standard mammography but may complement it.

Evaluation

The first step in seeking an evaluation for a breast problem is to speak to your regular physician. He/she will in most cases refer you to either a general surgeon, a breast surgeon, or a surgical oncologist. All of these physicians should be board certified in general surgery. Since breast problems are among the most common problems, a general surgeon frequently sees many such patients in his/her practice. A breast surgeon has a practice limited to breast diseases, or a special interest in breast diseases, and often has additional training specifically in breast diseases or surgical oncology. A surgical oncologist has additional training in many cancers, including breast, and may have a special interest in breast cancer. The decision about whom to see should usually be based upon the doctors available in your community and health care plan and upon recommendations of your personal physician.

On your initial visit, the physician will obtain your history and perform a physical examination. If mammograms have been done, it is important that you bring the actual mammogram X rays and written reports to the initial visit. Mammography centers will make copies if you so request or will in some cases release the originals. Old mammograms are also useful for comparison. If a biopsy has already been performed then it is also important that you bring the pathology slides (actual slides made from the tissue removed) and written report from the biopsy. You may obtain the slides by calling the pathology department of the hospital or laboratory where the pathology was performed. The pathology slides can then be reviewed to confirm the findings.

The evaluation may reveal that the breast abnormality has a low likelihood of being caused by a cancer, and your doctor may suggest a period of observation. It is extremely important that you return for a follow-up visit if this is what is recommended. You should schedule an appointment for the appropriate time. You must then be responsible for keeping that appointment. If an abnormality does not change or improves by the next visit, it can continue to be observed. However, if a more suspicious change were to occur, it might then be advisable to proceed with the next step, a biopsy.

BREAST BIOPSY

In other cases it might not be considered safe merely to observe an abnormality and a biopsy would be recommended. A biopsy simply means obtaining a specimen of breast cells or breast tissue and having a pathologist examine it on slides under the microscope. (A pathologist is the physician who reads the slides.)

Biopsies of Palpable Abnormalities (Abnormalities That Can Be Felt)

Fine needle aspiration biopsy: There are several different ways to perform biopsies. If your physician feels a lump during the office visit, a needle biopsy (fine needle aspiration, FNA for short) can be performed. A small needle is placed into the lump and a sample is obtained for examination under the microscope. It can give a rapid diagnosis but a negative test does not completely eliminate the chance that a cancer is present, because only a very small sample of cells is removed. If the clinical impression is benign, a negative result can give reassurance. However, if a lump is suspicious despite a negative needle biopsy, additional testing is required.

Excisional/incisional biopsy: Another way of doing a biopsy is to remove the entire abnormality (excisional biopsy) or a piece of the abnormality (incisional biopsy) surgically. This is done as an outpatient procedure.

Presurgical testing is often required several days in advance of the surgery date. Presurgical testing may include blood and urine tests and in some cases a chest X ray and electrocardiogram. On the day of surgery, an anesthesiologist is often present and often a sedative is given through an intravenous line to help make the patient comfortable. Then, after injection of a local anesthetic to numb the area, an incision is made in the breast and a piece of breast tissue is removed. The incision must be closed with stitches that either dissolve on their own or have to be removed in a week or so. Postoperative discomfort is often minimal and can be relieved with acetaminophen or a slightly stronger prescription medication. Complications are unusual but can include bruising or infection. In rare cases bleeding can cause a hematoma in the breast, which may require drainage.

Preliminary results on the biopsy can sometimes be found out the same day by doing a frozen section. This is a quick processing technique that evaluates a very limited part of the biopsy. The results are fairly accurate, but it is important to wait for the full processing of the biopsy for the final diagnosis. This may take several days. Some surgeons prefer not to order a frozen section, particularly for very small abnormalities.

Biopsies of Nonpalpable Abnormalities

There are several different methods to biopsy abnormalities found on mammograms or on ultrasounds. Since these abnormalities cannot be felt, special techniques are required. The choice of which method is best can be influenced by the characteristics of the abnormality and of the woman's breast.

Needle/wire localized biopsy: One way to biopsy an abnormal area seen on mammography (or on ultrasound) is to perform a needle or wire localized excision. In most cases, this is an outpatient surgical procedure. Presurgical testing is generally required several days before the planned surgery, just as with an excisional biopsy. On the day of surgery but prior to the patient's going to the operating room, the radiologist performs a procedure called a localization. A mammogram (or ultrasound) is done and after local anesthesia is injected, a small needle/wire device is inserted into the breast near the abnormal area. This wire will serve as the surgeon's guide to finding the abnormal area. Once the wire is in place, the woman proceeds to the operating room. As with the biopsies for palpable lumps, often an anesthesiologist is present and gives sedation intravenously. A local anesthetic is then injected and a skin incision is made. The area of breast tissue surrounding the wire is removed. It is important that a mammogram be taken of the specimen of breast tissue removed to ensure that it contains the abnormal area. For example, if microcalcifications were biopsied, they must be seen in the mammogram of the piece of breast tissue removed. In rare circumstances, the area can be missed. In this case, the surgeon will remove a small amount of additional tissue to find it.

Stereotactic biopsy: Remember that most biopsies done for mammographic abnormalities turn out to be benign and not caused by cancer. In recent years, several different types of procedures have been developed in an attempt to reduce the need for open surgical biopsies, and to make the biopsy procedure as simple as possible. One of these is called a stereotactic biopsy. A stereotactic biopsy is performed on a specialized mammographic table by a radiologist or surgeon trained in this technique. The woman lies facedown on the table with the breast hanging through an opening. The breast is then compressed as in a mammogram. Using a computerized digital imaging system, the abnormal area is located. Local anesthesia is given and a small nick is made in the skin. A special biopsy gun is fired into the area to take a small sliver, known as a core, of tissue. Several such cores are taken. The entire abnormal area is not removed and only a small portion is sampled. Not all women are candidates for this type of procedure. The breast must be large enough and the area to be biopsied cannot be too deep (close to the chest wall) or too superficial. The woman must not be pregnant because of the danger of radiation to the fetus.

The results from a stereotactic biopsy are very accurate; however, certain guidelines must be followed depending on the results. First, the results must be concordant with (in agreement with) the findings on the mammogram for which the biopsy was done. For example, if the biopsy was done for microcalcifications, then microcalcifications must be seen on pathology review. If they aren't seen, the biopsy is considered inadequate and it either must be repeated or a new biopsy must be performed by one of the other methods. If the results are clearly benign and are in concordance with the lesion biopsied, then a six-month follow-up mammogram is often recommended to ensure that no further change in the remaining area occurs. If a suspicious change were to occur on follow-up, a repeat biopsy or removal might be advised. If the biopsy shows any atypical cells, then the needle/wire localized biopsy is recommended to remove the area. If the stereotactic biopsy shows cancer, then the next step can be discussed with the surgeon, and a preliminary surgical biopsy has been avoided.

The risks of stereotactic biopsy are small, but include bruising and, far less commonly, infection or hematoma. It is highly unlikely, although possible, that a cancer would be missed by this procedure. It is extremely important to return for the recommended follow-up as assurance.

If the abnormality is visible or only seen by ultrasound, a similar type of procedure, known as an ultrasound guided core biopsy, can be performed. This is simply a biopsy done using the ultrasound during the biopsy to guide the physician to the correct spot. Several small samples are removed and the interpretation of the results, the recommendations for follow-up, and the risks are the same as for the stereotactic procedure.

A newer extension of the stereotactic procedure is called a mammotome biopsy. It is performed in a similar manner to the stereotactic procedure but it is possible to take many more cores of tissue by using a specialized biopsy instrument. The advantage of this procedure is that it allows many more cores of tissue to be taken through the same tiny skin nick and can lower the chances of obtaining an inadequate biopsy.

ABBI™ biopsy: Another very new option for biopsy is called an ABBI™ (Advanced Breast Biopsy Instrumentation) procedure. This procedure is a combination of the stereotactic and needle localized approaches. It involves use of a specialized mammogram table similar to that used in the stereotactic core biopsy procedure. It differs from the stereotactic procedure in that the entire abnormal area can potentially be removed in one piece. A small incision in the skin is required. A special biopsy instrument is used to remove a piece of breast tissue ranging in size roughly from the eraser on the head of a pencil to a wine cork. The advantage of the ABBI™ is that it is a single-stage procedure (localization and excision) and potentially allows the entire removal of the lesion. In contrast to the needle localized open biopsy procedure, the ABBI™ requires neither an anesthesiologist nor preoperative testing. There are some factors that limit the use of this procedure, similar to those limiting the use of the stereotactic biopsy. Since it is a biopsy procedure, if a cancer is found additional surgery will be required in most cases.

There has been some reluctance to recommend these newer and less invasive biopsy procedures. Physicians may be less familiar with and less comfortable recommending newer procedures. Patients are also sometimes reluctant to undergo a newer procedure, which may not have as much experience behind it as older methods. There is also a potential for misuse or overuse of these biopsy procedures in situations where they may not be the best approach or where a biopsy might not even be indicated. It is important that the appropriate indications for biopsy be followed. Certainly not all women are candidates for these procedures, and one approach may offer advantages over another in an individual situation. In certain other cases, any of the approaches could be used. It is important to know the options in order to make an informed decision about which one is best for you. If one is recommended to you over another, you should understand the reasons. After receiving your results, it is also important to follow the guidelines that determine the next step. If a six-month follow-up is recommended after a benign biopsy result, it is extremely important to return for that follow-up.

BENIGN DIAGNOSES

There are many benign or noncancerous conditions that can cause abnormalities in the breast, and they can sometimes be difficult to distinguish, without a biopsy, from cancers. The following are descriptions of some of these.

Fibrocystic disease, condition, or changes all refer loosely to painful and lumpy breasts. Benign breast disease and mammary dysplasia are two other terms often used. A large percentage of women experience such symptoms at some time during their life and so it seems inappropriate to call this a "disease." While fibrocystic changes can certainly cause pain, tenderness, and lumps, not all women with these symptoms have fibrocystic changes in their breasts. True fibrocystic changes can, however, cause lumps in the breast and abnormal findings on mammography. It is often not possible to distinguish fibrocystic changes from cancer without a biopsy.

Cysts, which may be a component of fibrocystic changes, are very common. These round, fluid-filled lumps are often multiple and can sometimes be painful. Sometimes they cause no symptoms at all and are only seen on mammograms. Simple cysts are smooth and thin-walled. Complex cysts may be filled with debris, have a thickened wall, or septations (separate pockets). If palpable, cysts can be drained in the office by inserting a small needle and aspirating the fluid. If they can't be felt, cysts can be drained using the ultrasound for guidance. Cysts do not always require drainage but may be drained if large and painful or if they appear complex on ultrasound. The association of a cyst with cancer is very rare so the fluid from simple cysts is not routinely tested. However, it is best to check the fluid from complex cysts or from cysts filled with bloody fluid. Cysts can sometimes come back after drainage.

Sclerosing adenosis is caused by a proliferation of lobular tissue which can cause a lump in the breast or calcifications on a mammogram. Biopsy is often required to differentiate from a cancer.

Fibroadenomas are firm, rubbery lumps that tend to occur in younger women. They can be multiple in ten to fifteen percent of women. They appear as solid lumps on ultrasound. If the clinical impression is strongly in favor of a fibroadenoma, observation with careful follow-up may be all that is required. Biopsy by one of the previously described methods may be needed, however, to confirm the diagnosis.

Fat necrosis can be mistaken for cancer since it can cause a lump or pain in the breast or an abnormal mass on a mammogram. There is a possible association with previous injury to the breast. Biopsy is often necessary to differentiate from a cancer.

Duct hyperplasia is seen when there is an increased number of cells within the ducts. Sometimes the cells can look atypical or slightly abnormal. These changes can cause a lump in the breast or abnormalities on mammograms. Lobular hyperplasia is similar and seen when there is an increased number of cells in the lobular units. Biopsy establishes this diagnosis.

Papillomas are warty growths that can occur within the duct system of the breasts. They are the most common cause of bloody nipple discharge but require biopsy to exclude cancer.

Duct ectasia is caused when the breast ducts dilate from stagnant secretions. Periductal mastitis results when inflammation occurs. It can cause nipple discharge, nipple retraction, lumps, or pain, and sometimes infections or abscesses ensue. Dilated ducts or calcifications can sometimes be seen on mammography, and there is often a characteristic appearance so biopsy is not always necessary.

Intramammary lymph nodes can cause nodules visible on mammogram and often have a characteristic appearance. Observation with follow-up is often recommended.

Phyllodes tumors can cause a firm lump in the breast. They are usually benign but occasionally malignant types can occur. Treatment is surgical removal.

"Why Me?": Risk Factors for Breast Cancer

The first question women ask when they find out they have cancer is, "Why me?" Unfortunately we don't have a definitive answer to that question. Many women react with, "But no one in my family ever had breast cancer." It's important to realize that the majority of women who develop breast cancer do not have a family history of the disease. In recent years a great deal has been discovered about the genetics of cancer. Most cancers result from defects or mutations in the normal genetic makeup of cells. But most of these changes are not passed on from parents to offspring because they don't occur in all cells of the body. They occur spontaneously in breast cells. Mutations can only be passed along to offspring when they occur in the cells responsible for procreation—the ova and sperm. Approximately 5 to 10 percent of breast cancer is believed to be genetically inherited. Because 50 percent of the genes come from the father and 50 percent from the mother, this form of breast cancer can be inherited from either side of the family.

The gene responsible for the majority of cases of inherited breast cancer has recently been identified and is called the BRCA gene. Women in whom there is a higher suspicion of having the inherited form tend to have breast cancer or relatives with breast cancer that has occurred at a younger age (premenopausal), in both breasts (bilateral), or they have a personal or family history of other cancers, particularly ovarian, colon, endometrial, and prostate. The most common gene responsible is BRCA1. The BRCA2 gene has also been identified. BRCA1 is a gene that is also strongly linked to the inherited form of ovarian cancer. Over fifty different mutations have been identified and each family has their own specific mutation. Specific mutations have also been seen in the Ashkenazi Jewish population. If a woman is found to test positive for the BRCA1 gene mutation, there is an estimated 85 percent lifetime risk of developing breast cancer and a 40 to 50 percent risk of developing ovarian cancer. On the other hand, if a woman tests negative, it does not mean she will not develop breast cancer. She still has a risk of carrying a gene defect that has not yet been identified or of developing breast cancer of the noninherited type.

Genetic testing is not a screening test to be used in the general population. Women who might consider having the test are those who actually have breast or ovarian cancer, especially if they've developed it at an early age, women with a family history of breast or ovarian cancer, women who have a blood relative with a known mutation, or women of Ashkenazi Jewish background.

Genetic testing itself carries a great many implications both for women who test positive and for their relatives. One issue relates to what to do medically for women who do test positive. Unfortunately, the best answer to this is not yet known. Close surveillance to detect cancer early and initiate early treatment is one possibility. Performing mammography at an earlier age and having more frequent breast examinations makes sense but no studies are available yet to show this is adequate. The extreme opposite is bilateral prophylactic mastectomy. We don't know, however, to what degree removing both breasts would actually be protective. A small amount of breast tissue is left behind with the standard mastectomy, so although it may lower the risk substantially, it probably doesn't completely eliminate it. Chemoprevention, or using some type of agent or medication to help prevent cancer, is also being investigated.

Another issue is what happens to a woman's ability to obtain medical and life insurance if she tests positive. If the insurance company pays for the test, do they have the right to know the results? If so, can they deny insurance based upon a positive test?

A third issue relates to a false reassurance if a woman tests negative. In addition, a woman testing negative may feel guilty if other family members test positive. There are many unresolved issues and questions that need to be carefully considered before going ahead with testing. Some of these will require legislative efforts to protect women who undergo testing. It is very important that a genetic counselor help guide the decision to proceed and be involved with counseling when the results are obtained.

Not everyone who has a family history of breast cancer will have the genetically transmitted form of breast cancer. Another 10 to 15 percent of women may indeed have a family history, but not have an identifiable genetic defect. We call this familial breast cancer. The risk for these women is higher than for women who don't have a family history and depends on the closeness of the family relationship. For example, a woman whose mother had breast cancer is at a higher risk than one whose aunt had breast cancer. However, the risk is not as high if the mother developed breast cancer postmenopausally.

There are many other risk factors that seem to be important in determining a woman's chances of developing breast cancer. But as with any risk factor, having these risk factors, or even having several of them, does not doom a woman to developing cancer. The following is a list of what is currently believed to increase the risk:

1. A prior personal history of breast cancer in one breast
2. Being of the female sex (although men get breast cancer too)
3. Increasing age
4. Early menarche
5. Late menopause
6. Having had no children (nulliparity) or having the first child after the age of thirty-five
7. Prolonged use of hormone replacement therapy
8. Prior breast biopsy showing any of the following:
   a. Sclerosing adenosis
   b. Papilloma
   c. Atypical ductal or lobular hyperplasia
   d. Lobular carcinoma in situ

9. Obesity

10. Higher educational status or family income

11. Urban residence

12. Prior exposure of the breast to radiation, e.g., exposure to atomic bomb blast or treatment of Hodgkin's disease (especially at a young age)

13. Moderate alcohol use

14. History of other cancers: colon, ovarian, endometrial

It is impossible to control some of these factors, such as when you start menstruating, and impractical to try to control others, such as how many children you have, in order to alter breast cancer risk. However, there are several things women can do that might help reduce the risk for breast cancer, including following a low-fat diet, regular exercise, limiting alcohol intake, and not smoking—all of which can help to improve health in many ways. Right now the best way available to help women who are at an increased risk for breast cancer is by trying to find it early if it does develop.

There are exciting new investigations into methods to prevent breast cancer. One national trial is being performed by the National Surgical Adjuvant Breast and Bowel Project (NSABP). The NSABP is a study group in the United States that has performed some of the pioneering investigations in breast cancer research and has helped to determine the way in which breast cancer is treated. One of their most recent trials is called the Breast Cancer Prevention Trial. Over a thousand women who have a certain calculated risk for breast cancer have been entered and randomly divided (to avoid bias) into two groups. One group received a pill called tamoxifen (to be discussed later in this chapter) and the other group received a placebo (nonactive drug). Preliminary analysis shows a significantly reduced chance of developing breast cancer in the group that received tamoxifen (see also raloxifene discussion, chapter 3).

Breast Anatomy

It's important that you understand normal breast anatomy and function to better understand what cancer means (see figure 10.2). Although it's often forgotten, breasts are functional organs of the human body. Their main purpose is the production of milk. A great deal of breast tissue is composed of fat, but to fulfill the very important function of milk production, the breast tissue is also composed of glandular elements. One of the main glandular components is the lobule, which is where milk is made. The milk then gets funneled to the nipple through a system of ducts, which are tiny tubelike structures. About fifteen to twenty main ducts empty at the nipple.

The development of these ducts and lobules depends on hormones in the body. During the normal monthly menstrual cycle, hormone changes occur that cause changes in the breast tissue. During the first half of the cycle, estrogen causes budding and proliferation of the ducts. During the second half, progesterone causes development of the alveoli (in the lobules), as well as an increase in the blood flow and swelling in the breasts. Many women become quite symptomatic and experience breast pain during this second part of the cycle right before menstruation starts. If pregnancy occurs, further changes occur to prepare the breast for lactation. When a woman goes through menopause, the normal glandular elements of the breast, which are no longer needed, shrink and get replaced with more fatty tissue. On mammography, the breasts often appear less dense with advancing age since X rays penetrate fatty tissue better.

Breast Cancer

Cancers result when the normal cells that make up the lobules and ducts become abnormal in appearance, number, and behavior. Cells that are ordinarily very uniform in size and shape take on a variety of different shapes and sizes. The controlling system of cells goes haywire and allows multiplication of cells that would not occur under normal circumstances. At some point, the abnormal cells can also break away from the breast and enter the bloodstream or lymphatic channels and spread to other parts of

Figure 10.2. Breast anatomy.

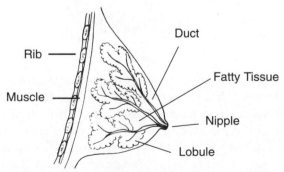

the body, where additional deposits of cancer can settle and grow. This is called cancer metastasis.

The very earliest type of breast cancer we can detect is what is called duct carcinoma in situ, or DCIS for short. DCIS means that the cancer cells arise from within the tiny tubes or ducts of the breast. However, the cancer cells are confined to the ducts only and have not broken through into the surrounding breast tissue. Hence we also call this type of cancer noninvasive, because it has not invaded into the surrounding breast.

Invasive breast cancer, also called infiltrating cancer, is the more common form of breast cancer. It occurs when the cancer cells break through the duct system and into surrounding breast tissue. Unfortunately, it is also the more dangerous form, since once the cancer cells break through the duct system, they can find their way into lymph vessels and blood vessels and travel to other parts of the body. Microinvasive breast cancer is a term that refers to the very earliest evidence of invasion that can be seen under the microscope. Much of what is seen in microinvasive cancer may be DCIS, but once microinvasion is present, the cancer is considered invasive. It may not behave quite as aggressively, although it still does have a small chance of spreading.

The most common type of invasive breast cancer is invasive ductal cancer. Invasive lobular cancer is less common. Other forms of breast cancer, which are even less common, are medullary, tubular, papillary, squamous, and adenoid cystic carcinomas. These are identified by certain characteristics under the microscope.

BREAST CANCER STAGING

Breast cancer and cancer in general are classified into stages to help determine how they will behave and how best to approach treatment. Breast cancer is staged according to the TNM system (see figure 10.3). T defines the size and local extent of the tumor in the breast. N defines the lymph node status, and M defines the presence of metastatic disease. Stages 0, I, II, III, and IV are determined by the T, N, and M characteristics.

Spread, or metastases, to lymph nodes is an important part of the staging. The main lymph nodes of concern are the axillary nodes located in the armpit, but other lymph node areas that also drain the breast are of concern as well (see figure 10.4). The risk for lymph node spread increases with the size of the tumor in the breast. Distant metastases refer to sites of spread beyond the lymph nodes. The most common sites where breast cancer can metastasize are the bones, the liver, the lung and pleura (lining of the chest cavity), and the brain. The risk for distant metastases increases both with the size of the tumor and the presence of spread to the lymph nodes. Unfortunately, there are times when even small cancers with negative lymph nodes can spread.

Primary Tumor (T)

Definitions for classifying the primary tumor (T) are the same for clinical and for pathological classification. The telescoping method of classification can be applied. If the measurement is made by physical examination, the examiner will use the major headings (T1, T2, or T3). If other measurements, such as mammographic or pathological, are used, the examiner can use the telescoped subsets of T1.

TX   Primary tumor cannot be assessed
T0   No evidence of primary tumor
Tis   Carcinoma in situ: intraductal carcinoma, lobular carcinoma in situ, or Paget's disease of the nipple with no tumor
T1   Tumor 2 cm or less in greatest dimension
    T1a   0.5 cm or less in greatest dimension
    T1b   More than 0.5 cm but not more than 1 cm in greatest dimension
    T1c   More than 1 cm but not more than 2 cm in greatest dimension
T2   Tumor more than 2 cm but not more than 5 cm in greatest dimension
T3   Tumor more than 5 cm in greatest dimension
T4   Tumor of any size with direct extension to chest wall or skin
T4a   Extension to chest wall
T4b   Edema (including peau d'orange) or ulceration of the skin of the breast or satellite skin nodules confined to the same breast
    T4c   Both (T4a and T4b)
    T4d   Inflammatory carcinoma

Note: Paget's disease associated with a tumor is classified according to the size of the tumor.

Regional Lymph Nodes (N)

NX   Regional lymph nodes cannot be assessed (e.g., previously removed)

N0   No regional lymph node metastasis

N1   Metastasis to movable ipsilateral axillary lymph node(s)

N2   Metastasis to ipsilateral axillary lymph node(s) fixed to one another or to other structures

N3   Metastasis to ipsilateral internal mammary lymph node(s)

Pathologic Classification (pN)

pNX   Regional lymph nodes cannot be assessed (e.g., previously removed, or not removed for pathological study)

pN0   No regional lymph node metastasis

pN1   Metastasis to movable ipsilateral axillary lymph node(s)

pN1a   Only micrometastasis (none larger than 0.2 cm)

pN1b   Metastasis to lymph node(s), any larger than 0.2 cm

pN1bi   Metastasis in one to three lymph nodes, any more than 0.2 cm and all less than 2 cm in greatest dimension

pN1bii   Metastasis to four or more lymph nodes, any more than 0.2 cm and all less than 2 cm in greatest dimension

pN1biii Extension of tumor beyond the capsule of a lymph node metastasis less than 2 cm in greatest dimension

pN1biv Metastasis to a lymph node 2 cm or more in greatest dimension

pN2   Metastasis to ipsilateral axillary lymph nodes that are fixed to one another or to other structures

pN3   Metastasis to ipsilateral internal mammary lymph node(s)

Distant Metastasis (M)

MX   Presence of distant metastasis cannot be assessed

M0   No distant metastasis

M1   Distant metastasis (includes metastasis to ipsilateral supraclavicular lymph node(s)

Figure 10.3. Breast cancer staging.

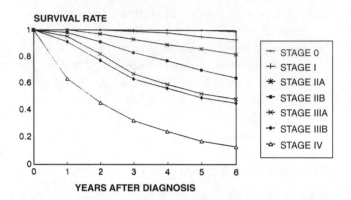

Relative survival rates according to stage of disease. Data taken from 50,834 patients listed in the Surveillance, Epidemiology, and End Results Program of the National Cancer Institute. Patients were diagnosed between 1983 and 1987. Stage 0 represents 4,601 patients; Stage I, 16,519; Stage IIA, 14,692; Stage IIB, 8,283; Stage IIIA, 1,656; Stage IIIB, 1,389; and Stage IV, 3,694.

STAGE GROUPING

Stage 0	Tis	N0	M0
Stage I	T1	N0	M0
Stage IIA	T0	N1	M0
	T1	N1*	M0
	T2	N0	M0
Stage IIB	T2	N1	M0
	T3	N0	M0
Stage IIIA	T0	N2	M0
	T1	N2	M0
	T2	N2	M0
	T3	N1	M0
	T3	N2	M0
Stage IIIB	T4	Any N	M0
	Any T	N3	M0
Stage IV	Any T	Any N	M1

*The prognosis of patients with N1a is similar to that of patients with pN0.

Used with the permission of the American Joint Committee on Cancer (AJCC®), Chicago, Illinois. The original source for this material is the *AJCC® Manual for Staging of Cancer*, 4th edition (1992), published by Lippincott-Raven Publishers, Philadelphia.

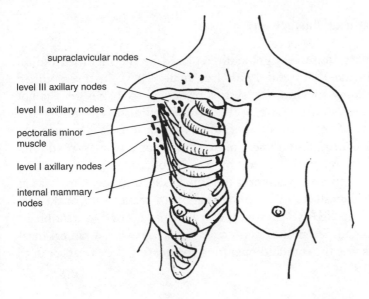

supraclavicular nodes

level III axillary nodes

level II axillary nodes

pectoralis minor
muscle

level I axillary nodes

internal mammary
nodes

Figure 10.4. Lymphatic drainage of breast.

SURGICAL TREATMENT OF BREAST CANCER

Radical Mastectomy

The surgical treatment of breast cancer has made a great deal of progress over the last century. At the turn of the 1900s many cancers were very advanced by the time they were diagnosed. Remember, this was before the advent of mammography. If a woman had a breast cancer the best chance for curing the cancer was to perform a very disfiguring operation called a Halsted Radical Mastectomy, popularized by a famous surgeon by the name of William Halsted. This operation involved removing the entire breast, the pectoral muscles under the breast, the skin over the breast, and the axillary lymph nodes. A skin graft was also necessary to cover up the defect that was left. Halsted's concept was that breast cancer started in the breast and spread in an orderly fashion from the breast to the lymph nodes, then systemically (or in other words, metastatically) to other parts of the body. If the entire breast and lymph node areas were completely removed, then the cancer could be cured. This was a revolutionary operation for its day because it was in fact able to cure some of the women with breast cancer who otherwise would have died. Unfortunately, the operation was very mutilating and many women were still not cured.

Modified Radical Mastectomy

The radical mastectomy was gradually replaced by the modified radical mastectomy in the 1940s and 1950s (see figure 10.5). In the modified radical mastectomy, much of the skin is preserved so a skin graft is not needed. The pectoralis major muscle is preserved also. The breast and axillary nodes, and sometimes the pectoralis minor muscle, are removed. It is not as disfiguring as a radical mastectomy, but a woman is still left without a breast. When this operation was introduced, there were many skeptics who questioned whether a modified radical mastectomy was as good as a radical mastectomy in controlling breast cancer. One of the earliest studies of the NSABP showed that it was just as good to treat breast cancer with a modified radical mastectomy as it was with a radical mastectomy.[2] This was the standard operation for treating breast cancer until well into the 1980s.

Figure 10.5. Modified radical mastectomy.

A. Area removed during surgery   B. Postoperative result

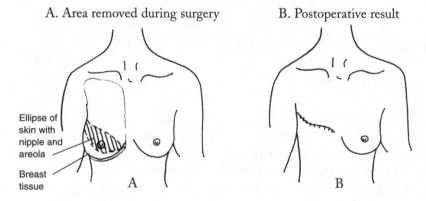

Ellipse of skin with nipple and areola

Breast tissue

A

B

Breast Conservation

As women and health care providers became more aware of the importance of early detection, and as mammography became widely available, many cancers were found earlier, at smaller and smaller sizes. The next natural question was whether it was necessary to remove the entire breast for a small cancer. Breast-conserving treatment was then evaluated.

Breast-conserving treatment generally includes three components: a lumpectomy, an axillary lymph node dissection, and radiation therapy to the breast. Lumpectomy is the most familiar term used in the United States. It means removing the cancer with a surrounding rim of normal breast tissue to ensure that all of the cancer has been removed (see figure 10.6). Partial mastectomy, segmentectomy, and quadrantectomy are other terms indicating breast-conserving procedures, and all generally involve removal of a larger amount of breast tissue. Sometimes an excisional biopsy can be considered a lumpectomy as long as there is an adequate margin of normal breast tissue around the cancer. In most cases, a formal lumpectomy will be needed after the biopsy. If there are cancer cells at the edge or margin of the biopsy or lumpectomy it must be assumed that cancers cells remain in the breast and additional surgery is usually advised. The goal of breast-conserving therapy is to provide good local control of breast cancer (which means treating it so it has a low chance of coming back in the breast) while leaving a breast that is cosmetically acceptable to the patient and the physician.

Figure 10.6. Lumpectomy and axillary node dissection.

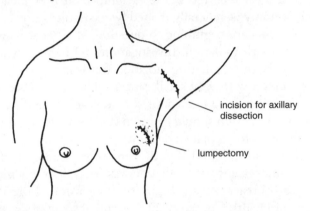

incision for axillary dissection

lumpectomy

The safety of breast-conserving treatment had to be proven before it could be recommended as an appropriate treatment for breast cancer. In the 1980s many groups in the U.S. and in other countries performed scientific studies to determine if breast conservation was equivalent to mastectomy for the treatment of breast cancer. The NSABP was one of the groups to do a study.[3] Women entering this study had to have cancers smaller than four centimeters in size. They were randomly assigned to treatment in one of three different groups. One group underwent a modified radical mastectomy. Another group underwent a lumpectomy with removal of axillary lymph nodes, and the third group underwent a lumpectomy with removal of axillary lymph nodes and additional radiation treatment to the breast after the surgery. The most important finding of the study was that at the end of twelve years, the survival results were not significantly different regardless of how the women were treated. Mastectomy was no longer necessary to cure women of breast cancer.

Another important finding was the importance of giving radiation therapy when a lumpectomy was performed. (Radiation will be discussed in more detail later in this chapter.) In the NSABP study, it was found that if radiation was not used, there was a 35 percent chance of the cancer recurring or coming back in the breast. Giving the radiation, which is a treatment directed at only the breast itself, significantly lowered the risk of local recurrence to 10 percent. In European studies, where the cancers treated were generally smaller than in the U.S. studies, the risk for local recurrence after breast conservation and radiation was even lower at 2 to 5 percent. Keep in mind that local recurrence is possible even after a mastectomy although the risk is quite small. A local recurrence after a mastectomy tends to be more difficult to treat and have a worse prognosis than a local recurrence after a lumpectomy. A local recurrence after a lumpectomy is generally treated by a completion mastectomy.

Doctors are beginning to question whether it is necessary to treat all cancers with radiation. Investigations are being performed to determine the safety of eliminating radiation for women over the age of seventy or for women with very small cancers. The studies are in progress and the results will not be known for several years. Therefore, until the answer is known, radiation should be given (unless a woman is participating in one of the investigational studies).

Besides the NSABP trial, many other studies confirmed the findings that lumpectomy with radiation was equivalent to a mastectomy for treating early breast cancers. In fact the conclusion of the 1990 National Institutes of Health Consensus Development Conference on the Treatment of Early Stage Breast Cancer concluded that "breast conservation treatment is an appropriate method of primary therapy for the majority of women with stage I and II breast cancer and is preferable because it provides survival equivalent to total mastectomy and axillary dissection while preserving the breast."[4]

Despite the clear evidence that lumpectomy with radiation is as effective as, if not a better treatment than, mastectomy, many mastectomies are still performed in the United States. Marked variation in the use of breast-conserving surgery has been found. In one study, it was disappointing to find that in some areas of the country, only 20 percent of cancers were treated by breast conservation in 1986,[5] while in other areas as many as 42 percent were treated this way. Another study looked at the use of breast conservation in women who participated in national trials that evaluated adjuvant therapy (chemotherapy and hormone therapy).[6] The hypothesis was that these women would have the benefit of the latest treatment recommendations. It was very upsetting to find that only 30 percent of women with early stage breast cancer were treated with breast conservation and that the majority of women were still being treated with mastectomy. Regional differences were found, as in the prior study. But other factors were also found that were influencing the use of breast conservation, factors that do not constitute sufficient basis for altering the recommendations for breast conservation. Some of these factors included the size of the cancer, whether there was lymph node spread, and the patient's age, educational level, and income level. Other potential reasons cited, though not evaluated by the study, included the type of hospital, the volume of breast cancer patients treated by the surgeon, the presence of and accessibility to a radiation facility, and the presence of geriatric services. Physician and patient bias and choice in the selection of mastectomy over breast conservation was also suggested but these factors are difficult to define; nevertheless, we could intuitively guess that these biases probably play an important role in the choice of treatment.

Although medical indications for choosing mastectomy over breast conservation do not account for the high mastectomy rates, there are some circumstances when mastectomy may be the recommended or preferred treatment:

1. When cancer is present in more than one location in the breast
2. For large cancers in relatively small breasts
3. When access to radiation therapy is limited
4. When cancers are diagnosed during certain times of pregnancy (radiation can cause birth defects)
5. When radiation therapy cannot be given for medical reasons
6. When the patient chooses not to have a lumpectomy (after complete explanation of the options)

It is critical that a woman be given a complete explanation of the treatment recommendations and also be given the opportunity to discuss the options of mastectomy or lumpectomy. There should be a clear understanding of the choices. If she is told that she is not a candidate for a lumpectomy then it should be absolutely clear why not. If a mastectomy is chosen or is necessary, then the option for breast reconstruction should be explained and considered (to be discussed later in this chapter).

Axillary Dissection

Lymph nodes are removed through a separate incision under the armpit (axilla) when a lumpectomy is performed or through the mastectomy incision when a mastectomy is performed. The part of the procedure in which the lymph nodes are removed is called an axillary dissection.

The axillary lymph nodes are divided into three levels or groups of lymph nodes determined by their location in relation to the pectoralis minor muscle (see figure 10.4). The standard axillary dissection removes level I and II lymph nodes. Individual lymph nodes are not removed; instead, a very specific area of fat containing the lymph nodes is dissected. It is up to the pathologist to dissect the individual lymph nodes from the fatty tissue and examine each one for cancer. At least ten to fifteen lymph nodes should be found when a standard procedure has been done but up to thirty are not unusual. The purpose of the axillary dissection is to determine if there is any spread of the cancer to the lymph nodes. Removing the lymph nodes surgically and examining them under the microscope is the only way to know if the cancer has spread to them. This knowledge is critically important. At the present time, the most important factor determining prognosis and the need for further treatment is whether the lymph nodes are cancerous. If they are, additional treatment besides the surgery is clearly recommended. If lymph nodes are not cancerous, other factors, such as cancer size, are used to determine whether additional therapy is indicated. However, removing lymph nodes may have consequences, including bleeding, infection, injuries to nerves traveling through the armpit, numbness behind the upper arm, fluid collections under the armpit (seroma), shoulder stiffness, and lymphedema (arm swelling). After removal of lymph nodes it is advisable to exert caution when doing anything that can injure the arm on the side of the surgery. Injury can increase the risk for infection and swelling. Avoid having your blood pressure taken, or blood tests drawn, or IVs placed on that side. With everyday activities, it is best to be cautious with manicures, gardening, and carrying heavy loads on the affected arm.

Research is currently under way to find better methods to detect spread to lymph nodes in order to reduce the need for axillary dissection.

A surgical procedure called the sentinel lymph node biopsy is currently being investigated. The sentinel lymph node should, in theory, be the first lymph node to receive lymph drainage, and therefore cancer spread, from the area of the breast where the cancer is located. If cancer is not found in the sentinel lymph node, then the rest of the lymph nodes in the axilla should also be free of cancer. Therefore, removal of the remaining lymph nodes would be unnecessary. If cancer spread is found, the standard axillary dissection should be performed to determine how many lymph nodes contain spread.

The sentinel lymph node biopsy procedure is performed by one of two methods, although some surgeons use both methods together. In one method, a blue dye is injected into the area of the breast where the cancer is located. The blue dye is absorbed into the normal lymphatic pathways of the breast and then travels toward the lymph nodes in the axilla. Several minutes after injection of the blue dye, a small incision is made in the axilla and the path of the blue dye in the lymphatic channel is followed until a lymph node is found. The first lymph node that stains with the blue dye is called the sentinel lymph node. That lymph node is removed and tested for the presence of cancer cells. In the other method, a very small dose of radioactive material is injected into the breast and a sensitive handheld detector is used to identify the location of the sentinel lymph node. An incision is made in the axilla over the area of radioactivity and the lymph node removed for testing. The sentinel node in this case is the lymph node that picks up the radioactive material first.

In most cases, one sentinel lymph node is detected, but in a small percentage two or even three sentinel lymph nodes may be found. However, one of the problems with the procedure is that in some cases it is not possible to identify a sentinel node. When a sentinel lymph node cannot be identified, the only way to determine if there is lymph node spread is by doing the standard lymph node dissection.

The sentinel node procedure is still in the testing phase to determine how reliable it is in finding spread of breast cancer to the axillary lymph nodes. It has the potential, however, for eliminating the need for axillary dissection in many women with breast cancer. It should only be performed by surgeons with special training in the procedure and presently is only used on an investigational basis.

Other newer imaging tests, such as the PET scan, are also being investigated as methods of detecting lymph node spread, but so far there are no tests as accurate as axillary dissection and pathologic examination of the lymph nodes.

RADIATION THERAPY

Radiation therapy for the breast is the standard treatment after a lumpectomy is performed for invasive breast cancer, and in most cases after a lumpectomy has been performed for DCIS. It does not routinely include treatment to the lymph node areas, unless extensive lymph node spread is present. Radiation to the chest wall is also recommended after mastectomy for certain more advanced cancers. Sometimes radiation is used for treating specific areas of cancer spread as well, such as bone metastases. It can help control pain at these sites.

Radiation therapy is a treatment using high energy beams to destroy cancer cells. The beams are generated from either a linear accelerator or a cobalt-60 source. Radiation dose is measured in units called gray (Gy). One gray is equal to 100 centigray (cGy). The dose used depends on the type of cancer and how much radiation the normal body tissues in the area of the cancer will tolerate. Normal body tissues can only tolerate a certain amount of radiation before they can become significantly damaged. Once the maximum dose is reached, no more radiation can ever be given. The dose that can be given in one day is also limited by the normal tissue. Therefore, it often takes several weeks to deliver the amount of radiation needed for cancer treatment.

Simulation is the process where the area to be treated with radiation is carefully mapped out. In order to ensure that the radiation is delivered to the exact area of body tissue with each daily treatment, tiny dots are tattooed on the skin.

Typical radiation given after a lumpectomy for breast cancer is given daily over five to six weeks. The entire breast that had the cancer is treated. The radiation beams are directed in such a way as to avoid damage to the underlying heart and lungs. The usual dose ranges from 45 to 50 Gy. In some cases a boost dose is also given. This is an additional small dose of radiation given just to the site of the lumpectomy itself. There is controversy about whether this is needed in every case.

Most women go through radiation therapy without much difficulty and are able to carry out many of their normal daily activities. Some women experience fatigue. Daily treatments do create an inconvenience for most women, but radiation centers appreciate this fact and try to make the timing and delivery of treatments as easy as possible.

Severe side effects from radiation are unusual. Mild side effects include a reddening of the breast, similar to that experienced with a sunburn. Sometimes the skin can peel, referred to as desquamation, and radiation therapy may need to be interrupted for a few days. Long-term side effects include swelling in the breast (especially for larger-breasted women); fibrosis, or thickening of the breast tissue and skin; discomfort and pain; hyperpigmentation, a darkening of the skin, which is more pronounced in darker-skinned women; and telangiectasias, which are small, thin, reddish lines caused by superficial blood vessels. Many of these changes improve with time, and it can take up to three years for the breast to reach its final appearance. Another possible problem after radiation to the breast is if subsequent surgery to the breast is required, it may take longer for the wound to heal, and there is an increase in the risk of a wound infection.

Other more serious complications from radiation are, fortunately, quite uncommon. Brachial plexopathy is a condition that can cause shoulder discomfort, weakness in the arm and hand, or paresthesias (different neurological sensations in the arm and hand). Radiation pneumonitis (lung damage) and heart damage are uncommon with the presently used techniques, but the possibility should be considered in a woman with preexisting heart or lung disease. Rib fractures are also unusual. The chance that radiation will cause other cancers is rare. The risk for lymphedema (arm swelling) is increased if the axilla requires radiation treatment.

The purpose of radiation therapy is to reduce the risk for local recurrence, the chance of cancer returning at the site treated. After lumpectomy, radiation therapy is very effective at doing this, as mentioned in earlier sections. For breast conservation, the other important goal is to leave a "cosmetically acceptable" breast. Factors that influence the overall cosmetic result include not only the radiation but the surgical procedure, the location of the cancer in the breast, and the size of the cancer in relation to the size of the breast. Only the woman herself can judge what is an acceptable cosmetic result. However, using their experience, the surgeon and radiation therapist can anticipate what the breast will look like afterward, given the individual patient's situation. Most women are pleased with the cosmetic outcome of the breast after lumpectomy and radiation therapy. Although the breast is never the same as it was before treatment, most women are eager to accept the results of breast-conserving therapy over the alternative of a mastectomy. (Breast reconstruction is discussed in greater detail later in this chapter.)

ADJUVANT THERAPY

As it was slowly realized that surgery alone did not cure every woman with breast cancer, the concept evolved that perhaps breast cancer didn't always spread in an orderly fashion. Perhaps it was a systemic disease right from the very start. Numerous investigations have been done to try to find other treatments to help improve the survival rate. Chemotherapy and hormonal therapies were developed and became part of the armamentarium for treating women with breast cancer.

In many cases of breast cancer, additional therapy after surgery is recommended. It is termed adjuvant therapy because it is being given in the absence of any known identifiable disease. It is given because there is a significant risk of undetectable or occult microscopic disease either in the breast or elsewhere in the body.

Radiation therapy can be considered an adjuvant therapy. Remember, unlike chemotherapy, radiation treats only the local area where it is directed. The use of radiation has no influence on the decision for using the other treatments of chemotherapy or hormone therapy (to be discussed below).

For the most part adjuvant therapy refers to either chemotherapy or hormone therapy. These treatments are directed at microscopic disease that may be present in any part of the body and they therefore treat the whole body. It is estimated that adjuvant therapy reduces the risk of these recurrences by about a third.

The decision for using adjuvant therapy is based upon features of breast cancer that are known to affect the outcome or prognosis of women with breast cancer. We call these features prognostic factors. The two most important prognostic factors, tumor size and lymph node status, are included as part of the staging system and are the main factors determining treatment recommendations.

Lymph node status is the most important prognostic factor. If cancer is found to have spread to the lymph nodes, then adjuvant therapy is clearly recommended. If the lymph nodes test negative for cancer spread, then the recommendation for adjuvant therapy depends on other factors.

The second most important prognostic factor is the size of the cancer. Virtually all women with cancers over 1 centimeter in size should be considered for adjuvant treatment. In borderline cases, other factors can be used to aid making the decision.

Prognostic Factors

- Lymph node status
- Tumor size
- Estrogen receptor status (positive more favorable than negative)
- Progesterone receptor status (positive more favorable than negative)
- Ploidy (diploid more favorable than encuploid)
- S-phase (low S-phase more favorable than high S-phase)
- Vascular invasion (if not present more favorable)
- Lymphatic invasion (if not present more favorable)
- Histologic and nuclear grade (low grade more favorable than high grade)
- Histologic tumor type (tubular, papillary and colloid more favorable)

- Her-2-neu
- p53
- Cathepsin-D
- EGFR

Chemotherapy involves the use of drugs to treat cancer. Most of these drugs are given intravenously, but some are taken orally. Several chemotherapy drugs are often given in combination to improve the effectiveness. The following are the common combinations of chemotherapy drugs used in breast cancer:

- CMF = cyclophosphamide, methotrexate, 5-fluorouracil (5-FU)
- CAF = cyclophosphamide, Adriamycin® (doxorubicin), 5-fluorouracil

The common side effects of chemotherapy are hair loss, nausea, vomiting, weight gain, premature menopause, lowering of blood counts (which can increase the risk for infections), heart dysfunction (particularly doxorubicin), and—very rarely but most seriously—death. The main side effect women tend to get most upset over is the temporary hair loss. No one looks forward to losing her hair, but many women try to make the best of the situation by experimenting with new hairstyles, wigs, or hats. Some women never get comfortable with this part of the treatment, but you must remember that it is temporary. Other women actually become quite brave and daring and show off their short hairstyle as their hair starts to return.

High-dose chemotherapy refers to chemotherapy given at four to ten times the usual dose. It is believed that a high dose is better for destroying cancer cells. Unfortunately, it is also quite toxic to normal cells, most notably the cells in the bone marrow that make normal blood cells. A bone marrow or stem cell (cells obtained from circulating blood) transplant is necessary to replenish these cells after this type of chemotherapy. Preliminary results are encouraging for improving the outcome of patients who have aggressive cancers. However, the complications of high-dose chemotherapy are substantial. Studies are ongoing to determine if it is any better than chemotherapy given at standard doses.

Tamoxifen is the other commonly used adjuvant treatment. It is sometimes used by itself or in addition to chemotherapy. Estrogen- and progesterone-receptor tests on the cancer help determine when tamoxifen should be used. Cancers that are estrogen-receptor-positive respond best to tamoxifen. Tamoxifen is usually given for two to five years. Not only does it reduce the risk that breast cancer will recur, but it also appears to reduce the risk of a woman's developing a new cancer in her other breast.

This preventative effect is why tamoxifen is being studied as a preventative treatment for women at high risk for breast cancer.

Tamoxifen is being investigated to see if it has other potential beneficial effects, such as protecting against osteoporosis and heart disease. The detrimental side effects may include hot flashes, nausea, vaginal dryness, blood clots, and depression. Many women, however, experience none of these at all. One more serious side effect is an approximately twofold increase in the risk for developing uterine cancer (overall less than 1 percent incidence in women taking tamoxifen). Women on tamoxifen should have a careful gynecologic exam and be monitored for this potential effect and report any abnormal vaginal bleeding to their physician. A woman who has had a hysterectomy can forget about this potential problem. The benefits in preventing recurrence of breast cancer are strongly felt to outweigh these risks, but a medical oncologist will need to discuss with a patient all of the risks and benefits prior to making the decision to proceed with treatment.

The general guidelines for use of adjuvant therapy are summarized in the following table:

	Estrogen-receptor-positive	Estrogen-receptor-negative
Premenopausal	chemotherapy +/- tamoxifen	chemotherapy
Postmenopausal	tamoxifen +/- chemotherapy	chemotherapy +/- tamoxifen

NEOADJUVANT THERAPY

There are certain breast cancers in which surgery may not be the best treatment to start with. In rare cases, breast cancer may have already spread to other organs by the time it is diagnosed. In this case it becomes more important to use chemotherapy, which will treat these other sites of disease (and the breast also) at the start.

Other cancers may be so advanced in the breast at diagnosis (locally advanced) without having evidence of spread that they are deemed inoperable because a surgical procedure could not remove all of the cancer. Treatment success has improved by starting with chemotherapy. The term for giving treatment prior to surgery is called neoadjuvant or induction therapy. There are several possible advantages to this approach. First, it allows the immediate treatment of cancer cells, which may have already spread. Second, it can be seen if the cancer responds to the chemotherapy. When chemotherapy is given after surgery there is no way of knowing if the chemotherapy being used is effective against a particular individual's cancer. Furthermore, if the cancer does shrink, surgery may become possible where it might not have been possible before. A rare type of cancer called inflammatory breast cancer is one of the special types of cancer that should be treated first with chemotherapy.

Newer investigations are also evaluating whether giving chemotherapy before surgery may be beneficial in other circumstances as well. For example, it may be possible to shrink a large cancer, which would have required a mastectomy, down to a smaller cancer, for which breast conservation could be considered.

DUCTAL CARCINOMA IN SITU (NONINVASIVE CANCER)

Ductal carcinoma in situ (DCIS), or noninvasive breast cancer, is becoming more common. The incidence of DCIS has increased by over 500 percent in the last twenty years.[7] The increase is attributed to mammography since DCIS often has a characteristic appearance on mammograms. About 30 to 40 percent of mammographically detected cancers are DCIS. However, DCIS can also cause a palpable lump in the breast or be responsible for nipple discharge. Cancers found in this very early stage are highly curable. Actually, prognosis is better than for many other common chronic diseases, such as diabetes. Since DCIS has not invaded into the surrounding tissue where the lymphatic pathways and blood vessels are located, it does not have the same ability to spread to other parts of the body the way invasive cancers can, although in rare cases this may happen.

The treatment of DCIS is not as clear as for invasive breast cancer because until recently it wasn't as common and studies weren't started until a few years ago. In the past, many cases of DCIS were treated by simple mastectomy, in which the breast is removed but not the lymph nodes under the armpit. Lymph nodes are not removed as part of the surgery for DCIS since the risk for lymph node spread is less than 1 percent. Simple mastectomy is able to cure about 98 percent of women with DCIS. With the trend toward breast preservation, however, it has become apparent that women with DCIS may have other options.

Lumpectomy, and lumpectomy with radiation therapy, are two other alternatives that have been used. Lumpectomy alone has been used as treatment for DCIS. The problem with lumpectomy is that cancer can return in the breast. If it does come back it may be in the form of DCIS. However, of more concern is the fact that when it does return, it can be in the form of invasive cancer, which then has the potential to spread.

Lumpectomy with radiation has been compared with lumpectomy alone in one randomized trial performed by the NSABP.[8] The results after eight years of follow-up showed a lower risk of having cancer recur in the breast if radiation is used in addition to lumpectomy. The risk of noninvasive recurrence after lumpectomy and radiation was 8 percent and after lumpectomy alone was 13 percent. The risk of invasive cancer recurrence after lumpectomy and radiation was 4 percent and after lumpectomy alone was 13 percent. Lumpectomy alone is being studied as a possible alternative for very small DCIS with certain specific features that indicate behavior that is less aggressive.

As with invasive cancer, many women with DCIS are still being treated with mastectomy. In one recent study, the use of breast conservation for DCIS was shown to have increased from 1983 to 1992.[9] As with invasive cancer, there were regional variations in how many women were treated with mastectomy; in 1992, the rate varied from 29 percent to 58 percent. There are some circumstances however, just as for invasive cancer, when a mastectomy is the preferred treatment (see page 299). If a mastectomy is chosen or is necessary, remember that reconstruction can also be performed.

LOBULAR CARCINOMA IN SITU

Another term associated with in situ or noninvasive breast cancer is lobular carcinoma in situ (LCIS). However, LCIS is *not* cancer. It was named LCIS before there was a clear understanding of what it was and how it behaved and, unfortunately, its name has led to a lot of confusion. LCIS does not cause a lump in the breast, nor does it cause any abnormal findings on a mammogram. It is, therefore, an incidental microscopic finding, detected when a woman has a biopsy for some other reason. For example, a woman is found to have a lump in her breast that, when looked at under the microscope, is clearly a fibroadenoma (a common nonmalignant growth). Next to the fibroadenoma, and totally unrelated to it, is a microscopic area of LCIS.

LCIS does not have the ability to spread to other parts of the body. The significance of LCIS, however, is that women who have this change in their breast are at an increased risk of developing a cancer of the breast at some time during their life. The cancer can develop anywhere in the breast or in the other breast as well. So we consider it a marker that indicates an increased risk of developing breast cancer. (The approximate risk is estimated to be about 1 percent per year.)

There are two options for treating LCIS. One is close observation with regular breast examinations and mammography in an attempt to detect a cancer early if it occurs. The other, more drastic option to consider is a bilateral prophylactic mastectomy to try to prevent the development of breast cancer. As mentioned earlier, this may not completely eliminate the risk and certainly is associated with great psychological distress in most women.

A third option has recently become available. As mentioned earlier, tamoxifen has been shown to lower the chance of developing breast cancer in women at high risk and may therefore be offered to women with LCIS.

Breast Reconstruction

Breast reconstruction should be offered to any woman contemplating a mastectomy. Reconstructions can be performed at the same time as the mastectomy, or at a later date, and are done by plastic surgeons. Performance of a reconstruction at the same time as the mastectomy does add significant time to the length of the operation, in addition to increasing the discomfort of the surgery and period of recuperation needed. However, it does have the advantage of the entire surgery being done under one anesthesia, during one hospitalization, and requiring only one postoperative recovery. It also has the psychological advantage of lessening the impact of having a mastectomy, since the woman will wake up with a new breast.

Different types of reconstructions can be performed, either by placement of implants, using tissue from other parts of a woman's body (flap procedures), or by combinations of the two. Implants are filled with saline (salt water) solution and are generally not filled with silicone anymore because of the concern that silicone may cause certain illnesses (further investigation continues in this regard). In some cases a temporary implant, called an expander, is put in at the time of the mastectomy. The expander is used to gradually stretch the skin of the breast so that later a permanent implant can be placed and have a more natural form. The plastic surgeon periodically instills saline into the implant during follow-up office visits by inserting a small needle through the skin and into a special port in the expander. When full expansion has taken place, the temporary implant is exchanged with the permanent implant in an outpatient surgical procedure.

The most common type of tissue reconstruction performed is called a TRAM flap (transrectus abdominal muscle flap, see figure 10.7). It is a procedure that moves skin, fat, and muscle from the lower abdomen to the chest in order to form a new breast. This procedure also adds the bonus of giving a "tummy tuck" as part of the procedure since the skin for the new breast is taken from the lower abdomen. Finishing touches, such as creation of a nipple and tattooing on an areola, are performed later in the office.

Other reconstructive procedures combine tissue transfer with implant placement. A latissimus dorsi flap is often combined with placement of an implant to achieve good cosmetic results. Keep in mind that in any breast reconstruction it is sometimes necessary to alter the opposite breast to achieve symmetry and optimal cosmetic results. Also, the final result is generally not achieved at the time of the first surgery. Several additional procedures are often required to give the reconstructed breast its final and optimal appearance.

Complications can also occur from breast reconstructive surgery, including bleeding, infections, problems with healing, and actual loss of the flap reconstruction in unusual cases. Smoking and other conditions, such as diabetes, can interfere with and affect the ability of the flap to

Figure 10.7. Tram flap reconstruction.

A. Incision lines   B. Postoperative result

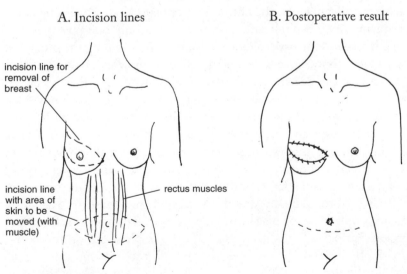

heal. Long-term problems such as implant leaks or ruptures and capsular contractures (scar tissue formation) or chronic pain are also possible.

If a woman is considering a mastectomy, it is wise to get an opinion from a plastic surgeon even if she doesn't think she is going to want a reconstruction. A normal reaction is to want to get the breast off and forget about it and not think about a reconstruction. Some women worry that a reconstruction will hinder their treatment. Others feel guilty about worrying about their appearance when they think the main concern should be to fight the cancer. Still other women feel they are too old to worry about their appearance. The reconstruction in the majority of cases will not interfere with further treatment, nor will it affect the outcome of the cancer. Furthermore, there is no strict age cutoff for reconstruction. A reconstruction can lessen the impact of losing a breast. It is important to have a frank discussion with the surgeon as well as the plastic surgeon before deciding what is best.

Other Therapies

A number of alternative approaches to treating cancer are also available outside of the standard medical community. Many of these approaches can be complementary to the standard medical care but should not be used as a replacement. A word of caution is warranted—many advertised approaches are not proven to be effective in large, scientifically performed studies. Everyone wants a quick, easy, "natural" cure for cancer. Many of the alternative treatments sound better than conventional medical care because they promise miraculous outcomes with no side effects. Discuss these with your medical oncologist. Chances are even if he or she is not totally familiar with the approaches, he or she can often provide counseling as to whether there is any risk to undertaking the alternative treatment.

Emotional and Psychological Issues

Emotional and psychological support is crucial for women diagnosed with breast cancer, and for their families. Fortunately, many channels for help are available. The American Cancer Society can assist in directing women to appropriate services. Many hospital-based and community-based support groups are available. The National Breast Cancer Coalition is a national advocacy organization for breast cancer patients and women at risk. They promote legislative efforts and encourage research funding and welcome new members.

Cancer Care, Inc., is a nonprofit organization dedicated to providing emotional support, information, and practical help to people with cancer and their loved ones. The agency also offers limited financial assistance for transportation to and from chemotherapy and/or radiation therapy, child care, and some other financial help. You may reach them through their national toll-free counseling line (1-800-813-HOPE). All of the agency's services are free of charge.

In addition, the National Cancer Institute has a cancer hot line, 1-800-4CANCER, which has been helpful for information about study protocols, new drugs, names of clinics and physicians in your local area, etc. Please see Appendix for other suggestions.

Conclusion and Future Directions

A great deal of progress has been made in the treatment of breast cancer, but unfortunately it remains true that many women still die from this disease. Early detection still offers the best hope for cure, and educational efforts to inform women must continue. But clearly early detection is not the final answer. Research is being conducted to determine the causes, particularly in regard to environmental factors. Investigations into methods of prevention are finally under way. Many discoveries are being made about the genetics of breast cancer, and future treatment could potentially target ways to correct these genetic defects. Improvements in the methods of detection, especially with regard to axillary node spread and imaging tests, are also being studied. We need improvements in treatment, such as elimination of unnecessary treatments in selected patients, and better and less toxic therapies for other patients. A great deal of progress has been made in the last thirty years, although for many it has not been fast enough, especially for those who have experienced breast cancer themselves or who have lost a loved one to this disease. It is often asked, why can we put a man on the moon and still not have a cure for breast cancer? I don't have a good answer, but the human body is far more complex than any mechanical object that can physically transport that body to the moon. Finding the cure for breast cancer will be a much greater triumph than setting foot on the moon.

Notes

1. S. L. Parker, T. Tong, S. Bolden, and P. A. Wingo, "Cancer Statistics, 1997," *CA: A Cancer Journal for Clinicians* (1997): 5–27.

2. B. Fisher, C. Redmond, E. R. Fisher, M. Bauer et al., "Ten-Year Results of a Randomized Clinical Trial Comparing Radical Mastectomy and Total Mastectomy with or without Radiation," *New England Journal of Medicine* 312 (1985): 674–81.

3. B. Fisher, S. Anderson, C. K. Redmond, N. Wolmark, D. L. Wickerham, and W. M. Cronin, "Reanalysis and Results after 12 Years of Follow-up in a Randomized Clinical Trial Comparing Total Mastectomy with Lumpectomy with or without Irradiation in the Treatment of Breast Cancer," *New England Journal of Medicine* 333 (1995): 1456–61.

4. NIH Consensus Conference, "Treatment of Early-Stage Breast Cancer," *Journal of the American Medical Association* 265, no. 3 (1991): 391–95.

5. O. C. Farrow, W. C. Hunt, and J. M. Samet, "Geographic Variation in the Treatment of Localized Breast Cancer," *New England Journal of Medicine* 326 (1992): 1097–1101.

6. K. S. Albain, S. R. Green, A. S. Lichter, L. F. Hutchins et al., "Influence of Patient Characteristics, Socioeconomic Factors, Geography, and Systemic Risk on the Use of Breast-Sparing Treatment in Women Enrolled in Adjuvant Breast Cancer Studies: An Analysis of Two Intergroup Trials," *Journal of Clinical Oncology* 14 (1996): 3009–17.

7. V. L. Ernster, J. Barclay, K. Kerlikowske, D. Grady, and C. Henderson, "Incidence of and Treatment for Ductal Carcinoma In Situ of the Breast," *JAMA* 275 (1996): 913–18.

8. E. Mamounas, B. Fisher, J. Dignam et al., "Effect of Breast Irradiation Following Lumpectomy in Intraductal Breast Cancer (DCIS): Updated Results from NSABP B-17," *Society of Surgical Oncology Cancer Symposium Abstracts* (1997): 7.

9. V. L. Ernster et al., "Incidence of and Treatment for Ductal Carcinoma In Situ of the Breast."

Chapter 11
OVARIAN CANCER—GETTING AN EVEN BREAK

Ovarian cancer is the most frustrating problem that any physician faces, because although it is highly curable in its early stages, it is rarely detected until it is far advanced. Ovarian cancer is a "hidden" cancer and is not associated with significant symptoms in its early stages. The result is that ovarian cancer is the fourth leading cause of cancer deaths in the United States. In 1997, approximately 26,800 new cases were diagnosed and 14,200 cases were fatal (SEER data). Every decade nearly 150,000 women at the height of their social and economic productivity die from this disease, making its diagnosis and cure one of the greatest challenges.

Cancer of the ovary is on the increase in the Western world, especially in highly industrialized countries. It seems to occur mainly among middle- and upper-class women. Women who have never married or have never borne children have two or three times the risk of developing this malignancy. On the other hand, women with four or more children have a lesser risk. It is even possible that pregnancy exerts a protective effect or, conversely, that an abnormality in ovarian function predisposes a woman to both infertility and ovarian cancer. Also, recent studies have shown that oral contraceptives offer some protection against ovarian cancer by shutting off ovarian function and allowing the tissue to rest. Giving the ovary a break from the repeated stimulation of "incessant ovulation" seems in some small way to reduce the cancer risk.

Back in the early eighties, Dr. Daniel Cramer of Harvard Medical School found that the use of talcum powder for dusting sanitary napkins or the external genitalia doubled the risk of developing ovarian cancer. In his study, women who used talc for both dusting activities were in an even higher risk group. The researchers did not investigate the use of talc on diaphragms, nor did they inquire whether women washed the talc off their diaphragms before using them.

Like asbestos, talc is a hydrous magnesium silicate, but it has a somewhat different structure. Talc may be contaminated with asbestos, although steps have been taken recently to ensure that talc contains as few contaminants as possible. During ovulation, when the surface of the ovary folds inward, the talc could be carried into the interior of the ovary and lead to the development of cancer. Dr. Cramer was quick to state, however, that he was not proposing talc as the only cause of ovarian cancer and that more studies would be done to clarify this possibility. I have always advised my own patients not to powder at all, or, if they must, to powder their genitals or diaphragms with cornstarch. It's cheap, effective, and may be less likely to cause problems. In 1997, another study implicated not only talc dusting of the vulva and perineum, but also feminine deodorant sprays.

Perhaps what is most important is, unlike the male, the female reproductive system is an open system. The vaginal opening leads to the opening in the cervix, which opens into the uterine cavity, then out to and through the open fallopian tubes and into the pelvic and abdominal cavity. It is theoretically possible for any substance applied to the perineum or placed in the vagina to wind up inside of the abdominal cavity. Sperm use this route, easily covering the distance to get into the fallopian tubes to fertilize the egg. Sexually transmitted diseases also enter the pelvis in this manner and cause terrible pelvic infections. It is not impossible that other substances, including carcinogens and viruses, could actively or passively wind up in the pelvic cavity where they could affect the ovaries. It is obvious that many more studies are needed.

Anatomy of the Ovary

The ovaries are paired, solid, slightly wrinkled, pink-gray bodies the approximate size of unshelled almonds, rarely bigger than one inch long in the postmenopausal woman. The ovaries are situated on either side of the uterus, behind or below the fallopian tubes. They are usually not symmetrical, the right ovary often being larger than the left. The ovary changes markedly in size, shape, consistency, and position during its lifetime. It is therefore important, when checking for abnormalities, to know the changes that occur in the ovary at different ages as well as within any given menstrual cycle.

In addition, the ovary undergoes a complicated development, for it arises from several different embryonic tissues. Each of the early tissues that composes the ovary retains its own potential to form a tumor. Therefore, many different cancer types can occur in this small organ, each type originating from its own cell line that dates back to the formation of the ovary itself. Consequently, there is no single "ovarian cancer." Instead, there is a long, complicated list of ovarian cancers, each with its own mode of spread and response to therapy.

MICROSCOPIC ANATOMY

Ovaries have an inner core, known as the medulla, and an outer cortex. There is no real capsule, but the surface of the ovary is covered by a mesothelial layer only one cell thick that is continuous with and resembles the cells that line the abdominal cavity. Below this layer are the tiny follicles—microscopic clumps of cells each encasing an immature egg, hormone-producing cells, and supporting cells.

The cells of the capsule of the ovary are quiet, up to the time of ovulation. Usually, a single egg and its follicle rise to the surface of the ovary, rupture through the surface, and the egg is released. To heal the tiny defect, the surface cells divide and fill in the defect and then sometimes are trapped beneath the surface of the healed site, causing a small inclusion cyst to be formed. Over many years and many ovulations, growth factors or lack of tumor suppressor genes may stimulate abnormal growth of these cells, which may lead to the most common cancer seen, i.e., epithelial cancer of the ovary. Besides epithelial cancers, which account for more than 85 percent of ovarian cancers, there are germ cell tumors that originate from the original tissues that compose the ovary and stromal tumors, that may produce hormones.

Symptoms of Ovarian Cancer

There are no specific early symptoms associated with ovarian cancer. Rather, the list consists of vague, insidious abdominal complaints that a woman usually attributes to anything but her ovaries. This lack of significant symptoms is a major contributing factor to late diagnosis and, therefore, poor prognosis of the disease.

The earliest manifestations are vague abdominal discomfort, dyspepsia, indigestion, gas with constant distension, flatulence, belching, a feeling of fullness after light meals, slight loss of appetite, and other mild digestive disturbances.

Women rarely feel discomfort from the ovaries themselves—they are fairly insensitive to distension, since they do not have a restraining capsule. Therefore, a tumor or a cyst can become large without the patient ever being aware of it (unless the increase in size occurs very rapidly). If the ovary were a sensitive organ, the diagnosis of cancer could be more easily made at an earlier stage. (The ovary, though it is not sensitive to distension, is exquisitely sensitive to squeezing or compression—a fact that is well known to physicians because their patients routinely complain about slight discomfort when their ovaries are lightly squeezed during a pelvic exam). Pain is, therefore, not commonly present unless an unusual problem occurs. For example, pain can occur if the ovary becomes heavy because of a dermoid, cyst, or other benign or malignant problem, and cuts off its blood supply as it twists and falls into the lower pelvis. The resulting pain can be extreme and of sudden onset. But otherwise, unfortunately, a tumor may grow to huge proportions before a woman seeks medical attention. All too often, she finally goes to her doctor because her abdomen has swollen to an embarrassing extent. By this time, the tumor may be very large and its weight may also be causing swollen ankles and varicose veins, much as pregnancy does. She may also complain about frequent urination.

There are, of course, ovarian enlargements that are not cancer. In young women, ovaries that are functioning at peak performance routinely enlarge every month as part of their normal hormone-secreting function. Most monthly fluctuations in ovarian size go unnoticed.

It is unfortunate that the symptoms of malignant ovarian tumors are the same as those produced by benign tumors. One of the problems when trying to diagnose ovarian tumors clinically is that, at least early on, the benign growths act very much like the malignant ones and vice versa.

If a woman complains of gastrointestinal symptoms that cannot be definitely diagnosed as originating from her stomach or intestines, she should have ovarian cancer ruled out by the appropriate examination and medical workup. Most doctors tend to ignore vague abdominal and pelvic symptoms, but these complaints should be taken very seriously. If you wait until the usual symptoms associated with ovarian cancer are present, for example, abdominal swelling, pain, weight loss, increased frequency of urination, or a mass that can be felt through the abdominal wall, the disease is usually far advanced. Even with extensive spread of the ovarian cancer within the woman's abdomen, the patient's only complaint may be abdominal enlargement or a sense of fullness low in the pelvic area.

Unlike the cervix, the ovaries are hidden within the abdomen and cannot be seen. So while the death rates from cervical cancer have fallen, ovarian cancer death rates have remained high.

Types of Ovarian Tumors

Some ovarian tumors have their origin in stromal tissue that keeps its capacity to produce female or male hormones. These are known as functional tumors, and are rare, accounting for only a small percentage of ovarian malignancies. Tumors producing estrogen (female hormones) may cause bleeding problems. Only 10 percent of malignant ovarian tumors disturb the menstrual rhythm or alter menstrual flow. Recurrence of monthly bleeding should alert a postmenopausal woman and her physician that such a tumor might exist. On the other hand, tumors that produce male hormones may bring an abrupt end to a woman's monthly period, cause her breasts to shrink, the hair growth pattern on her body to change to a male type, her clitoris to enlarge, and, later on, even cause her voice to deepen.

Masculinizing tumors arise in the ovary because in the course of its normal development, the ovary contains some testicular elements. These disappear with further differentiation of the ovary, but in many women, tiny remnants can remain. However, most ovarian tumors do not secrete hormones and so do not produce the symptoms that might alert a woman that a catastrophe may be brewing within her abdomen.

Other tumors derived from the germ cells (original cells) may contain bits and pieces of bone, teeth, or cartilage left over from the various embryonic tissues which originally got incorporated into the ovarian tissue. These are known as dermoid tumors and because of these inclusions, they show up easily on X rays and give clues to their nature. Most dermoids are benign.

The ovary is unique in that it not only gives rise to a number of different cancers, but is also the recipient of metastases from cancers in other parts of the body, particularly from breast, stomach, and colon. Colon cancer usually spreads to the ovary by direct extension of the tumor from the colon. Endometrial cancer (from the uterine lining) spreads through the open fallopian tubes onto the ovary. The method of spread from the stomach or breast is thought to be through the lymphatic or blood vessels.

Though the initial cancer may be only in one ovary, involvement of the opposite one occurs so frequently that the uterus and both ovaries are usually removed in most surgeries for ovarian cancer. (The uterus also often contains tumors that have come from other sites.)

Because the ovarian enlargement may be due to metastases or metastatic disease, any patient with a suspected ovarian mass should undergo a thorough preoperative evaluation to rule out a primary cancer elsewhere in the body. Women forty years of age and older comprise the high-risk group here, for increasingly as we age, cancers of all kinds become more common.

Ovarian growths may be either cystic (round in shape and filled with fluid) or solid, and both types may be either benign or malignant. Benign cysts change in size with the menstrual cycle and may be associated with alterations in the menstrual pattern. Often a benign cyst is a follicle that partly matured during the normal menstrual cycle but did not release its egg. These functional cysts usually disappear in one to two menstrual cycles. Cancers, on the other hand, tend to persist or to become larger. The rate of growth can range from extremely slow to very rapid.

Benign tumors, either cystic or solid, are most prevalent in the years preceding the menopause. Although cystic (fluid-containing) tumors may be either benign or malignant, the more solid portions that are mixed with the cystic elements, the greater the likelihood that the tumor will be malignant. Solid tumors (fibromas being the exception) usually possess some degree of malignant potential.

Although fewer than 4 percent of all ovarian tumors are solid, the majority of these are malignant in the over-forty age group. Two-thirds of these solid tumors are metastases from other sites, and, in fact, all tumors that metastasize to the ovaries are solid. A malignant solid tumor also tends to be bilateral, i.e., occurring in both ovaries.

The Search for Early Ovarian Cancer

With better public and professional education, more cases of ovarian cancer will be diagnosed while the disease is in an early stage. Although the overall prognosis for ovarian cancer is not good, it may surprise you to learn that women diagnosed with early ovarian cancer, stage I, have a five-year survival rate of 85 percent. The rate for stage II is 70 percent. Unfortunately, over 70 percent of women are diagnosed when they are in stage III or IV, when cancer has already spread within the pelvis, abdominal cavity, or to distant parts of the body such as the liver or lining of the lungs. These stages are the most difficult to treat and carry a poor prognosis.

The routine pelvic exam is our first line of defense and part of every woman's physical exam. During the exam, the external genitalia should be inspected for abnormal pigmented lesions, evidence of sexually transmitted disease, and chronic skin disease. If there is any doubt, a tiny biopsy can be taken. After noting the condition of the vaginal walls, routine Pap smears are taken. (Pap smears have been responsible for a marked decrease in the death rate from cervical cancer, but not ovarian cancer.) The next step, which is equally important, is the bimanual examination. Here the physician or nurse practitioner carefully feels the size and shape of the uterus and notes whether it is able to be easily moved back and forth. Next, he or she searches the pelvis to identify each ovary, its size and consistency. After changing gloves, a rectovaginal examination should be performed. By inserting the middle finger into the rectum and the index finger into the vagina, the more posterior aspects of the pelvis can be explored and the previous findings confirmed. At that same time, a tiny bit of stool or secretions on the finger of the glove that explored the rectum can be wiped onto a special paper. One to two drops of clear fluid from a dropper bottle are added and, if a blue color develops, it identifies that hidden, or microscopic, bleeding is present. This rapid test can help identify early colon cancer. Women have been educated about the importance of annual Pap smears. Too little time has been spent emphasizing the importance of the remainder of the pelvic examination, which can help detect uterine abnormalities and ovarian enlargement, and test for colon cancer.

Because of the nature of ovarian malignancies, the only hope for successful treatment lies in the early diagnosis and complete surgical excision of the tumor.

On physical examination the physician must always be alert to and suspicious of:

1. Any mass in the ovary.
2. Immobility of the ovary, as it may be caused by tumor adhering to adjacent organs. (The normal ovary can be easily moved up and down or side to side.)
3. Irregularity of the ovary with areas of increased hardness could be due to tumor.

4. Relative insensitivity of the mass. Normal ovaries are tender when palpated during the pelvic exam; ovarian cancers usually are not.

5. Increasing size of one or both ovaries above normal.

Knowing what to look for, however, will not suffice if the pelvic exam is not performed carefully. It is difficult to palpate the ovaries, and a small percentage of masses are missed by physicians. They should spend more time performing a thorough, careful, methodical pelvic exam. Doctors must also pay more attention to their patients' complaints.

In 1971, Barber and Graber made a suggestion for detecting ovarian cancer called the "postmenopausal palpable ovary syndrome." Their findings were based on the premise that the ovary shrinks with menopause and three to five years after a woman's last menstrual period, it should not be palpable to the examining physician. Consequently, they believed that an ovary that is palpable at this stage of life must have further workup to prove that a malignancy does not exist. They also believed that in postmenopausal women, unlike in younger women, there should be no cysts (due to ovulation) in the ovary.

But this concept was based on physical exam only. We now make use of ultrasound in patients at high risk or with abnormal or questionable pelvic examinations, or in obese patients where a good physical exam is just not possible. Not only can we be more accurate in our evaluation of the ovaries, but also we have learned some surprising facts about the postmenopausal ovary. One of those facts is that benign cysts can exist in the postmenopausal ovary, enlarge it, and make it feel abnormal on pelvic examination. If the cyst is simple (without solid areas or septations*), it can be followed carefully by ultrasound, color flow Doppler (see page 324), and blood tumor markers, first perhaps at six to eight weeks, then at three-month, six-month, and then yearly intervals. If all the studies remain normal, these patients can be reassured and surgery avoided. However, if any doubt arises, or if a blood test for a tumor marker (CA-125) is abnormal, it may be possible to remove the ovarian mass in its entirety through a laparoscopic procedure and get a rapid microscopic evaluation. On the other hand, if the patient is postmenopausal, has an elevated CA-125, and her ovary looks suspicious on an ultrasound or CT scan, after a complete workup for metastatic disease, an exploratory laparotomy will more often be the appropriate choice.

---

*Separations—thin, cobweblike membranes that divide the cyst.

GENETIC RISK FACTORS

In general, women have a one in seventy lifetime risk of developing ovarian cancer. However, the common epithelial cancers usually occur in women over forty and although the greatest number cluster around ages forty-five to fifty-five, the incidence peaks at eighty. To say it another way, the incidence at age twenty-five is only 1 in 100,000, but by age seventy-five to seventy-nine the incidence rises to 54 per 100,000. Therefore, yearly or biannual examinations become even more important as we age. While we would like to screen each and every woman with ultrasound and blood tumor markers for ovarian cancer, we simply do not have the money or precise tests to do it presently.

The large majority of ovarian cancer cases are not inherited and may be due to environmental causes. Less than 10 percent of women with ovarian cancer have a first degree relative (mother, sister, daughter) with the disease. However, women who are at genetically high risk usually tend to develop their cancers earlier than usual. As we learn more about genetic causes of cancer, we realize that there are three autosomal dominant syndromes where women inherit their cancer. They are hereditary breast-ovarian cancer syndrome, the most common; pure ovarian cancer syndrome, the least common; and Lynch syndrome II, where families have high rates of colon/rectal cancer that are related to increased risk for breast cancer, ovarian cancer, and uterine cancer.

Women who inherit a mutated form of BRCA1 are at increased risk for developing both breast and ovarian cancers. The breast cancer gene BRCA1 on chromosome 13 occurs in one woman in one thousand in the general population, but it occurs in one woman in one hundred in Ashkenazi Jewish women. Women who inherit this trait have greater than a 90 percent chance of developing either breast or ovarian cancer by age 70. There are also some families where breast, colon, and ovarian cancer are inherited as an autosomal dominant trait. Therefore, being aware of your family history is very important. Women who may want to consider BRCA1 testing are those who had breast or ovarian cancer before age forty, those with two or more first-degree relatives who had breast or ovarian cancer before age forty, and those who are related to women who have already tested positive for BRCA1.

It is important to realize that this kind of testing is new and may put you at risk for obtaining health, life, or disability insurance. It is hoped that in the near future, this will change. In addition, because of the psychological impact that testing can have, either with positive or negative results, counseling is necessary before and after testing. Much of the testing today is still being done under hospital-guided protocols.

If blood tests for genetic susceptibility are obtained, those who are determined to have hereditary risk may choose to talk to their physicians about having their tubes tied, for some studies have shown a decrease in ovarian cancer in women who have had this procedure. Additionally, birth control pills used for longer periods of time may reduce the risk of developing ovarian cancer. Because their risk is so high, women in this category should also talk to their physicians about prophylactic oophorectomy (having both ovaries removed) at thirty-five or after childbearing has been completed.

DIAGNOSIS OF OVARIAN CANCER

If your physician finds a mass on pelvic examination, or if you have persistent symptoms such as an increase in abdominal girth, bloating, fatigue, or change in bowel function, more accurate methods of diagnosis than history and physical examination are indicated. A full workup may be needed to differentiate between ovarian causes of distress, or functional bowel disorders, intestinal tumors, growing uterine fibroids, etc.

ULTRASOUND

One of the best and easiest methods of evaluating the ovaries is pelvic ultrasonography. Ultrasound uses painless, high-frequency sound waves to "visualize" organs inside the body. A small probe called a transducer sends sound waves into the body. The transducer also listens for returning echoes that are reflected off the internal organs. These echoes are converted by computer into a visual image on a television screen. Permanent film, photographs, or videotape records of the examination are made. Because there is no radiation involved in these examinations, they can be repeated as often as is felt necessary. Also, the studies are inexpensive compared with other methods of diagnostic imaging.

There are two types of pelvic ultrasonography used today. Sometimes both are used, and either has its own advantages.

The transabdominal ultrasound begins with a light application of oil to your abdomen. A small transducer is held gently against the skin sending, and listening for, sound waves. Often it is possible for you to watch the television screen as the technician or physician does the examination.

The advantage of the abdominal approach is that large uterine fibroids can be accurately measured, and kidney structures can be evaluated with a little extra effort when deemed necessary. However, ovarian detail is usually not as good as in transvaginal sonography. In addition, patients undergoing the transabdominal approach need to prepare for the exam by filling their bladder to capacity before the examination is done.

Transvaginal approach is newer and has improved our ability to evaluate the ovaries. In this method, a narrow, covered probe is inserted into the vagina (often by the patient herself). The top of the vaginal probe, in the vault of the vagina, lies closer to the ovaries than in the transabdominal approach. This results in greater detail of the ovarian characteristics. In women who have regular menses, it is best to schedule the examination at the end of the menstrual flow, when functional cysts are least likely to be present and thus less likely to confuse the radiologist.

Color flow Doppler, which evaluates the amount, direction, and rate of blood flow, is the newest development in ultrasound to give additional information about whether or not an ovarian mass is benign or malignant. Abnormal blood vessel growth and abnormal blood flow patterns, e.g., high velocity flow, are usually present with ovarian malignancy. Observing the combination of colored patterns of the blood flow and using computer calculations improves our ability to decide whether or not the ovarian growth is malignant. On the other hand, by showing that color flow Doppler studies are normal, and that the ovarian cyst is simple (without solid areas or septations), we have been able to follow many peri- and postmenopausal women without having to resort to surgery. It should be apparent that morphology and flow studies complement each other and serve together, along with tumor markers, to guide our decisions whether to continue to follow a woman with a subsequent ultrasound or to initiate surgical intervention.

Ultrasound is easy from the patient's point of view and has no contraindications. I tend to order pelvic sonograms freely and use them when I cannot be sure of my pelvic findings. Ultrasounds are also used serially, i.e., to follow a cyst over months, even over years, to ensure that its characteristics remain benign. They are also used to track the growth of uterine fibroids and measure the thickness of the lining of the uterus.

CT SCANNING

Computerized axial tomography (CT scan) is another method for evaluating the pelvis. This method does involve radiation as well as the risk of reaction to contrast dyes used orally or intravenously. This method is not used as a screening method due to that risk, and due to its high cost. Rather, its value lies in information it can provide in patients who are being monitored for spread of their ovarian cancer. With CT scanning, response to chemotherapy and/or surgery can be followed. Possible involvement of other organs such as the lung or the liver can also be evaluated.

MRI

MRI scanning can provide good, detailed studies of the pelvic organs and is sometimes helpful in differentiating between different types of benign growths of the ovary. For example, it can help differentiate as to whether the growth is a fibroid, a dermoid tumor, or endometriosis. Although no radiation is used, costs are very high.

PET

Positron emission tomography remains investigational to date. Its real use may one day be in detection of small areas of cancer that have appeared after initial therapy.

TUMOR MARKERS

One of the most exciting areas of research involves the effort to diagnose ovarian cancer by means of a blood test for substances called tumor markers. CA-125 is a tumor marker produced by 80 percent of epithelial cancers, the most common type of ovarian tumors. It is primarily used to follow women with diagnosed ovarian cancer for recurrence of their tumors after initial surgery or to follow their response to chemotherapy. However, its use for early screening for ovarian cancer is still not clear, for only half of the different types of ovarian tumors show this marker in the early stages when the cancer is still confined to the ovary. Elevated levels are also seen in other conditions such as endometriosis, pelvic infection, uterine fibroids, menstruation, and pregnancy. Therefore, premenopausal women are far more likely to have elevated levels due to nonmalignant conditions. In patients with elevated CA-125 who do *not* have cancer, the initial high level usually decreases over time. On the other hand, other cancers such as lung, breast, colon, and cervical cancer often show elevated CA-125 levels. Therefore, postmenopausal women with increased CA-125 levels who do *not* have pelvic abnormalities should be screened for other tumors that produce CA-125. Then, to confuse the subject further, some malignant ovarian tumors do not manufacture this marker at all. Therefore, used alone, for screening asymptomatic women, this test has less value than hoped. However, the test is especially useful and cost effective for high-risk women who should also be screened with ultrasound studies on some regular basis.

Other tumor markers exist, such as TAG-72, CA 19-9, and CA 15-3. Recently, more success in diagnosing ovarian cancer has been achieved by using a combination of CA-125 with one or two other markers: CA 15-3, TAG-72, M-CSF, or OXV1. Simultaneous testing may one day help avoid unnecessary surgery from falsely positive single-marker results and allow us to detect earlier smaller tumors.

GENETIC MARKERS

It is important to realize that over 85 percent of ovarian cancers are probably not inherited. The most commonly involved inherited problems surround the loss of normal function of the p53 gene, which is responsible for cell division and change. However, many other genetic markers are now being uncovered. Mentioned earlier, the BRCA1 and BRCA2 genes on chromosomes 13 and 17 respectively have been associated with inheritance of both breast and ovarian cancer. All normal men and women have a normal BRCA1 and BRCA2 gene. These genes stop abnormal growth of cells. If there is damage to the BRCA1 or BRCA2 gene, then their protective ability is lost and ovarian cells tend to multiply without control and cause cancer. The BRCA1 gene is a very complicated long protein. It took seventeen years to map (figure out the sequence of amino acids that make up this gene) and four years to clone (reproduce). However, following that, the BRCA2 gene took only one year to map and one year to clone. (The BRCA2 gene is also associated with cases of male breast cancer.) There are a large variety of mutations (mistakes) that can occur along this gene. Many of these are small, involving only a few amino acid sequences, and very hard to find; other mutations involve loss of nearly all of the gene.

It is possible to stain tissue for BRCA1. Normal tissue is darkly stained, showing the presence of BRCA1 in normal amounts. Cancer cells lose their BRCA1 activity and have little or no stain. If normal tissue is being invaded by a tumor, you can identify how far the malignant cells have invaded normal tissue by using these special staining methods.

These oncogenes (abnormal genes) cause ovarian cancer that occurs primarily in thirty to thirty-nine-year-old women, with less effect in forty to forty-nine-year-olds, and even less effect in those over fifty. As with breast cancer, women with abnormal genes tend to get cancers earlier. Blood tests for genetic susceptibility are not yet used on any routine clinical basis. However, along with counseling, they are available at most large hospitals for women with strong family histories of ovarian and breast cancer.

It should be clear by now that there is no single excellent test to screen the general female population for early detection of ovarian cancer. The best we can do today is to combine transvaginal ultrasound with color flow Doppler imaging and blood tumor markers, usually CA-125. This combination can be used and repeated if necessary at intervals to help diagnose early-stage or preclinical ovarian cancer in appropriately selected women. As is painfully apparent, additional research effort is needed to refine techniques to diagnose this cancer while it is in its early curable stage, or better yet, before it develops.

Surgical Diagnosis and Treatment

LAPAROSCOPY

Laparoscopy provides an opportunity for a direct view of the ovaries. Commonly called Band-Aid surgery, laparoscopy requires an incision about an inch long, made near the navel. The laparoscope is a tube slightly longer than a pencil, which is inserted into the abdomen. The laparoscope functions like a hollow fiber-optic flashlight, enabling the surgeon to see the ovaries and other internal organs. This is obviously an important alternative to full surgery for distinguishing benign uterine conditions and benign ovarian pathology from ovarian cancer. It can spare many patients with a pelvic mass the risk of more extensive abdominal surgery, for many of them have a benign disease that does not require it.

Laparoscopy is used in cases where the ovarian mass that has been identified preoperatively is likely to be benign. Done by a properly trained and credentialed surgeon, it can save a patient the longer recovery associated with a larger abdominal incision.

OPERATIVE LAPAROSCOPY

When indicated, the entire ovary can be removed for pathological diagnosis, or a bothersome cyst may be removed, leaving the ovary intact. This is accomplished by making additional tiny incisions in the pubic hairline and using operative instruments designed specifically for the procedure. If malignant changes are found, and if the surgeon cannot visualize all of the abdominal cavity, then depending upon the agreement or consent previously given by the patient, a new incision may be made and full surgical exploratory laparotomy may be done immediately. It is important to remember, however, that most ovarian masses, especially in younger women, are benign.

EXPLORATORY LAPAROTOMY

For women with suspicious pelvic and ultrasound findings, rising or abnormal tumor markers, or positive family histories and tumor-like findings, an exploratory laparotomy is often necessary. It is used for proper diagnosis, removal of the tumor, and for staging and determining the extent of spread of the tumor.

If the results of your workup point to a diagnosis of ovarian cancer, you must assume an all-out aggressive attitude to fight the tumor. The horizontal bikini-type incision (Pfannensteil incision) at the top of the pubic hairline that women have grown accustomed to for routine hysterectomy is probably not for you. Your surgeon will often choose to make a long vertical incision so that he can explore the entire inside of your abdomen, not just the pelvic portion.

I would also personally advise a patient of mine whose workup was highly indicative of an ovarian tumor to seek the services of a gynecologic oncology surgeon at a fairly large medical center. The gynecologic oncologist will have better training in cancer surgery than the general gynecologist and this may improve your prognosis. He/she will know that it is important to look under the diaphragm for tiny metastases; remove the omentum (the loose membrane covering the small intestine), which improves survival in patients with early ovarian cancer; biopsy the pelvic and para-aortic nodes; examine the lining of the entire abdomen for tiny metastases; and collect fluid within the pelvic or abdominal cavity. If none is apparent, he can then run sterile fluid over the area in order to collect cells for examination under the microscope, which will determine—even if there is no visual evidence of tumor—whether or not a microscopic tumor or tumors remain.

Because the surgery is often complicated and sometimes necessarily aggressive, your odds of survival are more likely to be improved if you use a gynecologic oncologist. He or she will have the experience it takes to remove large tumor formations or debulk them, leaving, in most cases, minimum residual or no visible remaining tumor. The less tumor that remains postoperatively, the better the prognosis. He will also head the team that integrates care. Such a team should also include a family doctor or internist, a medical oncologist (if the gynecologic oncology surgeon does not administer his own chemotherapy), and a pathologist.

Surgical Staging

Because survival rates in most ovarian malignancies are intimately tied into whether or not the tumor is confined within the ovary or has spread in a limited or widespread manner, the following table has been used for many years. Put together by the Cancer Committee of the International Federation of Gynecology and Obstetrics (FIGO), the following classifications are also the basis of treatment of the disease. Unless you have a keen interest, please skip to the bottom of page 330.

FIGO Staging System for Ovarian Cancer

Stage I   Growth limited to the ovaries

IA   Growth limited to one ovary, no malignant ascites.[1] No tumor on the external surface, capsule (covering layer of the ovary) intact

IB   Growth limited to both ovaries; no malignant ascites. No tumor on the external surface of the ovary, capsule intact

IC   Either IA or IB but with tumor on the surface of one or both ovaries, or with capsule ruptured, or with malignant ascites, or positive peritoneal cytology[2]

Stage II Growth involving one or both ovaries with pelvic extension

IIA   Extension and/or metastasis to the uterus and/or fallopian tubes
IIB   Extension to other pelvic tissues
IIC   Tumor with IIA or IIB but with tumor on the surface of one or
      both ovaries, or with capsule(s) ruptured, or with malignant
      ascites, or positive peritoneal cytology

Stage III Tumor involving one or both ovaries with peritoneal[3] implants
outside the pelvis and/or positive[4] retroperitoneal[5] or inguinal (groin)
nodes. Superficial liver metastasis alone also equals stage III. Tumor is
limited to the true pelvis, but with histologically proven malignant extension
to small bowel or omentum

IIIA   Tumor limited to the pelvis with negative nodes[6] but with
       microscopic spread onto the lining of the abdomen
IIIB   Tumor macroscopically (able to be seen with the naked eye)
       involving the abdomen but no single implant measuring greater
       than 2 cm; nodes are negative
IIIC   Abdominal implants greater than 2 cm in diameter and/or positive retroperitoneal or inguinal nodes

Stage IV Growth involving one or both ovaries with disease spreading
beyond the abdomen or invasion into the liver. If fluid is present around
the lungs, the fluid must contain malignant cells to put the case into a
stage IV category

---

[1]Ascites is an accumulation of fluid in the abdominal cavity which exceeds normal amounts.

[2]Positive peritoneal cytology refers to the fact that fluid sampled from the abdominal cavity is seen to contain cancer cells under microscopic examination.

[3]Peritoneal implants refers to areas where tumor has implanted (invaded) into the lining of the abdomen (peritoneum).

[4]Positive nodes are nodes that contain cancer cells.

[5]Retroperitoneal—behind the lining of the abdomen—closer to the back—very deep nodes.

[6]Negative nodes are nodes that do not contain cancer cells.

Remember, not all enlarged ovaries are dangerous. However, the following need to be thoroughly investigated:

1. Any ovary ten centimeters or larger in any age patient is dangerous. It is extremely rare to see functional (corpus luteum or follicle) cysts or even an endometriosis cyst of this size. Therefore, any cysts of this size would be highly suspect.

2. Any ovarian enlargement that occurs after menopause.

3. Any mass in the area of the ovaries in a woman of any age that progressively enlarges beyond five centimeters while under observation, particularly if it remains that size after her period. It is important to know that of cancers that are discovered in the ovaries, 95 percent are more than five centimeters in diameter. Therefore, the finding of a five-centimeter or larger ovarian mass on examination, especially in a woman over the age of forty, should require further evaluation for malignancy. Exceptions would be a five-centimeter cystic mass in a young menstruating woman, which may be a benign functional cyst. This should be treated with observation and/or hormonal therapy. However, if the follow-up ultrasound examination shows an increase in size, solid portions, or malignant characteristics, then further workup is indicated. Fortunately, in most young women these cysts usually disappear in two to three months.

4. Any persistence or new appearance of an ovarian mass while a woman is on an oral contraceptive.

5. Any pelvic mass must be considered to be an ovarian cancer until both ovaries are identified, or the mass is definitely seen on ultrasound or even laparoscopy and identified to be a fibroid or another benign problem.

MEIGS' SYNDROME

I must at least mention that sometimes all the classical signs of ovarian cancer are present, yet a benign tumor is found to be the culprit. This condition is known as Meigs' syndrome.

Usually the symptoms are ominous. The woman has increasing abdominal girth, often described as bloating, and her skirts and pants become tight. Her legs may ache and she may feel short of breath. Her physician finds a substantial amount of fluid accumulation within her abdominal cavity. Moreover, X rays may reveal that she also has fluid surrounding her lungs. The diagnosis must be made by a complete cancer workup and surgery. But the good news is that with Meigs' syndrome, the tumor that is removed is benign, and soon after it is removed, the fluid within the abdomen and lung cavity disappears.

Preoperative Evaluation for Women Where Ovarian Malignancy Is Suspected

A thorough preoperative workup and a physician with extensive experience in tumor surgery are essential for good results in these cancers.

Aside from physician and ultrasound examination, before undergoing abdominal surgery, women with a suspected ovarian cancer should have routine blood and urine tests for tumor markers. The following should be performed to rule out tumors elsewhere that may have spread to or from the ovary or may have even developed independently at the same time:

1. A chest X ray should be done to check the lungs.

2. A barium enema X-ray examination should be performed because of the high frequency with which colon cancer spreads to the ovary, and also because these women may have an increased risk of a second primary, i.e., two separate cancers.

3. CT scan or MRI of both pelvis and abdomen should be done.

Most patients, except for those with stage IA, will undergo chemotherapy after surgery to destroy residual cancer cells that might remain in the body. Even if there is a tumor so large that it can't be totally removed, surgery should remove or debulk as much of it as possible. This rids the patient of a large volume of cancer cells and gives chemotherapy the best of all chances to work. The anticancer drugs work by eliminating a certain percentage of cells during the various phases of their growth cycles. Therefore, results are best when fewer cells are physically present. The same process holds true for radiation therapy.

Reducing the volume of the tumor is important also because the tumor itself is an immunosuppressant agent, that is, it interferes with the patient's own immune system. Less tumor should mean less immune suppression, which should aid in restoring the patient's immune competence.

Therapy of Ovarian Cancer

Before chemotherapy is begun, if possible, all tumor that is visible should be removed from the pelvis and abdominal cavity. Chemotherapy is not indicated for stage IA, in which the cells retain somewhat normal characteristics, i.e., are well differentiated. However, the good news is that for more advanced cancers, multiple drugs are now available which increase life expectancy. This chapter cannot possibly cover all of the latest research in detail, nor would it be appropriate for a book of this kind. However, a once bleak subject is seeing some major turnaround as more effective drugs become available. Life expectancy as compared with a decade ago has markedly improved as study protocols have shown the advantage of new drugs and new combinations of drugs.

In 1989 paclitaxel (Taxol®) was isolated from the bark of the Pacific yew tree. Added to regimens already established, such as cisplatin, or used alone, it has brought new hope. Cisplatin and paclitaxel are an effective combination therapy for women with newly diagnosed stage III and IV cancer. In addition, a triple-drug therapy combining high doses of cyclophosphamide, paclitaxel, and cisplatin are being investigated at the National Cancer Institute and at Harvard. Another drug, topotecan hydrochloride (Hycamtin™), was recently introduced to prevent replication of the tumor cells. It may take years before its place is truly understood.

In addition, in cases where there is a genetic abnormality in the BRCA1 gene, researchers at Vanderbilt University are trying to suppress BRCA1-related ovarian cancer by introducing normal copies of the BRCA1 gene into the cancer. Restoring a normal BRCA1 gene will inhibit the growth of the cancer cells. This is currently limited to trials studying women who have failed chemotherapy. This method will be further tested across the country in phase two trials soon, where women who are less ill will be allowed to be treated.

Basically, the researchers are inserting the normal BRCA1 gene into viruses. Since viruses are very good at getting into cells, they simply take the accompanying normal BRCA1 gene with them. Liquid containing the virus is injected into the abdominal cavity. Then the liquid is sloshed around to coat the abdominal lining, which is often the site where ovarian tumor cells spread. Early results have been exciting, with slowing or decrease in growth of the tumors in a large proportion of the tumors.

Here is a therapy that will attack and help to normalize cancer cells by inserting a normal copy of the gene. This is exciting news!

Summary

Ovarian cancer presents a real problem for women and a real challenge to physicians. This chapter should make you aware of the problem and of the many symptoms that you might have been ignoring, but which might be significant. It was also written to get you to your doctor at least once a year, better every six months, for a pelvic examination if you are over forty. And if you are overweight or if your pelvic examination is unsatisfactory for any other reason, including your inability to relax your abdominal muscles during examination, get a pelvic sonogram. This simple test may give you and your physician the information that could set your mind at ease or begin a series of investigations. Ovarian cancer is not a pleasant subject, but it is one that should be part of your medical knowledge about your own body, for this information may truly save your life.

Chapter 12

CERVICAL CANCER—THE MOST SECRET SEXUALLY TRANSMITTED DISEASE

Some of the best news in women's health regards cervical cancer. Death rates from this disease have fallen 70 percent in the United States since the early 1950s when the Pap smear began to be widely used. This expanded testing coincided with the introduction of the "pill." This resulted in large numbers of young women who wanted to start birth control seeing their doctors and having Paps. Unfortunately, older, postmenopausal women did not have a similar impetus and did not gain equal benefits from this simple screening test, which has saved the lives of millions of women.

First, let us look at some important facts about Pap smears and cervical cancer:

1. Cancer of the cervix is a sexually transmitted disease. I'll tell you more about this later, but keep it in mind as you read through this section.

2. The Pap test is *the best screening test.* There is *no other test* that *can detect the presence of cell changes before a real cancer has begun.* This includes mammograms, tests for occult blood (blood that is present but not visible which may be associated with colon cancer) in the GI tract, and so on.

3. *The Pap test is not perfect.* I'll talk more about this as I move ahead.

Pap smears detect early changes in the cervical cells, often years before actual cervical cancer develops. By early diagnosis and treatment we actually prevent the cancer. Indeed, in other parts of the world, especially the undeveloped nations where facilities to perform Paps do not exist, cervical cancer still causes more deaths than any other cancer including breast cancer.

Worldwide there are about the same number of cases of cervical and breast cancer but most breast cancers occur in the industrialized nations while cervical cancer predominates in the undeveloped world. Unfortunately, in the United States, nearly five thousand women still die annually from this disease. Most of these cases occur in women who *do not have regular Paps*.

A 70 percent reduction in the incidence of this cancer over the past fifty years is a remarkable triumph. The tragedy is that five thousand women still die and our goal should be no deaths from this preventable disease. How do we continue to lower the rate of deaths from cervical cancer? You who are reading this book are probably in the age group at greatest risk. Peri- and postmenopausal women have the highest risk of developing cervical cancer. Yet, less than half of all women over age fifty-five had a Pap smear last year. The mean age of diagnosis in white women has been recently noted to be forty-seven and in black women, fifty-two. This slight shift toward a younger age is due to a sharp rise noted in the number of women under age thirty-five who are diagnosed with the disease. Yet many women in the fifty-plus age group feel that they're too old to get a Pap or to get cervical cancer and believe because they no longer are sexually active they're not at risk. Actually, one-quarter of the women diagnosed with cervical cancer fall into this age group. Among women who die of cervical cancer, four out of five have not had a Pap smear in the last five years.

Doctors recommend a yearly Pap beginning when a woman becomes sexually active or at age eighteen, whichever comes first. A recommendation from the American Cancer Society (ACS) states that "after three consecutive normal Pap smears, Paps could be done every three years or at the discretion of the doctor." This recommendation has confused many women and has led them to believe that the Pap and a yearly visit to their doctor are really not so important. This recommendation really relates to women who are presumed to be at "low risk," which means women who are in a totally monogamous relationship and have never had more than one partner (it also assumes that this one partner has also never had another partner).

I have long been upset that the ACS never cautioned women that they still need to go to their doctors on at least a yearly basis for a pelvic examination, whether they need a Pap or not. Observing the cervix and vagina and palpating the size and shape of the uterus and ovaries during an internal exam must be done at regular intervals whether or not a Pap is actually taken at the same time. Especially in the older patient, abnormal firmness or "grittiness" of the cervix may be a sign of early cancer. Increase in uterine or ovarian size is of great importance as well. Never confuse these two needs: You may or may not need a Pap, but you absolutely need a yearly or biannual pelvic examination.

Women who have had a hysterectomy are in another category. If you have had a hysterectomy for a malignancy, then your doctor will advise you on how often you should have a Pap smear. Usually, they will be done frequently at first and less frequently over years as the time from surgery lengthens. They are taken from the top or vault of the vagina with a cotton swab. On the other hand, if you have had a hysterectomy for benign reasons, there is disagreement about how often you need a Pap. Some doctors say once every three years, others, once a decade, and others have recently said "never." I believe that it is important to get the first Pap within the first year post-hysterectomy. (It goes without saying that a Pap should have been done within a few months prior to the surgery.) I recently did a Pap on a patient who had had a hysterectomy four months earlier for very large fibroids. Her Pap was unexpectedly positive for precancerous changes developing in the top portion of her vagina. All of her previous preoperative Paps were normal. She had this small area removed by a gyn-oncologist as an outpatient procedure and is fine. If she had waited three years or longer, she would most likely have developed a large, possibly invasive cancer.

I also feel it is necessary to return for routine gynecologic care after hysterectomy for benign causes. If ovaries are left in, they must be checked every six to twelve months to help ensure that there is no abnormality brewing. If a patient is very overweight, an ultrasound examination can be done.

Some women in the past have had supracervical hysterectomies. That means that although the upper portion of the uterus was removed (the part within the abdominal cavity), the cervix (the portion within the vagina) remains. (In chapter 13 on hysterectomy, page 385, you will find that this procedure may be making a comeback.) If the cervix remains, then normal guidelines for Pap smear intervals should be followed.

In either case, the interior of the vagina should be examined visually for tissue dryness, redness, etc. Then, carefully, the doctor should use a gloved finger to go over the vaginal walls to make sure they are smooth and without roughness or irregularity due to tumor formation. A rectovaginal exam to feel for pelvic or rectal abnormalities and to check stool for occult blood should also be performed at this same time.

Furthermore, for women with a cervix, I can make an even better case for a yearly Pap. There are some countries, especially in the Scandinavian areas and Iceland, that support nationwide planned and controlled screening programs. In these countries virtually every woman has a Pap smear on a regular basis. Although longer intervals between smears may be acceptable in these circumstances, in our country, where screening tends to be opportunistic (that is, smears are only done if you choose to go for them), the importance of regular and frequent screening must be constantly emphasized.

The Pap smear is not one hundred percent perfect. Few things in life are. The Pap is no exception. Paps can miss cancers. These results are called false negatives, i.e., the patient has a problem, but the Pap misses it. There will be false-negative Paps, but by coming back three years in a row and having three consecutive Paps, this error will be picked up and Paps become almost one hundred percent efficient.

WHY DO PAPS MISS CANCERS?

You could be part of the problem. Here's how to help your health care provider: Avoid having your Pap done if you are menstruating. If there is only minimal spotting, it might be all right, but excess red blood cells can make your Pap difficult to interpret. Do not use vaginal creams or lubricants for at least forty-eight hours prior to your appointment. Avoid intercourse for that same time. Also, do not douche; it washes away the cells that we are trying to capture for the slides. It also washes away secretions that enable us to make a diagnosis of infection. Do not insert a tampon for twenty-four hours prior to your appointment, as the tampon collects cells and secretions. This results in sampling errors because fewer cells are able to be picked up on the Pap smear. Sampling error is responsible for nearly 70 percent of the false-negative results—the cells that we want to identify are just not on the slide. Doctors should instruct patients prior to their visit. If a patient appears in the office with a vagina full of antifungal cream, she should return at a later date for her Pap.

The person who takes the smear may be part of the problem. His or her training and familiarity with cervical anatomy may play a part. The Pap should be taken from an area of the cervix called the transformation zone. Being able to identify this area is important for taking a good Pap. This area is where the squamous (flat, plate-like) cells of the outer portion of the cervix meet the columnar (tall, column-like) cells that line the opening of the cervix. It is at this junction where column-like cells become most active and actually transform into squamous, or plate-like cells. Because cellular activity is greatest here, these cells are more vulnerable to viral and other carcinogens. Therefore, this area is where precancerous changes are most likely to begin. In young women, the transformation zone extends farther out on the cervix—it actually covers a larger area—especially when women are pregnant or on oral contraceptives. If these cells develop abnormal characteristics, they may be on their way to malignancy unless they are carefully followed or removed by some type of therapy. As a woman becomes postmenopausal, the transition zone regresses from the outside of the cervix to within the opening of the cervical canal and becomes smaller in area.

Letting the cells dry on the slide before spraying them with fixative can be a problem as well. Doctors used to take one sample from the cervical opening, roll the collected material on one slide, and spray it. Then a second specimen was taken from the outer portion of the cervix and rolled onto a second slide and sprayed. Now, to save money, almost all women have both samples placed on one slide. Making two steps takes more time before spraying the cells. If a doctor is working without a nurse, if a health provider is slow or not aware of the importance of immediately plating and preserving the cells by spraying them, then detail may be lost and false negatives become more likely.

If too few cells wind up on the slide, or if the doctor lumps all of the cells in a thick blob, there will be problems for the cytologist who has to read these slides. If you have ever actually read Pap slides, you quickly appreciate how important technique is. Each nurse who works with me is specifically instructed how to make slides for proper Paps. I always tell them to spread the cells out as evenly as possible over the entire slide to give the cytologist who reads it the best possible chance to see individual cells.

The Pap smear improved some years ago when the cotton swab was replaced by a small brush, the endocervical brush, that more efficiently picks up cells from inside the cervical mouth. Because more cells are picked up by this simple mascara-wand-like device, more cells wind up on the slide.* However, both the wooden spatula that is used to pick up cells from the outer portion of the cervix and the brush are thrown into the trash still containing many more cells than they have deposited on the slides. This realization is leading to a new means of cancer detection, i.e., using a liquid collection system. With this method, the brush used to

*On the downside, sometimes the tiny bristles cause slight bleeding.

obtain the smear is swished in a small container of liquid fixative to remove all of the cells. The liquid and the cells it contains are sent to the lab, where red blood cells and white blood cells and debris will be filtered out. Then the clean cells can be placed evenly on a slide.

Viral typing for human papillomavirus, known as HPV, can also be done from the same specimen, if indicated. There are many types of HPV. Some low-risk types are types 6 and 11. The most common high-risk HPV viruses are numbered 16 and 18. HPV 31, 33, and 35 are called intermediate-risk. High-risk HPV viral types are most often found in women with the most abnormal Pap smears and in the majority of women with cervical pre-cancer and cancer. The amount of this cancer-causing virus present could also be evaluated, as could the presence of other sexually transmitted diseases. Such total information could help predict a woman's risk of developing cervical cancer. This will be a routine test in the not too distant future. One day soon, these liquid specimens may run through a chamber where the cellular contents in the liquid will be analyzed by automated special computerized systems, much as blood counts are done today.

Currently, there are rules and regulations for labs that read Pap smears. All labs must rescreen 10 percent of all the "negative" slides. This is normally done by pathologists or cytologists. Computerized machines have recently been approved by the FDA to check quality control at some laboratories. They are known as the AutoPap 300 QC System and PapNet. The AutoPap system rescreens 100 percent of the Paps and selects a certain percentage for the cytologist or pathologist to rescreen. The PapNet makes digitized images of the slides. It images 128 of the most abnormal-looking cells on each individual slide and records them on videotape. To avoid false negatives, these tapes are then reviewed by the same cytologist/pathologist who read the original Pap smear. Both methods have been shown to have the capability of decreasing the number of false-negative Paps reported. (Other reports have shown that having two cytologists read the Pap gives similar results.) However, as you may suspect, both devices can add from five to forty dollars to the price of a Pap. This amounts to more than it costs to have a cytologist review all the slides a second time.

Even after the "negative" slides have been picked out by the machine, a pathologist or cytotechnician still has to make the final decision on whether or not a slide is abnormal. It seems to me that the easiest course would be to use these computers to screen out the easy, run-of-the-mill, majority of normal Paps and leave just those that are abnormal for the pathologist to review. This might make the most economic and timesaving sense and may well be the wave of the future, but even the computer screen is not one hundred percent effective.

If you have always had a normal Pap, if you have been in a long-standing, monogamous relationship or have not been sexually active for many years, and if you can swear that your partner has never strayed (including a lesbian partner), then the following is not for you and you should go on to the next chapter. (However, you may wish to read on just for the information you may obtain.)

This might be a good place to say something about lesbians and their need for Pap smears. All lesbians need yearly Paps, period—even the 10 percent who state that they have never had relations with a man. Abnormal smears most likely result from the fact that HPV can be shared, transmitted through sexual activity, from one woman to another. Information from the National Lesbian and Gay Health Association in 1996 showed a 34 percent incidence of HPV in a Seattle lesbian population. Bacterial vaginosis and HIV-AIDS are also risk factors for cervical cancer. Actually, the risk for HIV in this population is higher than for other women in general, at least in the San Francisco area. Though lesbians were often regarded as the group with the lowest rates of sexual infection, this may no longer be true; with them as with everyone else, much of the risk depends upon social behavior. Lesbians who go to gay bars, have more partners, use intravenous drugs, and have unprotected sex with men will be at higher risk than a woman in a long monogamous relationship with her female partner. It seems the same rules apply to homosexuals or heterosexuals.

Smoking, having HIV, being on immunosuppressive drugs for kidney transplants or Hodgkin's disease, having been exposed in utero to DES (diethylstilbestrol), and having other sexually transmitted diseases all increase your chances of having an abnormal Pap.

What are other factors that put you at risk for abnormal Paps (or developing cervical disease related to HPV infection)? They begin with early age of first intercourse. During teenage years, when cervical cells are undergoing very active division and transformation, they are more susceptible to damage by viral carcinogens. Exposure to cigarette smoking at the same time may enhance these viral effects. Common sense tells us that early adolescence would be a bad time for sexual activity as it would make contact with possible carcinogens more likely. It also follows that having more than one sex partner increases your chance of catching an infection. However, there are cases where it is known for certain that the woman had only one sex partner, yet developed cervical cancer. This has to do with the concept of the "dangerous male" originally proposed by my friend, Dr. Albert Singer of London. While my patients are sure whom they have slept with, it is much more difficult to know with whom your partner might have slept. And so, if you are unlucky enough to sleep with a man who may have contracted one of the more virulent cancer-causing HPV-type viruses, it is possible that sleeping even with only that one high-risk partner will get you into trouble.

The other bad news is that condoms may not be protective. While latex condoms seem to protect against the HIV virus, the condom does not cover the base of the penis or the scrotum where the cancer-causing papillomavirus may also live. And let's be honest, there is often genital contact between partners before condoms are used. Condoms are not perfect either and tear from time to time. For better protection, a woman could try the female condom, which covers the vulva when used properly.

The spread of HPV virus is the reason for women getting cervical cancer when their husbands have been seeing a prostitute or other women on the side. In countries where males are openly permitted to be promiscuous and prostitutes are often part of their lifestyle, the incidence of cervical cancer among monogamous wives is high.

In the beginning of this chapter, I gave you the bad news that cervical cancer is a sexually transmitted disease. Unfortunately, this is probably true for 98 percent of cases. This fact has been suspected since a doctor by the name of Rigona-Stern examined death records in Verona, Italy, in 1842. For well over a century, and recently intensified with better epidemiological data in the last fifty years, we have been searching for the culprit—the agent that is sexually transmitted. Currently we put most of the blame on the human papillomavirus. Even today there is still no sure way to protect yourself from this virus. Worse, if you are postmenopausal and entering a relationship, remember that decreasing estrogen levels cause the vaginal lining to thin. As a result, the lining is more prone to small rips and cuts which can increase the risk of infection. Lest you think this news is shocking and just discovered, I would like to insert a few lines from my book, *No More Menstrual Cramps and Other Good News*, published in 1980:

> Although there are various theories, cervical cancer is thought
> to be a sexually transmitted disease. It is almost never found

in virgins or nuns, and is most often found in women who have had sexual relations at an early age or who have had multiple partners. One reason for the first cause seems to be that the cells of the transformation area of the cervix (where cervical cancer almost always begins) are especially active during adolescence and pregnancy. During this active period, the cells are especially susceptible to stimuli that can cause cell transformation.

. . . A higher incidence of cervical cancer is found in women who are married to men who have cancer of the penis. Another researcher, Kessler, found that the incidence of cervical cancer in the second or in a few cases in the third wives of men whose first wives had developed cervical cancer was 3.5 times higher than it should have been.

These facts should be carefully explained to our daughters. Looking at sex as a means of contracting cancer is not a happy thought. As I said in 1980, "It is one of the best reasons that I can think of for saying 'no' to boyfriends. Five minutes of pleasure is not worth chancing years of problems."

More recently some studies suggest the possibility that the virus can be transmitted through inanimate objects such as wet towels that have been shared, underclothing that has not been properly washed, or even speculums that have not been properly cleaned in your doctor's office. Although these possibilities exist they are rare at best. Infection by direct sexual contact is by far the most important route of transmission.

What about the detection of the virus on the male partner? First of all, it is important to know that any time there is a change in sexual partners, there is risk to both partners. Either could bring a new variant of the HPV virus to the bedroom. If he has visible warty-like growths on his genitals, these should be looked at by an expert. Such warts may shed virus (or could even represent an unrecognized cancer of the penis). If there are no visible growths, it may be a waste of time to search for lesions. You can be infected when nothing is visible because he may still be able to shed virus after his immune system has gotten rid of the visible wart. Furthermore, it is also now known that HPV can be harbored in an invisible state on the man's genitals. Years ago, we sent many male partners to urologists. Presently, unless there are visible lesions, this practice is rare.

Why has this information been such a deep, dark secret? This information has been around for years and years. I wanted to write a book on the subject in 1981, but felt the world was not quite ready. I have believed for two decades now that there is a conspiracy of silence surrounding this information. The fact that sexual activity among heterosexuals can cause cervical cancer is very bad news—news that is not commonly known except among gynecologists. But even gynecologists have never come out publicly and warned their patients about this potential problem. In fairness, however, it didn't become clear until this past decade that the actual culprit involved was HPV.

But now we must spread the news. And what is good for the goose is good for the gander. A male also must become concerned about his future. One day he will find his true love. Would he want to give this virus to her? Men need to know that their sexual activity during youth may result in guilt-filled lovemaking one day in the future. These are the unfortunate truths that should underscore today's sexual education. Unless there is a major reversal in our society's morality, men must take proper responsibility for their role.

One more note: HPV may also cause anal cancer. A study from Sweden and Denmark found that 84 percent of men and women with anal cancer had tumors that tested positive for high-risk types of HPV, mostly HPV-16, which is known to cause half of all cervical cancers.

Women with promiscuous partners are at increased risk, as are those with a higher lifetime number of sexual partners (ten or more), earlier age at first intercourse, a history of anogenital warts, and a history of anal intercourse. It is also possible that the virus may spread during routine toilet habits.

Preventing HPV infection could therefore help prevent cervical, vulvar, and anal cancers. With time, we will hopefully be able to prevent these sexually transmitted viral agents that cause a variety of diseases, from HIV to cancer.

Also, women who smoke are more likely to get cervical cancer than nonsmokers. A tobacco-specific carcinogen has been found to be significantly increased in the cervical mucus of women who smoke. One more reason to stop smoking.

ABNORMAL PAP SMEARS

If you have ever had an abnormal Pap, you may be interested in the following section, which explains the new way Paps are reported. On the other hand, this section is rather dry, but may give you a greater appreciation of what your Pap really means. Many women are requesting a copy of their Pap report but most don't understand the words. Worse, physicians are confused since there has been a change in the terminology by which Paps are reported. It used to be a simple Class I–V, with Class I being normal and Class V being the worst. To better describe the cellular changes that occur in the progression to cervical cancer, the more descriptive Bethesda System was developed in 1988 by the National Cancer Institute and then modified in 1991.

Remember that whatever system is used to report Pap smears, the result of the reading is completely dependent upon the knowledge, training, and subjective interpretation of the individual who is looking at the smear. Studies have shown that even a well-trained cytologist may interpret smears differently at different times. (This occurs most often with smears that are in intermediary categories and rarely with those that are normal truly or obviously cancerous.)

I will try to make this simple. The first change made on all Pap reports was that the condition of the smear be noted, i.e., whether infection, discharge, or other elements hide abnormal cells from view. Also, if the slide does not contain enough cells or if they had not been properly preserved, the report suggests that the Pap be repeated.

The Numbers Game

Let me try to use some simple numbers to help keep this example clear. If we assume that we have done Pap smears on 100,000 women, then 90,000 (90 percent) will be Class I or "within normal limits." Basically, the old Class I Pap now is described simply as a Pap that is within normal limits or one that has some benign changes, usually due to the presence of infection. This is an easy category and one that almost everyone agrees upon. As cells become less typical, there can be increasing confusion in their description.

Let's try to overcome that confusion:

If 90,000 smears are "normal," then 10,000 are *not normal* and require classification.

TABLE 12.1. CYTOLOGIC FINDINGS, EXPECTED DISTRIBUTION (N=100,000)

	N	% abnormals	% overall
NORMAL (I)	(90,000)		
NOT NORMAL	(10,000)		
BENIGN CELLULAR CHANGES (IIR)	(5,000)	50	5
EPITHELIAL CELL ABNORMALITIES	5,000	50	5
ASCUS (II)	(2,000)	20	2.0
AGUS (II)	(500)	5	0.5
LGSIL (II-III?)	(2,000)	20	2.00
HGSIL (III/IV?)	(400)	4	0.4
CA (V)	(30)	0.3	0.03

In the Bethesda System classification, about 5 percent of smears (5,000) are described as having "benign cellular changes," which means that the cells have been altered by the presence of local vaginal infections due to yeast, trichomoniasis, herpes, or other benign infectious conditions that can be treated locally. Other conditions, such as normal physiological tissue repair, vitamin deficiencies, or other noncancerous types of changes, are also included. These were included in the old Class II, which formerly denoted these benign cellular changes along with many other changes that I'll continue to describe.

After eliminating the 90,000 normals and the 5,000 benign abnormalities, we are left with 5,000 abnormalities that can now be grouped in what are called "epithelial cell abnormalities." This group contains the smears that truly require further attention. Within this group, there is a subgroup, only 30 of 100,000 smears (0.03 percent), that cytologists agree are the old Class V "cancer cells."

"Low-Grade Squamous Intraepithelial Lesion," or LGSIL

There are about 2,000 of the 100,000 smears (2 percent of all smears reported) that have clearly defined characteristics that fit into a group that is now described as "low-grade squamous intraepithelial lesion" or LGSIL.

LGSIL includes Paps that were previously labeled "mild dysplasia," which include:

• the old Class II category with cell abnormality caused by infection or inflammation

• the old Class III category where cell changes are caused by "condyloma" (wart, i.e., HPV-virus infection), but the cells do not have premalignant characteristics

Although the Pap smear is called LGSIL, after complete testing with colposcopy and biopsy about 10 percent will be shown to have a more advanced condition, that is, "high grade."

"High-Grade Squamous Intraepithelial Lesion," or HGSIL

About 0.4 percent, or 400, of the 100,000 Pap smears are reported as "high-grade squamous intraepithelial lesion." These reports were formerly in the old Class III or IV groups. This is a category in which agreement between cytologists is high and in which the potential for future malignancy is likely. Fortunately, this is a relatively uncommon finding.

ASCUS and AGUS—New Categories

If at this point you added up all of our numbers, you would find that there are clear reports in nearly 97.5 percent of patients. There are then about 2,500 of the 100,000, or 2.5 percent, that show some atypical changes that are less clearly defined. In order to avoid overlooking something that could be a problem, a *new category was created* (along with LGSIL, HGSIL, and cancer), the group of *epithelial cell abnormalities*. Epithelial cell abnormalities are divided into two subgroups: (1) ASCUS (atypical *squamous* cells of undetermined significance), which involves 2,000, or 2 percent, of smears, and (2) AGUS (atypical *glandular* cells of undetermined significance), involving 500, or 0.5 percent, of all smears. This last category refers not to abnormalities in cervical squamous cells, but to abnormalities in the column-like secreting cells that line the cervical canal above and inside the cervical opening. (Both of these types of cells were included in the old Class II category, which also included abnormalities caused by infection and inflammation.) Therefore, the new Bethesda System classification is more descriptive and more exact.

What does "atypical squamous cells of undetermined significance" really mean? Because the name is so long, this category is called ASCUS. As noted, about 2 percent of smears (but in some laboratories as many as 5 percent) fall into this category. *All of these Paps need follow-up.* The patient must either return for a repeat Pap or go on to more definitive procedures such as colposcopy. Again, this decision must be based on the advice given by the pathologist regarding the Pap smear findings and health professional's clinical findings.

The National Cancer Institute has recently sponsored a major national study to help determine the best possible management of these relatively minor abnormal smears (the ASCUS and the LGSIL groups), which comprise the overwhelming majority of all the epithelial abnormalities reported. Unfortunately, because of the size of the study and the need to assess long-term outcomes, it will take about five years to get answers. In the meantime, many of you will have these minor abnormalities and will require care. If the ASCUS report contains a good description from the pathologist, appropriate evaluation can be taken more readily. For example, if he states that the cellular changes are due to infection or lack of hormone, then a repeat Pap after treatment is complete or in six months appears to be the most reasonable action. If, however, the pathologist states that dysplasia is present, then consideration for HPV testing, colposcopy, or just repeat smears might be the best course of action.

Therapy

Benign cell changes: Recommended therapy or follow-up when there are benign cell changes: If the changes seen in the cells seem to be due to infection, then the infection should be treated and the Pap repeated in two to three months.

If there is simply a lack of estrogen, the postmenopausal patient can be treated with an intravaginal estrogen cream or the Estring™ ring for three to five weeks and the Pap repeated. In most cases the Pap reverts to normal and long-term oral or vaginal estrogen therapy may be considered if appropriate. If the new Pap is not normal, then colposcopy is indicated.

If inflammation but no infection was noted on initial exam, and no infection seen on repeat exam, then the Pap can be repeated in four to six months. If the Pap is still abnormal the patient may be advised to have a colposcopy but this should rarely need to be done.

For pregnant and postpartum patients, or for women who tend not to show up for repeat visits, decisions may be made on different bases.

LGSIL, low-grade squamous intraepithelial lesions (or the old Class III): This report does not mean that you have a life-threatening disease. It is important to remember that *the Pap smear is a screening device to find women who need further evaluation. The final diagnosis must always be made by biopsy.* This can be done by simply seeing the abnormal area on the cervix that is causing the abnormal Pap and doing the biopsy, or most commonly by doing the biopsy with the help of a magnifying binocular lens called a colposcope. (Unless there is a grossly visible abnormality, all biopsies should be taken using colposcopic guidance.)

The good news is that those women with the least amount of abnormality (called CIN I) have a lesion that usually goes away without therapy. The problem is that LGSIL can also be associated with a variety of abnormalities, which can only be defined after biopsy. LGSIL may reveal HPV disease, or there could be more abnormal diagnoses that have the potential to become cancer sometime in the future. So if you have a diagnosis of LGSIL on your Pap smear, at present you should have colposcopy and possible biopsy to find out what this diagnosis really means, in your case. Your diagnosis can be further defined by HPV testing, which can help to differentiate high-risk from low-risk situations. HPV testing reduces the subjectivity in the testing process.

The national study that I mentioned above may finally show that testing with repeat smears, doing HPV testing, or other intermediary steps may be preferable to more invasive methods.

HGSIL, high-grade squamous intraepithelial lesions: This Pap report suggests that there are increasingly abnormal changes in the cells, but all changes are confined to cells that lie in the superficial layers of the cervix. Unless you have this problem, stop before you read farther, because this will be useless, soon-forgotten information.

HGSIL must be evaluated by colposcopy to see the extent of the lesion and to identify those areas that must be biopsied. High-grade disease always requires treatment (usually done on an outpatient basis) to prevent the development of invasive cancer of the cervix. This class includes what used to be called in-situ cancer of the cervix. In-situ cancer does not invade but remains confined to the superficial cell layers of the cervix and does not spread beyond the cervix.

In rare cases, the Pap report of HGSIL is actually found to be associated with invasive cervical cancer. This is the first time we have used the term *invasive cancer*. It has a special meaning: It means that the cancer is no longer confined to the superficial layers of cells, but has invaded beneath the basement membrane. (The basement membrane is a tissue landmark seen with the microscope and represents a barrier between the actively growing cells and underlying tissue that contain blood vessel and lymph channels. The barrier prevents spread.) Once this landmark structure is no longer intact, invasive cancer occurs. Cancer cells can then invade, grow, and expand their way into the interior tissues of the cervix and from there can grow down into the vagina or up into the uterus, bladder, or rectum. Once the cancer is within the interior of the cervical tissue, it can make its way into lymphatic and blood vessels, and to distant lymph nodes or other organs.

Invasive cancer of the cervix: As previously described, the last cytologic category is reserved for the relatively rare invasive cancers and is the old Class V. Most of these cancers are visible to the naked eye during pelvic examination. Here there is good agreement among cytologists. Fortunately, these are found in only 30 of 100,000 smears (0.03 percent). It must be stressed that *any visible abnormality* seen on pelvic exam should be biopsied whether or not the Pap was normal.

Over 90 percent of these cervical cancers arise just as we described above, from the flat squamous cells that cover the outer portion of the cervix. However, there is another category called "adenocarcinoma" of the cervix. This cancer stems from the column-like secreting cells that line the cervical canal. These cancers tend to have a somewhat worse prognosis only because the early stages of the cancer tend to be hidden up inside the cervical canal. When diagnosed these cancers are often already in an invasive state. Recent studies suggest that the increased use of the endocervical brushes that are used for obtaining Pap smears may increase the ability to diagnose such cancer at an early stage.

Women with invasive cancers, either squamous carcinoma or adenocarcinoma, usually have symptoms. They have bleeding after intercourse, irregular vaginal bleeding, and/or bloody, foul-smelling vaginal discharge. Pain is rare, usually associated only with advanced cases. And that is the reason why the Pap is so important. The cervix has few nerve endings that conduct pain. Because of this, a cancer can get started and grow and grow without the woman having any pain or discomfort. That is the reason to come to your doctor, because like many other diseases including heart attack, or fracture from osteoporosis, there are often no warning signs.

For just a moment, let's take a look at a simile developed by Dr. Richard Reid of Detroit. It may help you understand the whole cancer process better. He noted that the growth and development of cervical cancer can be likened to the growth of weeds. It is necessary to have "seed," a "soil," and in addition, growth depends upon the presence of "fertilizers" or "weed-killers." In scientific terms, the seed, or initiator, is the HPV virus. The soil, fertilizer, and weed-killers would be the "tissue type," the "tumor promoters," and the "tumor suppressants." As previously noted, there are high-risk, intermediate-risk, and low-risk forms of this virus, just as there are

TABLE 12.2. THE ORIGIN OF CERVICAL CANCER

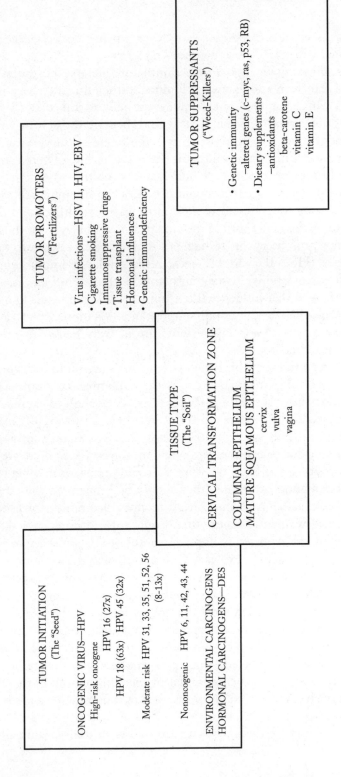

TUMOR INITIATION
(The "Seed")

ONCOGENIC VIRUS—HPV
High-risk oncogene
HPV 16 (27x)
HPV 18 (63x)   HPV 45 (32x)

Moderate risk HPV 31, 33, 35, 51, 52, 56
(8–13x)

Nononcogenic   HPV 6, 11, 42, 43, 44

ENVIRONMENTAL CARCINOGENS
HORMONAL CARCINOGENS—DES

TISSUE TYPE
(The "Soil")

CERVICAL TRANSFORMATION ZONE

COLUMNAR EPITHELIUM
MATURE SQUAMOUS EPITHELIUM
cervix
vulva
vagina

TUMOR PROMOTERS
("Fertilizers")

• Virus infections—HSV II, HIV, EBV
• Cigarette smoking
• Immunosuppressive drugs
• Tissue transplant
• Hormonal influences
• Genetic immunodeficiency

TUMOR SUPPRESSANTS
("Weed-Killers")

• Genetic immunity
  –altered genes (c-myc, ras, p53, RB)
• Dietary supplements
  –antioxidants
      beta-carotene
      vitamin C
      vitamin E

bluegrass seeds and crabgrass seeds. Seventy percent of cervical cancers are associated with HPV-16 as an initiating factor.

The soil, or tissue type, is either immature metaplastic epithelium (the cervical transformation zone), columnar epithelium (the tissue inside the cervical canal), or mature squamous epithelium (the tissue that covers most of the cervix, the vaginal canal, and the outer lips of the vulva). The tissue at greatest risk from the virus is the tissue of the cervical transformation zone. This is the soil that is the most "fertile." There is ten to one hundred times *less* risk of developing cancers on the other tissues. Growing grass on these vaginal and vulvar tissues can be compared to growing grass on your concrete sidewalk or driveway—it's difficult to do, but if there are cracks in the surface the crabgrass may still grow in those cracks.

Tumor promoters (or "fertilizers") include other virus infections such as herpes (HSV II) and HIV, cigarette smoking, immunosuppressive drugs (corticosteroids), tissue transplants, hormonal influences, and some genetic factors that influence tissue immunity. Much less is known about the "weed-killers"—the tumor suppressants. Vitamins, foods, and genes that may act as tumor suppressants are actively being investigated by many researchers today.

The importance of this little simile is to allow you to focus on the fact that a lot of things must go wrong at the same time for a cancer to develop, and that infection with HPV alone is not enough to cause a cancer.

It must also be recognized that cancer related to HPV can occur at other sites in the female genital tissues—the vulva and the vagina—but one hundred times less frequently than on the cervix. If there are growths such as warts or moles on the vulva or in the vagina, or in other areas that are irritated and not healing, they should be brought to the attention of your doctor as soon as possible. It is not uncommon for older, postmenopausal women to ignore these conditions for long periods of time. They should be reported promptly. In addition, the presence of persistent burning or itching of the vulvar skin (outer lips) that does not respond relatively quickly to simple treatments must be carefully checked to be sure that there are not early cancers developing.

As mentioned earlier, most treatments for cervical lesions are simple office treatments that do not require hospitalization or general anesthesia. The abnormality can be destroyed by freezing, electrical or diathermy heating, or by a laser beam, which can vaporize away the abnormal areas. Other treatments may be excisional in that they cut away the abnormal tissue by using a knife, an electrosurgical cutting tool, or a finely focused laser beam.

Cervical cancer treatment currently costs $6 billion annually in the

United States. Several drug companies are already working on vaccines to prevent cervical cancer. Having a vaccine to prevent viral infection in both men and women would save untold suffering in the U.S. In developing countries where cervical cancer is a major cause of cancer deaths, thousands of lives could be saved. In addition, work is under way to develop vaccines to treat the HPV virus once it has already invaded the cervix. Infected cervical cells show abnormal proteins on their surface. Therapeutic vaccines would increase the woman's own immune cells' ability to recognize these proteins and kill cells that have them. Trials are already under way.

Although most of this information may seem complex, these are facts you should be aware of so that if they should involve you, you can explore the information in a more knowledgeable fashion with your health care provider. Or you may simply decide to pass this chapter on to your younger sister, daughter, or mother.

Chapter 13

HYSTERECTOMY—WHEN TO SAY NO, WHEN TO SAY YES

The thinking was: "Why would any normal, sane woman who has finished her family want a uterus anyway?" Competent, conscientious physicians were positive that hysterectomies were a boon to womankind.

And so it followed that until recently, only a small percentage of the hysterectomies proposed by gynecologists were justified. Many women had surgery for uterine fibroids that caused no symptoms, or for bleeding problems that needed medical therapy, not surgery.

Fortunately, the number of hysterectomies decreased and reached 5.8 per 1,000 women in 1992. As women are becoming more knowledgeable about their bodies and more educated, the rates of hysterectomy decrease. My previous books were written to educate women so they could know when hysterectomy surgery was appropriate. I like to think that the books were instrumental in decreasing the rate of hysterectomy in this country.

Definitions

Hysterectomy is a major surgical procedure, and any major surgery carries with it the risk of death from the surgery itself, from anesthesia, or from postoperative complication.

Today, hysterectomy remains one of the most frequently performed operations. *Hysterectomy or total hysterectomy* refers to removal of the entire uterus and sometimes, the attached fallopian tubes as well. The ovaries remain. Less often, a *partial or subtotal hysterectomy* is done. In this procedure, the upper part of the uterus is removed, but the cervix is left intact. *Radical hysterectomies* are done as part of endometrial or cervical cancer surgery. Here the entire uterus, a small portion of the upper vagina, lymph nodes, and supporting ligaments are removed. A *hysterectomy with unilateral or bilateral salpingo-oophorectomy* (complete hysterectomy) refers to the removal of the uterus and one or both ovaries and fallopian tubes (salpingo-oophorectomy).

Nearly 1,700,000 women underwent hysterectomy between 1988 and 1990 according to the National Hospital Discharge Survey. Ovaries were also removed in 37 percent of women under the age of forty-five and in 68 percent of those women over forty-five. Interestingly, the rates of hysterectomy vary from state to state, from the east coast to the west coast, and from north to south. Some of that variance depends on whether there are more gynecologists in a given area, as well as the prevailing local surgical philosophy. We see this variance in medical therapy as well. Women on the West Coast are treated with hormones for menopausal symptoms three times as often as women on the East Coast. I truly doubt that women on the West Coast have three times more hot flashes! Well, women in high hysterectomy-rate areas don't have three times more fibroids and bleeding problems either, but there may be more gynecologic surgeons available, or the doctors may be more aggressive due to local training and philosophy.

After a hysterectomy, your belly might never be the same. While complications of surgery such as fever, infection, and bladder and bowel perforations are not uncommon, most women do not have life-threatening complications. However, even a week or a month post-op, late complications such as adhesions, which cause pain or intestinal obstruction and create other misery, may occur. Unoperated abdomens are generally less troublesome to their owners.

Nonetheless, there are major reasons for having a hysterectomy. Let us be clear about the *indications for hysterectomy, where almost everyone agrees:*

1. Cancer of the uterus, ovaries, or vagina (only rare exceptions)
2. Obstetric hemorrhage, where hysterectomy is done to save the woman's life
3. Cancers or infections of nearby tissues which have spread to involve the uterus
4. Large fibroids, causing symptoms of pressure or *bleeding that cannot be medically controlled*

5. Uterine prolapse, the medical term for a uterus that has dropped from its normal position. Indications here would be complete prolapse, that is, where the entire uterus is protruding outside the vagina. It may be possible to treat lesser degrees of prolapse by other means. (See the urinary incontinence chapter.)

Beyond this list, there is much less agreement on exactly what conditions require hysterectomy. Interestingly, hysterectomy for cancer accounts for only 10 percent of hysterectomies. Now we can begin to discuss the most common *benign* problems that often result in hysterectomy. In descending order, they are uterine fibroids, abnormal uterine bleeding, endometriosis, uterine prolapse, chronic pelvic pain, ovarian masses, urinary stress incontinence, adenomyosis, and last, chronic pelvic infections.

Actually, hysterectomy for *benign* gynecologic problems is not an easy subject. In fact, although it is one of the most common surgeries, there is still much controversy surrounding proper indications for when it is appropriate and when it is better and safer simply to ignore the problem. Here is information to help you make your decision, so that you do not bleed too long and become anemic and need transfusions, or grow fibroids that are too big for newer, easier surgical techniques. On the other hand, you don't want to have surgery for a condition that might go away in time on its own. The remainder of this chapter will try to help you make that choice.

Fibroid Tumors

In my previous book, I wrote:

> Actually, most women are surprised when the doctor says, "Hmmmmm, you have fibroids," during a pelvic examination. "Really? I feel fine, I don't have any symptoms." "Well, don't worry, just come back in three to six months, and I'll check again." And that's all there is to it. You have joined the ranks of those who have a fibroid uterus.

A fibroid is a benign tumor, in fact, the most common benign tumor of the uterus. Fibroids account for one-third of all hysterectomies. Although we still don't understand why they appear, because they rarely appear before the age of puberty or enlarge after menopause, they are probably linked to the hormonal stimulation of estrogen produced in the reproductive years. In fact, they increase in frequency as we get into our forties. So, by the time a woman is in her forties, she has a 25 to 40 percent chance of being the owner of one or more. For some reason, black women have an even higher incidence. Autopsy data show that nearly 50 percent of women have fibroids, most of whom never knew it.

Fibroids, or leiomyomas, are solid, benign growths of tightly compacted muscle and fibrous tissue within the muscular wall of the uterus, enclosed in a capsule that separates them from the surrounding tissue. There are usually several, though they may occur singly. From their site within the muscular wall (*intramural* fibroids) they may expand, pushing muscle aside, either in the direction of the outer surface of the uterus (*subserosal* fibroids) or, more rarely, toward the inner lining of the cavity of the uterus (*submucous* fibroids). Submucous fibroids expanding just beneath the endometrium may be responsible for excessive bleeding during periods, because they distort the lining of the uterus and/or decrease the ability of the uterus to contract during menstruation. Some women have gushes so heavy that they become anemic.

DIFFERENT TYPES OF FIBROIDS

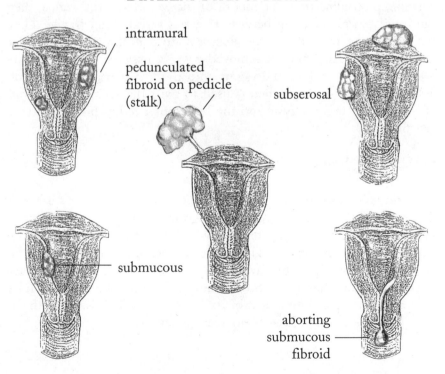

intramural

pedunculated
fibroid on pedicle
(stalk)

subserosal

submucous

aborting
submucous
fibroid

Types of Fibroids

Submucous Fibroids

Fortunately, this placement of fibroids is least common. Even though most women who have fibroids have few symptoms, the uterus does not seem to tolerate submucous fibroids as well as fibroids in other positions. Severe menstrual pain can sometimes result as these fibroids are the object of uterine contractions pushing as if trying to expel them. Furthermore, because of their location, they cannot be felt by the physician. Fortunately, they can be easily spotted by pelvic ultrasound. Remember too that submucous fibroids can cause heavy or gushing-type bleeding but generally do not affect bleeding patterns (bleeding between menses or shortened intervals between menses). Bleeding pattern changes are usually due to hormonal imbalances or, on rarer occasions, to cancer.

Not only do submucous fibroids cause trouble as they sit beneath the lining of the uterus, but also, sometimes, these fibroids assume a stalk and, as the stalk lengthens, creep into the uterine cavity. Then they may poke down through the cervical opening, which opens. In this exposed position, protruding from the mouth of the womb into the vagina, they can cause terrible bleeding because they are vascular and fragile. They can usually be removed in the doctor's office if the stalk is slender enough. Otherwise, they are removed using a hysteroscope, an instrument that is inserted via the vagina into the uterine cavity to provide light. Another instrument then is used to twist the stalk of the fibroid off its base, or it is cut away and the base cauterized to prevent further bleeding.

Subserosal Fibroids

Still other fibroids may start off beneath the outer lining on the surface of the uterus. Some of these continue to grow and project outward until their only connection to the uterus is by a slender stalk that contains the blood supply to the fibroid. These rare fibroids may "float" within the pelvis and be confusing to physicians, who must carefully differentiate them from an ovarian tumor. Sometimes, such a fibroid may twist on its stalk and create pain due to loss of its blood supply and tissue death. In all my years of practice, I have only seen this twice.

Degenerating Fibroids

Other fibroids, even those within the uterine wall, may also degenerate—probably due to an alteration in blood supply. This often occurs in pregnancy, though I have seen a small number of women in their fifties who have had such an episode. The patients complain of pain and uterine contraction. On physical examination, the fibroid is found to have become softer, and tender. Luckily, many of these simply get better on their own, but accurate diagnosis by ultrasound or even MRI is necessary. (See leiomyosarcoma, below.)

Before leaving the subject of fibroids, I need to address one other area. Fibroids rarely enlarge in women on hormone replacement or low-dose birth control pills because the dose of estrogen is so low. Any fibroid that does increase in size while the woman is on hormone replacement should be checked for possible malignant transformation to a leiomyosarcoma (see below).

In general, I give hormone replacement to postmenopausal patients whose fibroids are or have shrunk to approximately ten weeks' size. Nearly all of these patients note that their fibroids continue to shrink. And it follows that in perimenopausal women with fibroids, low-dose 20 mcg birth control pills or birth control pills that contain only progestin may be just the ticket to decrease heavy flow. Here again, the woman should be monitored with ultrasound.

Fibroids must be differentiated from pregnancy, the usual cause of increasing uterine size. They also must be differentiated from adenomyosis (see page 379). On rare occasions they must be differentiated from malignant fibroids called leiomyosarcomas.

Leiomyosarcoma of the Uterus

These are rare malignant tumors that occur in less than 0.5 percent of fibroids. Their incidence is only 0.67 per 100,000 women. They can arise directly from the muscle of the uterine wall, or from an existing fibroid. Those that are confined within the fibroid have the best prognosis. If the sarcoma (cancer) is confined to the uterus, survival is still good in most cases. Either way, continued monitoring postoperatively is necessary to be aware of recurrence. Furthermore, because fibroids are estrogen dependent, premenopausal women with leiomyosarcomas will have their ovaries removed at the time of their hysterectomy and generally will not be able to take hormone replacement therapy.

Leiomyosarcomas may cause pelvic or abdominal pain, pressure on the rectum or bladder, or abnormal bleeding. However, most women have few symptoms. Preoperatively the patient is often assumed to have a fibroid. Suspicion may arise if there has been a rapid increase in size of the "fibroid." However, because malignant change is so rare, chances are greater than *99.5 percent* that your fibroids are benign. And that is why for the most part (unless there is rapid increase in the size of a fibroid, which is often solitary), watching and observing fibroids is worthwhile because most often surgery is not indicated and not necessary.

FIBROID SIZE

That is why it is so important for you to keep track of the size of your uterus. How else will you know if there has been a change? Therefore, don't settle for a doctor's knowing "hmmmmmm" as you are examined. Speak up and ask just how large your uterus is. The measurement should be reported to you in terms of how enlarged your uterus is in relation to a pregnancy. Doctors understand and can compare notes that way. This is important and useful information to a doctor who is seeing you for the first time.

For example, if you can tell him that your uterus contains fibroids and has been enlarged to twelve weeks' size for the past five years, and he then finds your uterus is still twelve weeks' size, that is very reassuring. On the other hand, if your uterus was normal size just six months ago, this could be a significant finding. And because "the size of an orange or grapefruit often varies with the price you pay," get a scientific answer. A twelve-week uterus is just that and can be confirmed on ultrasound.

PRESSURE PROBLEMS

Fibroids may create one other problem, especially if they are large. They may exert pressure on the bowel or the ureters (the tubes that carry urine from the kidneys to the bladder). This pressure can prevent the kidneys from emptying properly. Over time, it is possible to destroy kidney function. Therefore, in women with large fibroids, the ultrasound technician should take the time to check the kidneys for signs of hydronephrosis (swelling), i.e., signs that urine cannot freely flow out from the ureters or kidneys. If this occurs, although it is rare even with large fibroids, it may mean that surgery is necessary in order to preserve kidney function.

ULTRASOUND, THE MOST IMPORTANT EXAM

It is important to remember that the most accurate way of following a fibroid is by ultrasound examination. Serial ultrasounds can tell better than your doctor's fingers whether a fibroid has grown or shrunk since the last visit. Ultrasound should be utilized primarily when your doctor feels there may have been some change or to gauge the extent of the change or, as very often happens, to get a good measurement in a patient who is unable to relax well or who is overweight, making the physical exam difficult. Ultrasound should be used anytime the doctor is unsure, or unable to do an accurate exam of the uterus and ovaries.

In addition, a new technique called a saline infusion sono-hysterogram (SIS) can be easily performed. A small amount of fluid can be instilled into the uterine cavity through a tiny catheter placed through the opening in the mouth of the womb immediately prior to performing the ultrasound examination. The fluid slightly distends the cavity of the uterus so that the walls separate, making it easier to spot submucous fibroids or polyps.

Fibroids normally appear on ultrasound as uniform structures. If they appear to have a cavity, this can occasionally be an ominous sign, as it could mark a rapidly growing tumor with a decaying interior. Or it could be just a simple cyst inside of the fibroid. Such findings, because they are unusual, give an impetus to a surgeon or a patient to consider surgery. On the same note, fibroids that grow *after* a woman is postmenopausal must also be considered abnormal unless she is on unusually high doses of estrogen.

IS SURGERY NEEDED?

Years ago, the thinking was that a woman needed surgery if her uterus increased beyond the size of a sixteen-week pregnancy, because there was simply no way to feel her ovaries because her oversized uterus was in the way. Now, in the age of the transvaginal ultrasound, we can see the ovaries in most cases and may choose to watch and wait. I have watched women with up to twenty-weeks'-sized fibroid uteri, but nearly all of these women have been in their late forties or early fifties and had *no* significant symptoms. Most never needed surgery.

The majority of women with symptomatic fibroids tend to be perimenopausal. As their high levels of estrogen fall at menopause, their fibroids and uterus almost always decrease in size. Therefore, if you are perimenopausal and can hold off, it is likely that menopause will make surgery unnecessary as your fibroids shrink.

GnRH Agonists, or a New Means to Shrink Fibroids

A synthetic peptide known by trade names as Lupron® (which is injectable), Synarel® (a nasal inhaler), or Zoladex® (a subcutaneous implant) induces a postmenopausal low-estrogen state by turning off pituitary drive to the ovary. The resulting lack of estrogen tends to shrink the size of fibroids, resulting in a 30 to 50 percent loss of volume. Side effects include loss of menses (which may be good), hot flashes, and vaginal dryness. Bone loss will occur if the drug is continued for more than two to six months.

It is important to understand that a thirty-six-year-old woman with a fourteen-weeks'-sized uterus is very different from a forty-nine-year-old with a fourteen-weeks'-sized uterus. The forty-nine-year-old will probably go into menopause in a year or two and her fibroids will shrink spontaneously. The thirty-six-year-old has years to go before menopause. Until then, it is likely that her fibroids will continue to grow and create problems. On the other hand, if there are no symptoms, the wait can be easy. She may only have to put up with a rounded lower abdomen. I might consider giving each of these women a GnRH agonist, if either had a major complaint, but for different reasons.

For the younger woman: By shrinking the size of fibroids, these medications make surgery easier, and give additional surgical options such as a laparoscopic or vaginal approach rather than open laparotomy. These approaches mean less blood loss, smaller incisions, less time in the hospital, less suffering, earlier recovery, and in the long run they save dollars.

GnRH agonists improve anemia by stopping menses. Prior to the time of surgery, this has several advantages. It decreases the need for transfusion, lets the patient build up her own blood, and enables surgery to be scheduled when the patient is no longer anemic and is in better health. At the time of surgery it decreases blood loss. These medications are commonly used for three months prior to hysterectomy or myomectomy (removal of fibroids) surgery.

For the older woman: Because of their action, a GnRH agonist might just be the ticket to provide a few months' reprieve that will take a fibroid-troubled forty-nine- or fifty-year-old woman into her menopause. This may provide an option, other than surgery for bleeding or other problems that develop just prior to menopause.

For special cases where a woman is doing well on a GnRH agonist and it seems that prolonged therapy would be beneficial, "add-back" therapy can be done. This simply means adding replacement doses of estrogen or estrogen and progesterone-like medication while keeping the woman on the GnRH agonist. This technique is usually done to avoid the development of osteoporosis.

No Free Lunch: Postponing Surgery

But as your mother taught you, "There is no free lunch." Making the decision to wait is not always as easy as it seems. No one can guarantee that everything will be all right if you wait. Surgeons imply that if you have your hysterectomy now, you won't have to worry anymore. If you choose to wait, some doctors or even family members will surely make you feel uncomfortable with your decision. Also, you have to continue to have close follow-up with physical and ultrasound exams. Sometimes, CT scans or MRI may be needed. Final decisions most often rest with how much nuisance the fibroids are causing in terms of bleeding, pressure symptoms, their rate of growth, or suspicions of malignant change. For some women, emotional aspects regarding the loss of their reproductive organs are the most important deterrent. The bottom line is, unless you have major problems such as severe anemia from uncontrollable hemorrhage, hydronephrosis from large fibroids, etc., you must remember the important truth that *surgery is always available, if and when other measures fail.*

I would not be honest if I did not add that among those women who suffer from fibroids, many say postoperatively that having their hysterectomy was the best decision they ever made. They are no longer anemic, no longer afraid to go out of the house on the first days of their menses, no longer troubled by having to urinate every hour, and newly able to get into slim skirts; these are definite lifestyle advantages that should not be forgotten. I should also add here that if these women plan to take hormone replacement in the future, they will not have to worry about monthly periods, unexpected bleeding, or progesterone-type side effects.

The only women in my practice who have been genuinely unhappy and regretted their hysterectomies have been women who felt they were pressured into the decision. They felt that the surgery was done without good reason—that their hysterectomy really didn't have to be done. On the other hand, women who participated in the decision making and were knowledgeable and understood their options were, to a woman, satisfied—indeed happy—with their results. In cancer cases, where decisions are black and white, surgical decisions are usually obvious. In most cases, however, gray areas having to do with fibroids and bleeding problems predominate. Happily, for some women, major surgery can now be performed in much less traumatic ways. These newer surgical techniques will be discussed next.

Myomectomy

Myomectomy means removal of the fibroids while leaving the uterus intact. The solitary floating fibroid on a long stalk is obviously the easiest to remove, and this can frequently be done through the laparoscope. However, occasionally, the stalk is thick or located near the fallopian tubes or large blood vessels. In such cases, there may be advantages to open surgery. Often this type of fibroid does not have to be removed at all.

Otherwise, in my opinion, removing fibroids should be reserved for women who would like to preserve their childbearing capability, or who insist on preserving their uterus. Even in these women, there should preferably be one or just a few fibroids and they should be fairly easily accessible.

It is important to realize that *nearly 25 percent of women undergoing myomectomy will need a second operation, to remove new fibroids, or to remove the entire uterus.* Postmyomectomy, patients with many fibroids are left with a uterus that may not function well. Those who do become pregnant often need a cesarean section if scars are extensive, otherwise rupture of the uterus during labor and delivery is possible. Women may be advised to wait a few months after myomectomy before trying to become pregnant.

Myomectomy surgery takes longer, is more difficult to perform, results in more blood loss, and is more dangerous than ordinary hysterectomy. Two of my patients having the procedure done by gynecologists in New York City wound up needing over ten units of blood each. Whether it was bad luck or bad surgery, I don't know. For the most part, myomectomy surgery results in more postoperative pain and complications. Worse, new fibroids or fibroids that were not removed may grow, only to enlarge the uterus again.

My patients who require myomectomy in order to become pregnant are generally referred to gynecologists who specialize in infertility. These doctors are best able to counsel and predict the patient's odds for getting pregnant and carrying the pregnancy and whether or not the surgery would really be beneficial in the long run. Furthermore, they may be more likely to be better educated in hysteroscopic techniques for eliminating bothersome submucous fibroids embedded just under the inner surface of the uterine cavity. These are cut away in a fashion that is something like peeling an onion, layer by layer, away from the muscular uterine wall where it is embedded. (See hysteroscopy, page 382.)

Ovaries: In or Out?

This question almost always arises when a hysterectomy is suggested. Unless there is a malignancy present, where the ovaries are removed to keep the tumor from spreading, you should have major input in this decision. There are no specific age guidelines for keeping or removing ovaries, but most doctors agree that if you are postmenopausal, ovaries should be removed.

The other important consideration is whether or not you have a family history of ovarian cancer. If you have two first-degree relatives (a mother, sister, or daughter) or one first-degree relative along with a second-degree relative (such as a grandmother, for example) with ovarian cancer you may be at increased risk, especially if that cancer occurred when they were less than thirty-five years of age. We are all now familiar with Gilda Radner's sad story and the fact that ovarian cancer may run in families. That information must be shared with your doctor and, if appropriate, with a geneticist. It is now possible to test for genetic problems. The results of testing may alter your choice, so family history is important to consider when making your decision. If you turn out to have the BRCA1 or BRCA2 gene, you may want to consider having both ovaries removed after you have completed your childbearing or at the age of thirty-five. (See page 322 in ovarian cancer chapter for longer explanation.)

Actually, the risk of developing ovarian cancer will be no higher than for a woman who has not had her uterus removed, but it is important that you remember that the threat of ovarian cancer increases each year as we age. Statistics predict that we could prevent three thousand deaths from ovarian cancer a year by doing prophylactic oophorectomies (removing ovaries prophylactically) at the time of hysterectomy. So, to some, it often seems foolish to leave a potential problem, when uterine surgery is necessary anyway, and ovarian function is over, or nearly over. Yes, it is true that ovaries secrete some reduced levels of male hormone for as long as five years after menopause, but this may not be reason to keep a potential source of problems.

Furthermore, because about one-third of the blood supply to the ovaries comes from the uterine artery, which is severed at the time of hysterectomy, this decrease in blood flow to the ovary may predispose it to cyst formation or early ovarian failure. Though benign, ovarian cysts can be the source of worry and sometimes result in a second surgical procedure. And because of adhesions from the first surgery, second surgeries may be more difficult and dangerous.

If you are forty-seven or older, are having symptoms of perimenopause, and are scheduled to have a hysterectomy, I would most often advise ovarian removal. Even at forty-six? A lot depends on my patient's emotions around the issue. Family history (i.e., when your mother or older sister went into menopause) and how regular menstruation has been for the past few months can be helpful when trying to calculate just how much longer normal ovarian function might last. In addition, blood tests for FSH and estradiol can be obtained on day 3 of menses as an elevated FSH often portends that menopause will occur soon. (See page 18 in the perimenopause chapter.)

Generally, younger ovaries have more years left to contribute female and male hormones. Removing both ovaries before the onset of menopause will immediately bring on menopause. This will increase the risk of heart attack, stroke, osteoporosis, etc., unless you begin hormone replacement. Removing your ovaries prior to menopause will often mean that you will need to begin estrogen replacement with pills or a skin patch. You may even be tempted to add back a small amount of testosterone. That's all a small bother. But you'll probably be on hormones sooner or later, so in many cases, it may just mean that you've started earlier by a year or so. However, if you are in your thirties or early forties, it would almost always be best to try to keep your ovaries.

On the other hand, if ovaries are left intact, it means that you must return to your doctor on a yearly basis to have your ovaries checked to make sure that they are normal. Physical examination, with or without ultrasound, should suffice. Besides, you should be seeing your physician at regular intervals anyway.

For the woman in her perimenopause facing hysterectomy, I would like to add once again that because the blood supply to the ovaries is thought to be compromised as a result of surgery, ovarian function may end sooner than it would have if no surgery had been done. The second point is that the perimenopausal ovary is in a descending spiral of function with extreme fluctuations in estrogen production. Estrogen levels can be extremely high, especially if ovarian cyst formation occurs. Many of these cysts occur during the perimenopause as the result of abnormal follicle development. I am somewhat concerned that these high levels of estrogen that are unopposed by progesterone may have adverse effects on breast tissue.

Dysfunctional Uterine Bleeding (DUB)

DUB is abnormal bleeding from the uterus that is not associated with a tumor, inflammation, or pregnancy. It refers to any abnormal bleeding for which no organic cause can be found. Eighty-five to 90 percent of such cases are due to lack of ovulation. In the remainder, ovulation has occurred, but the life span of the corpus luteum may be either shortened or prolonged, or other problems might exist.

Doctors use several medical terms to describe the many different bleeding patterns that occur. You may see them written on your insurance forms and should know what they mean:

Menorrhagia: Normal cycle, but with flow that is excessive in amount or duration.

Menometrorrhagia: Prolonged uterine bleeding occurring at completely irregular intervals.

Polymenorrhea: Normal flow with cycles occurring at less than 21-day intervals (from first day of flow to first day of flow).

Metrorrhagia: Excessive flow that is acyclic, i.e., occurs at irregular but frequent intervals.

Other common problems include light bleeding or spotting prior to menses in a normal ovulatory cycle, or bleeding that occurs in midcycle with ovulation. Women who have spotting with ovulation generally have had this pattern for most of their lives. The spotting is caused by a slight fall in the estrogen level that occurs with ovulation. Some patients, however, may think that they are having a period every two weeks, especially if there is bleeding at midcycle, rather than spotting. Reassurance is the only required therapy. Sometimes this bleeding can provide a convenient way to determine the time of ovulation for conception or contraception. Some women also have pain associated with ovulation. This is known as mittelschmerz. It is caused by the egg popping out of its follicle accompanied by follicular fluid and tiny amounts of blood that spills upon and irritates the abdominal lining.

Similarly, women with light premenstrual spotting generally have always had this pattern. Some, however, may develop it when they reach a certain age and then the pattern will persist for years. After ruling out other problems, I tell such patients that their menstrual pattern has simply "changed" and not to worry.

On the other hand, if you have abnormal bleeding and wind up with a biopsy, it is really important that you understand the pathology report. If you receive anything other than a normal report, you will want to know just how much you need to worry. In most cases, after reading, you will realize that it's not very much. First, it's important to quickly review the basic monthly cycle of the endometrium.

THE NORMAL MENSTRUAL CYCLE

Estrogen stimulates the activities that occur in the first half of the monthly cycle, when the cells of the uterine lining increase in number and glands begin to grow. This is known as the *proliferative phase* of the monthly cycle.

Ovulation occurs at midmonth (approximately) and triggers the second or secretory phase of the cycle. Ovulation cues the ovaries to create a "corpus luteum," which secretes a second female hormone, progesterone, and this phase of the cycle continues under the control of both estrogen and progesterone. The uterine lining now prepares for the possible implantation of a fertilized egg; glands increase in number and secrete sugar-containing substances to nourish the implanting egg. Since this part of the cycle is triggered by ovulation, *production of progesterone occurs only when ovulation has occurred.* If the egg is not fertilized, estrogen and progesterone levels rapidly fall, and the superficial portion of the endometrium disintegrates. The cells and blood that composed the lining become the bloody discharge of the menstrual period. Bleeding stops as platelets form plugs in vessels and release substances that constrict the tiny blood vessels. Only the innermost or basal layer of the endometrium does not slough. It remains and forms the base for the growth of the new lining each month.

If you are having irregular periods that are increasingly heavy it may be necessary to have a biopsy. If it is at all possible, your in-office biopsy should be scheduled late in the cycle when you are premenstrual. In that way, more endometrial tissue is present and it can be determined whether or not you have ovulated. If proliferative endometrium persists at the end of the cycle (rather than a secretory lining), then you have not ovulated (see chapter 1). For women with infertility, it is also possible to tell when ovulation occurred and whether or not the second half of the cycle is normal. On the other hand, there are rarer cases where the woman is ovulating but still has DUB. This can be due to a corpus luteum that lasts too long or, more commonly, that quits too quickly. Short luteal phases result in more frequent bleeding, whereas long luteal phases can delay menses by a week to months.

TREATMENT OF DUB—STOP THE BLEEDING FIRST

After documenting that there isn't an anatomic cause for the bleeding, and in some cases, after doing a biopsy, a progesterone-type drug is usually given to stop the bleeding. To do this, 10 to 30 mg of MPA or 5 to 15 mg of norethindrone acetate (Aygestin®) may be prescribed immediately and then should be taken daily until the flow stops. Then, if the initial dose was high, the dose is decreased slowly. This lower dose is then maintained until the woman's next menses is due or for 21 to 25 days or more. At that point, the medication is stopped and the patient has her menses.

NORMALIZING BLEEDING PATTERNS IN WOMEN WITH ABNORMAL BLEEDING

To re-create or reestablish her former 28-day cycle, she will wait 18 days after her last pill, then take her PLM for 10 days. She should continue her schedule of "18 days off, 10 days on." With time, this schedule sets up almost an exact 28-day cycle. And it works! Other doctors may choose 12 to 14 days on PLM and fewer days off, depending on the woman's diagnosis. Still others simply tell their patients to use a progestational agent for the last 10 to 12 days of their predicted cycle, after which they should expect their menses.

In more stubborn cases, when women are bleeding very heavily or cannot tolerate the side effects of MPA, I have found that norethindrone acetate (Aygestin®) works better. It is less often used because it has slightly more adverse effects on lipids than MPA depending on relative doses. However, it stops bleeding faster. And although it is more potent in its ability to stop bleeding, it has milder side effects (less bloating and less mood changes) than MPA. This medication comes in 5 mg tablets. In a woman with heavy bleeding that needs to be stopped, 15 mg is given immediately. Most women will note a decrease in bleeding, or no bleeding within 24 hours. I then instruct her to continue reducing the dose by one-half to one tablet after each 48 to 72 hours where no bleeding has occurred. Then, when she is on only one tablet, she continues this dose for 20-plus days. In a case where bleeding has been heavy, and the woman anemic, I like to extend this time to give her more time to recover from her blood loss and build up her own iron stores. After her next period, she may continue cycling with 10 to 12 days per month of 2.5 or 5 mg of norethindrone acetate, as long as seems prudent. She can continue for 3 to 6 months, then be taken off and observed, or depending on circumstances, this regimen can be continued up to the time of menopause.

How will you know when you are menopausal? Simply: If after three cycles of MPA or norethindrone acetate, there is no flow after discontinuing the drug, then you are probably menopausal. The lack of flow indicates that you are not producing sufficient estrogen to build an endometrial lining. Therefore, when you go off the MPA or norethindrone acetate, there is no lining to slough, and therefore, no menstruation.

Another way to treat DUB is with low-dose birth control pills. Oral contraceptives contain doses of estrogen and progesterone-like medication that are large enough to override the body's own hormonal system. They provide a balanced hormonal influence on the endometrium and bleeding stops. Young women with irregular or heavy menses are frequently offered birth control pills first, often without a full work-up, because younger women are less likely to have polyps, cancer, or other serious problems. Perimenopausal women should have a work-up to rule out organic causes of abnormal bleeding. If no abnormalities are found, then low-dose birth control pills can be prescribed if the woman is not a smoker and has no other contraindications.

One more important point: If bleeding patterns do not become normal on progesterone-type medication or birth control pills, a pelvic sonogram or hysteroscopy must be done. *Failure to revert to normal bleeding patterns after two to three months of treatment means that a diagnosis was missed, that there is an anatomic abnormality such as a submucous fibroid or polyp, cancer, etc., and that the bleeding is not due to DUB.*

Therefore, if there is any question, a pelvic sonogram will easily rule out ovarian cysts and other culprits. On the other hand, younger women are more likely to be bleeding from complications of pregnancy, a missed spontaneous abortion, ectopic pregnancy, a copper-containing IUD, or von Willebrand's type of coagulation disorder. (However, women with coagulation defects often have giveaway clues such as a history of bruising, bleeding gums, or nosebleeds.)

Further investigation may even prove that the cause is thyroid disease, submucous fibroids, endometrial polyps, or other pathology. Only after pathology and pregnancy have been ruled out can you assume that the bleeding is caused by hormonal imbalance.

As you can see, *DUB is not a specific diagnosis. It is the term used to denote abnormal bleeding patterns after anatomic causes of bleeding have been ruled out.* This is especially important in the perimenopausal woman, for one-third of all adenocarcinomas (uterine cancers) occur in this age group. For perimenopausal women, a full workup, endometrial biopsy, and ultrasound should be done before a diagnosis of DUB is given. Having ruled out all organic causes, your physician can feel free to treat you with progesterone-like medication or birth control pills.

"Precancerous Conditions": Are They Just Another Excuse for Hysterectomy?

In both of my previous books I described what is seen under the microscope when the normal endometrial lining of the uterus progresses through increasingly abnormal stages to endometrial cancer. There has been a change in the pathological terms recently. If you are having abnormal bleeding and have had a biopsy, it is important to read the following section. You need to understand the terms that appear on your biopsy report so that you can assess, along with your physician, the need for medical or surgical therapy or, if you are on hormone replacement, the need to alter, or stop, your hormone therapy. If you are not having problems, skip this section and go on to page 376, where the chapter continues.

UNDERSTANDING YOUR ENDOMETRIAL BIOPSY REPORT

Much of the following material is taken from Drs. Robert J. Kurman and Henry J. Norris in *Surgical Pathology* as well as my original chapters:[1]

Hyperplasia, Simple or Complex

Overgrowth of cells of the lining of the uterus is called hyperplasia. *Simple or complex hyperplasia is an innocuous response to unopposed estrogen stimulation, and by itself is not an early form of endometrial cancer.*

This abnormality occurs when ovulation does not occur for several months or when a woman on hormone therapy forgets several months of her progesterone-type pills. Cells and glands accumulate and begin to look slightly crowded under the microscope; however, *the cells themselves appear to be normal.* Complex hyperplasia occurs when there is longer unopposed or uninterrupted estrogen stimulation. Cells and glandular structures, although normal in appearance, are more crowded.

Atypical Hyperplasia, Simple or Complex

This condition shows cells that have great variation, from normal cells to cells that initially appear bizarre or cancerous. There are fewer characteristics that are usually associated with estrogen activity. Individual cells divide faster and are less well differentiated. A study by the above authors showed that of 170 women with simple atypical hyperplasia, 8 percent progressed to cancer while 29 percent of those with complex atypical hyperplasia progressed to cancer, because both glandular crowding as well as cellular abnormality are present.

Let us now try to see what difference age makes with the same diagnosis, according to Kurman and Norris:

Women in Reproductive Ages (Forty and Younger)

Simple or complex hyperplasia: Most women who are forty or younger and have short-term hormonal disorders are at low risk for developing endometrial cancer. In this age group, simple or even complex hyperplasia can almost always be treated with progesterone-type medication. Surgery, other than in-office endometrial biopsy, can almost always be avoided unless the woman has persistent bleeding or happens to be in a high-risk group because of obesity, or has problems such as polycystic ovarian disease (a condition where ovulation rarely occurs) or a positive family history of uterine, breast, or colon cancer. Women with this type of endometrial hyperplasia who are not treated may progress to a diagnosis of cancer, but the process takes approximately *ten years.* Therefore, there is a long time to detect, think about, and treat the condition. Furthermore, the *process must go through atyp-*

ical hyperplasia before actual cancer develops. Simple or complex hyper-plasia *without atypia* (atypical hyperplasia) can easily be treated with progesterone-type preparations and is not a reason to rush into hys-terectomy.

Atypical hyperplasia: Should atypia be present in this young age group, better intrauterine sampling of tissue should be done with an in-hospital D&C (dilation and curettage) or a Vabra aspiration. (The Vabra is a more thorough office procedure biopsy method than simple "Pipelle" suction method.) Women who desire a child must immedi-ately attempt to become pregnant after PLM reverts the lining to nor-mal. If pregnancy ensues, the high progesterone levels of pregnancy itself will be beneficial. Then, after delivery, close scrutiny must begin again. These patients must understand and be willing to be closely fol-lowed for any recurrence of the hyperplasia. Most elect to have a hys-terectomy after delivery. On average, it takes *four years* to progress from atypical hyperplasia to obvious endometrial cancer.

Perimenopausal Women (Forty to Fifty-five Years Old):

Simple or complex hyperplasia: Most women in this age group have problems stemming from anovulation, similar to the younger women in the paragraphs above. These women are at low risk for developing cancer. In hyperplasias without atypia, women without risk factors are treated with progesterone-type therapy and followed with office biop-sy until the endometrium has returned to normal. They then can be monitored with transvaginal ultrasound but usually biopsy is also indi-cated.

Atypical hyperplasia: With atypical hyperplasia, there is increased likelihood that a cancer may have been missed, even on D&C. Even so, 60 percent of cases go away *without* therapy; however, close follow-up (every three months) must be done. If the abnormality persists or worsens, although there is less danger generally than in older women, hysterectomy may have to be done.

It is essential that you and your doctor understand that even after the endometrium has reverted back to a normal secretory endometrium after you've taken a progesterone-like medication, the same underlying hor-monal problem that brought on the hyperplasia will generally not go away and still exists. *When the progesterone-like medication is discontinued, in most cases, the abnormal process will begin again* unless regular ovulation resumes because (1) a medical problem that has been corrected, for example, hypothyroidism; (2) a major mental trauma that has now been overcome, or (3) menopause, which has occurred.

The biggest mistake I see is that doctors stop progesterone-like medications after reversion to a normal biopsy. They seem to forget that these perimenopausal women will rarely ovulate and produce progesterone again on a regular basis. These women should therefore continue their progesterone-like pills for ten to fourteen days each month until they become menopausal! (Or they may try an every-other-month or an every-third-month regimen, *depending on the seriousness of their original pathological diagnosis.*)

Other doctors may offer low-dose oral contraceptives to nonsmokers, once the abnormality has reverted to normal. A progesterone-containing IUD called the Progestasert® is another option for women who do not want to take oral progestins; however, it must be changed once a year. (A new progesterone-type IUD that lasts for several years will be available soon.) While finely milled natural progesterone, i.e. micronized progesterone, is a more "natural" alternative, there is no study that shows that it is effective in these circumstances, and therefore it should *not* be used.

Some women cannot tolerate progesterone-type medications. Sometimes too, bleeding can be heavy, sudden, and force the surgical choice. If a woman elects to keep her uterus, she will need to be closely watched for years by in-office biopsies and/or transvaginal ultrasound. Some women find this unnerving. Therefore, therapy must be individualized for each woman.

Postmenopausal Women (over Fifty-five Years Old)

Postmenopausal women who have abnormal bleeding have an increased risk of having uterine cancer and/or its precursor, atypical hyperplasia. Therefore, they need immediate evaluation. The older they are, and the farther they are from menopause, the more urgent the situation. A transvaginal ultrasound to rule out uterine as well as ovarian abnormalities can be done first and followed by an in-office biopsy or D&C.

If there is no atypia, these women can be given MPA or other progesterone-type medication for fourteen days out of each month and then undergo additional biopsies to *ensure that the abnormal lining has reverted to normal.* In these women, their source of estrogen may be due to obesity and the increased conversion of androstenedione to estrone that occurs in their peripheral fat (see chapters 1 and 2). Transvaginal ultrasound can be used for later follow-up as several studies have shown that if the lining of the uterus measures less than five (some say four) millimeters in thickness (in women not on hormone replacement), there is little chance that a cancer exists. However, if there are *any* doubts, biopsy should be done.

For postmenopausal women with atypical hyperplasia who are on estrogen therapy without progesterone-like medication, just stopping the estrogen will usually result in a reversal of the process, although it would seem wise to cycle such a woman on MPA or other progesterone-like medication until withdrawal bleeding stops and a normal biopsy is obtained. (Menopausal therapy using properly balanced estrogen and progesterone does *not* increase the risk of uterine cancer.)

For women who are postmenopausal and have a diagnosis of atypical hyperplasia, hysterectomy is the treatment of choice. For those women who are poor surgical risks because of coexisting medical problems, Megace® (megestrol acetate), a long-acting progesterone-type medication, can be used to avoid surgery in the majority of patients.

One additional point: Atypical hyperplasia is a premalignant lesion that can be very confusing for the pathologist. If he is not very experienced in reviewing such slides, he may overread (overreact) and call the condition adenocarcinoma (cancer), or underread and not cause the gynecologist enough concern. It is a good idea to *have the pathology reviewed by an expert in all cases labeled atypical hyperplasia.*

Remember: All of the hyperplasias above must be followed up until the endometrium reverts back to normal or hysterectomy is done.

After trudging through all of the above, as you see, there are a great many opportunities to detect, treat, and most often reverse these conditions. Furthermore, as I have often said, uterine cancer does not just sneak up one day and bite you. The warning signs are usually there for a long time, and tissue is easily sampled. Your major responsibility then is simply to pay attention to your body, see your physician regularly, and report any unusual bleeding patterns. Remember too that there are always exceptions. Older women who have a closed cervix due to changes with aging may have uterine cancer and never bleed. The bottom line is to see your doctor for regular visits!

The following are, then, additional generally agreed upon indications for hysterectomy:

1. Complex hyperplasia that recurs after treatment
2. Atypical hyperplasia in postmenopausal women
3. Atypical hyperplasia in perimenopausal women

4. Certain cases of bleeding from blood-clotting abnormalities or leukemias—when medical or hormonal therapies fail

Endometrial Cancer

Endometrial cancer is now the third most common type of cancer in women, usually striking at age fifty to sixty. The incidence is 25 per 100,000 per year in women of all age groups but rises from age thirty-five on, reaching 75 per 100,000 by age fifty and increasing to a peak of 125 per 100,000 at age seventy-five. Because the proportion of women over forty-five is increasing in the United States, we are seeing an increasing number of cases.

Since a major cause of hyperplasias is prolonged unopposed continuous estrogen stimulation without the modifying effect of progesterone, conditions associated with continuous estrogen states such as polycystic ovary syndrome, estrogen-secreting ovarian tumors, chronic lack of ovulation, and infertility are risk factors. Hormone replacement therapy without progesterone is a well-known problem. However, age is still the prime risk factor. Obesity can also be added to this list, for women who are 30 percent overweight double their chances of getting endometrial cancer. Diabetic women, hypertensive women, and women with a family history of endometrial, breast, or ovarian cancer may also be at increased risk.

Although endometrial cancer is seen in a greater number of women than either ovarian or cervical cancer, it has a lower death rate. This is primarily because it has early warning signals.

The most common early sign of endometrial cancer is unexplained bleeding. Approximately 80 percent of patients with uterine cancer have this experience. Premenopausal women with endometrial cancer often have unusually heavy flow during their menses or have abnormal bleeding patterns with breakthrough bleeds occurring anytime in their menstrual cycle. In postmenopausal women, bleeding may occur in the guise of light spotting, a pink discharge, or a return of "menses." As a general rule, the farther past menopause the patient is, the more likely it is that her bleeding spells endometrial cancer. The rule is simply that *any bleeding that occurs more than one year after the last menstrual period is cancer until proven otherwise.* Also, women who have been on hormone replacement without monthly bleeds for years who suddenly have vaginal bleeding also must be proven not to have cancer. Of course, there are other reasons a woman might bleed postmenopausally, including endometrial hyperplasias, polyps, ovarian or vaginal tumors, atrophic vaginitis, or even an unexpected pregnancy. The woman who still has regular monthly bleeding and is older than fifty-four or fifty-five may also be at higher risk for this cancer.

Prognosis of this cancer depends upon the grade of the tumor (how abnormal the individual cells look), how far the tumor has invaded into the muscular wall of the uterus, and whether or not the cancer has remained confined within the uterus, or spread to other parts of the pelvis or via the lymphatics or blood vessels to more distant sites of the body.

If the tumor is confined to the innermost layers of the uterine wall, surgery may be curative and no further therapy may be necessary. If there is extension of the cancer more than half of the way into the uterine wall, or down the endocervical canal, or if the cancer has spread outside the uterus, then radiation therapy and/or chemotherapy will probably be offered to the patient. The good news is that 75 percent of cases are found early, while they are still confined to the uterus. This is, of course, because uterine cancer usually causes bleeding, and that early warning sign brings most women to their physician while their disease is still in a curable stage.

A detailed discussion regarding therapy of this cancer is beyond the scope of this book. In cases when a malignant diagnosis is anticipated, it is ideal to have the surgery done by a gynecologic oncologist. These physicians specialize in gynecologic cancer surgery, and are aware of all the latest surgical procedures that can give a patient the best possible outcome. They will remove the uterus and ovaries. They will then look and feel for any enlarged lymph nodes. Because the tumor grade (how abnormal the cells look) and the depth of invasion of the tumor into the muscular wall of the uterus correlate with prognosis and metastasis, a frozen section is done during the time of surgery. A frozen section is a process wherein a small slice of tissue is frozen and looked at under the microscope. This occurs during surgery so that the result will guide the extent of the remainder of the surgery and give the patient the best outcome.

If on frozen section there is less than fifty percent invasion into the uterine muscle and the tumor is grade I, nodes will generally not be removed unless they are enlarged. When there is fifty percent or deeper invasion of the tumor into the uterus, or the tumor is grade II or III, nodes will be automatically removed. In addition, the entire abdominal cavity and surface of the liver, colon, and intestine will be carefully observed for any signs of spread. If needed, these surgeons have the skills to go ahead and debulk large tumors, and resect diseased intestine. In many hospitals, an ob/gyn will start the surgery, but have a gyn-oncologist stand by, in case a cancer is present. If that happens, the specialist takes over and completes the surgery along with the ob/gyn.

See your doctor early, relieve your mind: Some cases that seem to portend disaster may turn out to have a pleasant ending. One of my patients in her early seventies stated that she'd had a tiny amount of bleeding the previous day. I gave her an immediate appointment, and then I examined the napkin she had wisely saved. I tested the reddish-pink stains on the napkin with my office kit and found they indeed were positive for blood. Examining her vaginal canal and urethral orifice as well as doing a rectal and checking for blood, I could find no clinical or chemical evidence that there was any blood present. Taking a second look, I noted a small swelling of her right labia and the telltale red dot. Her bleeding had obviously come from a cyst that ruptured and bled and was now nearly invisible. Happy patient, happy doctor, happy ending.

It is important to realize that seeing your doctor as soon as possible may not only lead to early diagnosis, but may also turn up an unexpected anxiety-relieving result that can prevent days, weeks, even months of worry.

More Reasons for Hysterectomy

ENDOMETRIOSIS

Endometriosis is a disorder where the cells of the endometrial lining flow out of the uterus via the fallopian tubes during menstruation. This has actually been seen during surgical operations and is thought to be the way these cells and tiny amounts of endometrial tissue make their way into the pelvis and implant themselves onto the ovaries, lining of the pelvis, bowel, etc. Then, because the endometrial implants continue to function, they actually cycle as the ovarian hormones wax and wane, breaking down and bleeding. Implants on the ovary can grow, bleed, and result in large "chocolate cysts." (The name comes from their brown color and is due to the presence of old blood.) Adhesions can also form and cause minimal or dense matting of one organ to another, causing pain. Some women suffer from severe menstrual pain. Other women have pain with intercourse. This occurs especially with deep penetration and may last several hours afterward. Rarely, endometrial tissue can spread to remote sites in the body, such as the lung. It is thought that this spread is through lymph channels or blood vessels.

Endometriosis is one of the most common problems women experience. It occurs in approximately 10 percent of all women, and in 30 to 50 percent of infertile women. Therapy for this condition depends mostly on a patient's symptoms, age, and desire for pregnancy. In women past their childbearing years who have marked pelvic pain, complete hysterectomy is often done. For younger women wishing to preserve their pelvic organs, laparoscopic destruction using laser techniques is possible in many cases. GnRH agonists or danazol are often prescribed for three to six months preoperatively to decrease the size of the implants. Low-dose oral contraceptives or high-dose progesterone-type therapy are other popular alternatives.

Adenomyosis

Adenomyosis is defined as infiltration of the uterine wall by endometrial glands. It is usually seen in women over the age of forty who have given birth to more than one child. Generally, the uterus becomes rounded into a globular shape and enlarges. Women often complain of menstrual pain that starts with the first day of flow and ends with the last. They also may suffer from heavy flow.

Until recently, this diagnosis was usually made after hysterectomy when the uterus was opened. Now transvaginal ultrasound can often tip us off that there are endometrial-like structures within the muscular wall. MRI is even more reliable but, as you are well aware, very expensive. As many women who actually have this problem have no complaint, it is hard to know just when it is a correct indication for surgery. This abnormality may run in families. So, if your mother or sister had a hysterectomy, you may wish to obtain and check their pathology report.

Atrophic Endometrium

For reasons not well understood, an atrophic endometrium remains thin, cannot regenerate, and often tends to bleed simply because of fragile, leaky blood vessels. This type of lining seems to have lost its ability to regrow. It can be a reason for hysterectomy.

CHRONIC PELVIC PAIN (WITHOUT OBVIOUS CAUSE)

Women with noncyclic pain that lasts for more than six months may decide to have a hysterectomy. Such cases make up about 10 percent of the benign indications for surgery. There seems to be little agreement as to whether or not the surgery is beneficial. Some studies show that pain persists even *after* surgery in nearly a quarter of these women. Therefore, a very careful workup should be done prior to any surgery.

It is very difficult for a woman to distinguish whether pelvic or abdominal discomfort is coming from a gynecologic problem or inflamed intestines or bladder problems. Therefore, a gastroenterologist and urologist should also be consulted. An orthopedist should also be seen to rule out back problems that might cause pain to be referred to the pelvic area. In other cases chronic pelvic pain stems from previous physical or psychological trauma such as sexual abuse or undiagnosed depression. For these reasons, a psychiatric consult may also be a good idea. Sometimes, drugs such as amitriptyline can be used with almost miraculous pain relief. This drug, originally used in the treatment of depression, has recently been found to interrupt pain neurotransmitters. It also helps patients get to sleep and sleep well, which also helps to alleviate pain. It is a shame to go through a major surgical procedure only to have pain continue to persist, or have a new complaint take its place. So, remember to do all of your homework first.

Techniques for Diagnosing Endometrial Abnormalities

THE D&C

For the most part, in-office procedures are preferable. However, some women require in-hospital D&Cs. In some women who are past menopause or who have never given birth vaginally, the cervical opening may be very small and too tight to allow even a tiny instrument to pass through. Using an instrument to open and widen the cervical canal is painful, so for these women, a Pipelle or Vabra office procedure is not possible and a D&C is usually necessary. Most often the procedure is done in an outpatient setting, except when there are medical concerns or malignancy or major hemorrhage is present.

General anesthesia or regional-type anesthesia (which numbs the body below the waistline) can be given or a local anesthetic can be injected into the cervix. If a local injection is used, usually it is given in conjunction with intravenous sedation or medication for pain.

The next step is to dilate the cervical canal. The cervix is dilated by passing a sound (a smooth, tapered instrument with a blunt, rounded end) into the opening of the cervix. First a very tiny sound is used, then subsequent sounds with progressively larger diameters are used until the desired dilation is obtained. Then the sound is inserted until it gently touches the top of the inside of the uterus. This measures the depth of the uterine cavity. After that, another instrument, a spoon-shaped curette with a sharp cutting edge, is used to strip away the lining of the uterus and any polyps that may be present. Then the tissue is put into a preservative and sent to the pathology lab where it will be cut, stained, and put onto slides to be examined under the microscope.

Although you will be sent home as soon as you have recovered from the anesthetic, you may continue to have some cramping and some light bleeding. Should fever, heavy bleeding, increased abdominal pain, or odorous vaginal discharge occur, contact your doctor immediately.

Because the D&C removes tissue that has accumulated, it can be therapeutic in itself and stop heavy bleeding, especially in cases where the woman has built up a thickened lining. However, remember the advice from page 374: The problem will probably recur in time if the hormonal imbalance is not corrected medically.

Suction Endometrial Biopsy

Unless there are specific problems that require an in-hospital D&C as described above, most patients and doctors prefer the convenience of an office procedure, with its lack of anesthesia risk, and relative low cost compared with a bill for anesthesia, hospital fee, and surgical fee.

The office procedure takes only two to three minutes. It's effective and quick. There are nicer things to do on a sunny day . . . but it's over before you know it. The procedure can diagnose endometrial cancer or hyperplasias with more than 85 percent accuracy. (This compares favorably with a 97 percent accuracy reported for the in-hospital D&C.) Furthermore, this simple procedure is usually all that is necessary to make a diagnosis and establish a basis from which to treat most women knowledgeably. The one problem with the technique is that growths such as polyps or submucous fibroids may remain unknown. (However, pathology reports often reveal that there are cells present that may originate from polyps.)

With a perimenopausal or postmenopausal patient who has abnormal bleeding, there is not a lot of room for guesswork. An accurate pathological diagnosis must be established and cancer ruled out so that specific treatment can be undertaken. The office biopsy can be repeated some months later to follow up on her therapy and to make sure that her endometrium reverts to normal.

For woman who are older and are bleeding postmenopausally, a biopsy can result in a false negative report. Because the cervical canal lengthens postmenopausally (reverting back to prepubertal uterine proportions), occasionally the physician does a suction biopsy, but does not really enter the uterine cavity. Consequently, the doctor extracts no tissue or insufficient tissue for diagnosis. In this case, a D&C, sometimes with ultrasound guidance, can more accurately obtain needed tissue for diagnosis. On the other hand, sometimes the patient has bled because of an "atrophic endometrium" where there is just not any tissue to obtain. In these cases, often no tissue is obtained with either office aspiration or D&C.

There are a variety of suction methods. Most use a hollow, tiny plastic tube with a tiny plunger. After obtaining an informed consent, where the patient is informed about the rare possibility of infection or perforation, the doctor swabs the cervix with a Betadine (iodine) solution and passes the small sterile instrument into the cervical opening. After gently guiding it into the uterine cavity, the doctor starts suction by pulling back on the tiny plunger inside the tube, or in some cases, suction can be created from a syringe or suction machine connected to the tube. The tissue is aspirated from the endometrium into the tube (or collecting device if a suction machine is used). By rotating and moving the little hollow tube up and down inside of the uterus, it is almost always possible to get a good sample of endometrial lining. The tube with its contents is withdrawn from the uterus at the end of the procedure. The same plunger that created the suction is now used to push the biopsy contents out into a small bottle of preservative. The empty plastic device is then thrown away. In all cases, the tissue is sent to the pathology lab, where it is stained and examined microscopically.

The discomfort of an office aspiration is very fleeting in most cases. Within two to three minutes afterward, most cramping is gone. Almost all of my patients have left the office smiling. Honestly! I pointed out to one of my patients after her follow-up aspiration that she was smiling and she laughed. I told her, however, that she must tell her husband that she had "major surgery" today, and couldn't possibly be expected to make dinner.

HYSTEROSCOPY

The hysteroscope is an instrument with a fiber-optic light source that illuminates the interior of the uterine cavity. Miniaturization has also enabled a lens or videocamera to peer into the illuminated area. By introducing fluid or carbon dioxide gas into the uterine cavity, the doctor can obtain a better view. He or she can then use tiny instruments to remove polyps and submucous fibroids.

The advantage of being able to see, rather than scraping the interior of the uterus blindly, is that the doctor can identify congenital abnormalities of the uterus, determine whether the entrance to the fallopian tubes is open and unobstructed, and can see and remove multiple polyps or see how far an endometrial abnormality extends. Although more invasive than a simple D&C, the technique allows newer procedures—some too new to have good statistical data (such as endometrial ablation with roller balls)—to be done at this time. It also allows the excision of submucous fibroids that poke into the cavity from beneath the endometrial lining.

ENDOMETRIAL ABLATION

Roller-ball technique, or endometrial removal with a resectoscope, is faster, cheaper, and less invasive than hysterectomy and may in the future be a good alternative for women who do not want a hysterectomy and have a negative workup for cancer, yet have uncontrolled bleeding. Because no incisions are necessary, women often go home the same day as their surgery. The technique is also preferred for those women in poor medical condition who cannot tolerate more extensive surgery. In this procedure, most of the endometrium is removed down to the basalis or deep layer. Some women never bleed again after the procedure, while others have light or more normal flow. To date, because the procedure is so new, we are still uncertain as to how to monitor patients for—and diagnose—endometrial cancer. It would make sense that a woman's risk would lessen after such a procedure, but the risk will not be zero.

Even newer techniques will allow doctors to destroy the endometrium in their offices without the use of a hysteroscope. These simplified techniques include a balloon-type structure that is filled after being placed inside the uterus. Then it is heated by microwave as it lies against the endometrial lining for a few minutes. Quick and effective, it should soon make its way to this country and may be another good choice for women with DUB. Other balloons will have surface electrodes to deliver electric current. This will destroy the uterine lining. Others may work by freezing the tissue. Soon, women will have faster, more efficient, and cheaper ways to rid themselves of heavy menstrual bleeding. And there will be less reason for hysterectomy.

How Should Your Hysterectomy Be Done?

If you need surgery, there may be another choice to make: whether to have abdominal, vaginal, or laparoscopic hysterectomy. Years ago there were studies that showed that women had fewer complications when the vaginal route and antibiotics were used rather than the abdominal approach. Historically, the vaginal approach has been used when ovaries were not going to be removed, or for women who had premalignant disease of the cervix. It was especially useful when a dropped bladder or rectum needed to be repaired because the hysterectomy was done in conjunction with that procedure. On the other hand, the abdominal approach is the standard. It is often used when there are large uterine fibroids, when severe endometriosis or infection is present, and in most pelvic surgery for malignancy.

However, perhaps the best surgical news is that of laparoscopy, often called Band-Aid surgery. A small incision (which can be covered with a Band-Aid) is made in the umbilicus and a laparoscope (a long tubelike telescope that you can see through) is passed into the abdominal cavity. In order to facilitate visualization, gas is added to distend the walls of the abdominal cavity. A diagnostic laparoscopy means that the pelvic contents are just looked at in order to make a diagnosis. However, most often, operative laparoscopy is done. This might include removal of the uterus, ovaries, or both; removal of endometriotic adhesions by laser or cautery; tubal ligation or tubal surgery, etc. Most often two small additional incisions need to be made just above the pubic hairline, along with a tiny incision in each lower portion of the abdomen to provide small openings for the instruments used for the surgery itself.

The major benefit of this procedure is that postoperative pain is much less and recovery time is much shorter. The usual large abdominal incision causes more problems contributing to recovery time than the surgery itself. And that is why patients who have laparoscopic surgery do so well. I was able to talk our well-trained gyn-oncologist into a laparoscopic procedure for my last patient who had an endometrial cancer. Because of her favorable workup, we were aware that this was a very early cancer. I reasoned that if there was any sign that all was not well, the laparoscopic procedure could immediately be terminated and an open abdominal procedure substituted. As suspected, the patient was in a very early stage of the disease and went back to work two weeks after her surgery.

One caution: Because not every gynecologist is well trained in laparoscopic surgery, it is important to know if he or she is credentialed for doing laparoscopic surgery. Call the hospital and ask, or specifically ask your doctor.

One last thing: There are new drugs available called GnRH agonists that can shrink large fibroids in premenopausal women. Generally, they are given for three months prior to surgery as a monthly injection or a daily nasal spray. Basically, they produce a postmenopausal state. Because the fibroids are deprived of their estrogen stimulation, they shrink, although not all fibroids are so obliging. As you may realize, heavy bleeding usually is also controlled. But sometimes bleeding is increased in the first two weeks of therapy, so patients have to be selected carefully. With the use of these drugs, even women with larger fibroids are now sometimes able to have them removed with a laparoscopic procedure.

You should know about your doctor's training. Doctors who have trained more recently may be more comfortable with laparoscopic techniques. Sometimes, because laparoscopic hysterectomy normally takes more time, the shorter open procedure may be picked. Sometimes that's for the doctor's schedule, sometimes it's because the patient is not a good candidate for a longer anesthesia.

Is There Sex after Hysterectomy?

Sex posthysterectomy doesn't seem to change for the vast majority of women. Women who are premenopausal and also had their ovaries removed will notice vaginal dryness unless the hormones are replaced. Even a woman with contraindications to hormonal therapy can use lubricants or moisturizers. Or she might be able to use tiny amounts of estrogen cream or the Estring™ ring, both of which lubricate the vagina well but allow only small amounts of estrogen to be absorbed.

Some women may notice the loss of uterine contractions during orgasm. But many more women can get back to enjoying a better sex life without pain and discomfort from endometriosis, fibroids, etc. Also, often there is relief that pregnancy worries are gone. Furthermore, sex lives that were ruined by constant bleeding now can bloom again. In thirty years of practice, with nearly a third of my patients coming to me having had a hysterectomy in the past, I have found that the number of sexual complaints is minimal, and usually those who complain feel they were "talked into their surgery" without other options discussed or tried.

In rare cases where extensive surgery was necessary and the vagina shortened, deep thrusting during sex can be painful. But those patients have been limited to those who needed major repair of their bladder after previous surgery and some patients with cancer who required radiation therapy.

Some women would like to leave the top of their vagina and cervix intact for sexual reasons, yet need the upper portion of their uterus removed for fibroids, bleeding, or other *non*cancerous conditions. In the past, supracervical hysterectomy was done simply to save time, but the technique may find its way back into some popularity. However, women who choose this procedure must be aware that they still have a cervix, which means that they must continue to get routine Pap smears. Whether maintaining the cervix helps a woman's sexual response is unknown.

Final Advice

I hope that this chapter has given you the information you need to make or wait on a surgical decision. Some of it should just be common sense. If the surgery is for large fibroids and you find yourself hemorrhaging every month and you are forty-two, hysterectomy may be the sanest way out. You will most likely have another eight to ten years of the problem, which will probably only get worse. On the other hand, with the same circumstances, if you are forty-eight or forty-nine, you may get by with good medical therapy until menopause comes along.
To summarize then:

- Know how often your particular condition might lead to cancer.
- Know what the medical alternatives to surgery are.
- Become familiar with minor surgical alternatives to complete hysterectomy that may treat the condition.
- Be aware of your age and probable length of remaining ovarian and menstrual function and make that part of your surgical decision.
- If you do have a cancerous condition, try to locate a gyn-oncologist to do your surgery.

The good news is that the rate of hysterectomy has decreased as women are becoming more outspoken and more knowledgeable about their bodies. More good news is that male and female physicians today seem to be more empathetic and willing to listen. And so we are making progress.

Note

1. Robert J. Kurman and Henry J. Norris, "Endometrial Hyperplasia and Related Cellular Changes," in *Blaustein's Pathology of the Female Genital Tract*, 4th ed., ed. Robert J. Kurman (New York: Springer-Verlag, 1994).

Final Words

This is the time to take stock of your life so that you may look forward to many years of excellent health. It is time to stop bad habits, such as smoking or excessive alcohol intake, and take care of medical problems that could in any way detract from your health in the future. Prevention is the key. Take care of yourself. Get enough sleep, rest when you are tired. Too many of us go on when we need to stop. It is not a crime to lie down for thirty minutes in the afternoon.

Worry about only those things that you can directly affect. Do what you can without causing yourself physical and emotional harm. Stick up for yourself and your needs. Then, give yourself a pat on the back. Chronic diseases (and women suffer from more chronic diseases than men) come from stress and overdoing what might otherwise be a good thing. Regard this time as an entry into a long period of maturity. Think about how much you really have to work, want to work. If you do not work and are bored or unfulfilled, think about going back to school. Take classes you never got a chance to take before. Try painting, music, art history, or Japanese. Or fulfill your life by taking courses to allow you to get a better-paying or more satisfying job.

Plan your lifetime ahead as you would plan a garden, filled with things you love, balanced with tasks you must do. Beautiful gardens do not bloom unless the soil has been worked, the seeds planted, and the weeds discarded. The sun is always there to warm the earth, and the rain to provide life-giving moisture. Similarly, your sun and rain—the knowledge and insight you have acquired from years of living—are always there to guide you. During your early years you "worked the soil," "planted your seeds," and now you should enjoy nature's reward—the full flowering of your life.

I wish you much success in your endeavors, much happiness, love, and peace in your life, and—basic to all that we do and ever hope to do—good health.

PENNY WISE BUDOFF, M.D.

Appendix

Here is a list of resources that may be useful to you.

The North American Menopause Society
P.O. Box 94527
Cleveland, Ohio 44101-4527
Telephone: (216) 844-8748
Fax: (216) 844-8708
E-mail: nams@apk.net
Web site: http://www.menopause.org

The North American Menopause Society (NAMS) was started almost a decade ago by Wulf Utian, M.D. He opened the first menopause clinic in Cape Town, South Africa, many years ago, and then came to this country and with great foresight founded this society. The organization has a multidisciplinary membership of physicians, nurses, psychologists, researchers, and others with an interest in menopause. Its ever growing annual meetings bring accurate, well-balanced information to health professionals and to the public.

NAMS, a nonprofit organization, provides information about menopause, menopause centers, physicians treating menopausal women, suggested readings, brochures, etc.

National Cancer Institute (NCI)
Office of Cancer Communications
Building 31, Room 10A 18
Bethesda, Maryland 20205
Telephone: 1-800-4CANCER or (301) 496-5583

Free information about cancer, mammography facilities, community resources, experimental protocols, free brochures, etc. Phone representatives answer your questions and help with referrals. Physicians also may call the institute for up-to-date information. Phone hours: Monday–Friday 9:00 A.M.–4:30 P.M.

American Cancer Society (ACS)
ACS National Office
1599 Clifton Road NE
Atlanta, Georgia 30829-4251
Telephone: 1-800-ACS-2345

The ACS has many programs to help the woman with breast cancer from Early Support, where "friends" are provided to help a woman before and through her surgery; Reach to Recovery, where women visit other women with breast cancer; Road to Recovery, which provides transportation and other help to cancer victims; Man to Man, a program for men with prostate cancer and their wives; and smoking cessation programs. Limited financial assistance is available for medical appliances, etc.

The National Alliance of Breast Cancer Organizations (NABCO)
9 East 37th Street, 10th Floor
New York, New York 10016
Telephone: (212) 889-0606
Fax: (212) 689-1213

The National Alliance of Breast Cancer Organizations (NABCO), a nonprofit organization, is a resource for information and education about breast cancer. Its resource book lists hundreds of local support groups, cancer centers, other organizations, etc.

Cancer Care, Inc.
1180 Avenue of the Americas
New York, New York 10036-0263
Telephone: 1-800-813-HOPE
E-mail: info@cancercareinc.org
Web site: http://www.cancercare.org

Cancer Care, Inc., is a nonprofit organization that provides counseling and referrals nationally. Its main offices are in New York, New Jersey, and Connecticut. All of its many services, counseling, transportation, and support groups are free of charge.

Susan G. Komen Breast Cancer Foundation
Web sites: www.breastcancerinfo.com
          www.raceforthecure.com
          www.komen.org

This site contains information on breast health, information for breast cancer survivers and their families, and allows women to share their personal experiences with breast cancer.

Bonne Forme vitamins and skin care products
    by Penny W. Budoff, M.D.
Long Island, New York
Telephone (worldwide): 1-800-426-0034 for free brochure

About the Author and the Contributors

When we walk into a doctor's office, the first thing we all do is study the diplomas on the wall. Therefore, the purpose of this "About the Contributors" is solely to present you with the fine educational credentials of the wonderful contributors of this book.

Penny W. Budoff, M.D.

Penny Wise grew up in Endicott, a small town in upstate New York. At fifteen, she won a four-year early admissions Ford Foundation scholarship, skipped her last two years of high school, and went to college. Her first biology course at the University of Wisconsin persuaded her to pursue a career in medicine. She spent her last two years of college at Syracuse University and then attended the State University of New York Upstate Medical Center at Syracuse. She met and married Seymour L. Budoff at the end of her junior year in medical school. At the end of her internship they moved to Woodbury, Long Island, New York. There she opened a practice out of her home while raising her two children, and conducted her seminal research on menstrual pain. These early studies led to publications in *The Journal of Obstetrics and Gynecology*, *The Journal of the American Medical Association*, *The New England Journal of Medicine*, and *The Journal of Reproductive Medicine*. These publications led to many invitations to lecture around the world. In 1978, her award-winning speech in Berlin at the International Women's Medical Association meeting encouraged female physicians to use television and other media to educate women about health issues. In 1980, she wrote *No More Men-*

strual Cramps and Other Good News, and three years later, *No More Hot Flashes and other Good News,* a *New York Times* best-seller. Because of her concern about women's nutrition, in 1982 she formulated the first vitamins for women by age in separate day and night formulations. Her vitamin and skin care company is named Bonne Forme (pronounced *bun form*), which means "in good shape" in French. Then in 1985, she opened the Penny Wise Budoff, M.D. Women's Medical Center, an independent multispecialty center for women. *Newsweek, Time,* and many women's magazines featured articles about her center, which quickly became the model for many other women's centers in this country. In 1992, the center became part of North Shore University Hospital and is presently known as North Shore University Hospital Women's Healthcare at Bethpage. She is listed in *Who's Who.*

Jeffrey Budoff, M.D.

Dr. Budoff is an orthopedic surgeon with two fellowships to his credit, one in sports medicine and one in hand surgery. He graduated Harvard University cum laude, Cornell University Medical College with AOA honors, a residency in orthopedics at the University of California, Irvine; a sports medicine fellowship at Arlington Hospital, Georgetown University; and a hand and microsurgery fellowship at Pacific Medical Center in San Francisco. Jeff is currently specializing in surgery of the upper extremities (shoulder, elbow, wrist, and hand) and knees. He is practicing with Palm Beach Orthopedic Associates, West Palm Beach, Florida.

Erna Busch, M.D.

Dr. Busch graduated Phi Beta Kappa from Rutgers University, then attended the University of Medicine and Dentistry of New Jersey. She completed a five-year residency in surgery at St. Vincent's Hospital and Medical Center in New York, then a fellowship in Roswell Park Cancer Institute in Buffalo in thoracic surgery, followed by two years of fellowship in general surgical oncology, which included training in breast, gastrointestinal, and head and neck cancers. Unlike many breast surgeons who were general surgeons and decided to do breast surgery instead, she was trained as a cancer surgeon. She is practicing at North Shore University Hospital in Manhasset, New York.

Howard Fillit, M.D.

Dr. Fillit graduated cum laude from Cornell University, then received his medical degree from the State University of New York Upstate Medical Center. He has been on the staff of New York Hospital–Cornell Medical Center, the Rockefeller University, and The Mount Sinai Medical Center. He has received numerous grants and awards, both public and private; has published over 200 articles, abstracts, and books related to aging and other fields; and is the editor of the leading international *Textbook of Geriatric Medicine and Gerontology*. He has lectured throughout the world on aging and Alzheimer's disease. Currently he is the corporate medical director for Medicare at NYL-Care Health Plans (a subsidiary of New York Life Insurance Company). He is also Clinical Professor of Geriatrics and Medicine at The Mount Sinai Medical Center in New York City.

John R. Miklos, M.D.

Dr. John R. Miklos received his medical degree from the Medical University of South Carolina, and completed a residency in obstetrics and gynecology at Hahnemann University in Philadelphia. He completed his two-year fellowship in urogynecology and reconstructive pelvic surgery at Good Samaritan Hospital in Cincinnati, Ohio. A member of the American Urogynecological Society and Fellow of the American Board of Obstetrics and Gynecology, Dr. Miklos is a widely published author and lectures to patients and physicians alike. Specializing in laparoscopic surgery, he has a private practice in Atlanta, Georgia, and operates at Northside Hospital and several of the city's leading hospitals.

Lawrence R. Lind, M.D.

Dr. Lind graduated from Haverford College then received his medical training at Cornell University Medical College. He completed a residency in obstetrics and gynecology at North Shore University Hospital–New York University Medical Center and fellowship training at Harbor–UCLA Medical Center–UCLA School of Medicine. He is presently chief of the Division of Urogynecology/Pelvic Reconstructive Surgery and Associate Residency Program Director at North Shore University Hospital, Manhasset, New York. Dr. Lind is involved extensively in research to improve treatment of incontinent women and has received numerous awards for excellence in teaching.

James Simon, M.D.

Dr. Simon received his medical degree from Rush Medical College and completed his residency in obstetrics and gynecology at the George Washington University Hospital. He completed his fellowship training in reproductive endocrinology and infertility at Harbor–UCLA Medical Center. Dr. Simon then became Assistant Professor of Obstetrics and Gynecology at the Jones Institute for Reproductive Medicine in Norfolk, Virginia. He later served as Chief of the Reproductive Endocrinology and Infertility Division at the Georgetown University School of Medicine. The list goes on and on. To sum up, he has been selected as one of the "Top Washington Physicians" and "Best Doctors in America." He is currently Clinical Professor of Obstetrics and Gynecology at the George Washington University and has a private practice in Washington, D.C.

Stuart Weinerman, M.D.

A graduate of Yeshiva College in Manhattan, Dr. Weinerman then went to Albert Einstein College of Medicine and did a residency in internal medicine at North Shore University Hospital, followed by an endocrinology fellowship at New York Hospital and Memorial Sloan-Kettering. He is presently head of the metabolic bone unit at North Shore University Hospital and practices at the North Shore University Hospital Women's Health Services in Bethpage, New York.

Index